Nobody Ever Told Me
(or My Mother) That!

Everything from Bottles and Breathing to
Healthy Speech Development

Nobody Ever Told Me (or My Mother) That!

Everything from Bottles and Breathing to Healthy Speech Development

by Diane Bahr, MS, CCC-SLP, NCTMB, CIMI
Author of *Oral Motor Assessment and Treatment: Ages and Stages*
(Allyn & Bacon, 2001)

All marketing and publishing rights
guaranteed to and reserved by:

Sensory World
www.SensoryWorld.com

2000 East Lamar Boulevard Suite 600,
Arlington, Texas 76006
Phone and fax (888) 507-2193
www.SensoryWorld.com
E-mail: info@SensoryWorld.com

Cover design: TLC Graphics
Interior design: Publication Services, Inc.

ISBN 13: 978-1-935567-20-2

Dedication

To all of the children and families with whom I have had the pleasure to work, particularly Cris, Tony, and baby Anthony, who helped me gain momentum in writing this book. A special thank-you to the lactation consultants at Greater Baltimore Medical Center (Cindy, Dee Dee, Marla, and Peg), who sent many babies my way and constantly inspired me. To my husband Joe, who provides me with continuous support and caring. And to my daughter Kim, who taught me about babies in the first place.

Advance Praise for *Nobody Ever Told Me (or My Mother) That!*

"Diane, you've got a gem here…your book is a well-organized resource that is chock full of new information and ideas in an easy-to-read format. It's an extremely valuable book—valuable to parents who are troubled about their child's feeding or speech difficulties and don't know where to turn, and valuable to speech therapists who seek sensible and practical answers to apply in their own therapy. Thank you for your creation and compilation of this highly useful material!"
Char Boshart, MA, CCC-SLP, Speech Dynamics, Inc

"This book provides a wonderful resource, full of beneficial information and practical ideas to support our international community of parents. Diane shares the secrets of her expertise and experience, providing us with a guide to best practice in the areas of feeding and speech development for infants and young children. Her dedication to writing this for parents is a gift to all of us, parents and professionals alike."
Mari Caulfield, Speech and Language Therapist, Galway, Ireland

"This much-needed book helps parents identify possible feeding and speech problems early and provides a wealth of practical advice and strategies from infancy up, to help secure the best possible prognosis for the child's future development. It's a treasure for anyone that cares for children."
Lisa Geng, Coauthor of *The Late Talker: What to Do If Your Child Isn't Talking Yet* and President of The Cherab Foundation

"What an informative book! Whether you are searching for everyday activities you can use to encourage your child's feeding, speech, and mouth development, or you are interested in exploring the mechanics of these skills, this is great resource, filled with nuggets for parents and professionals."
Dr Debra Jervay-Pendergrass, Linguist, Speech-Language Pathologist, Early Language-Literacy Consultant, and Director of the "First Stories" Project

"Diane's book is great, and should be in every parent's hands! There is no other reference for helping parents understand the connection between feeding, speech, and mouth development. Finally—a comprehensive, invaluable resource with the practical information parents need for one of their top parenting concerns: successful feeding!"
Nina Ayd Johanson, MS, CCC-SLP, CEIM, Feeding Specialist and Certified Educator of Infant Massage

"It has been my pleasure to work with Diane to more effectively help babies with breast-feeding difficulties. My hope is that this book will foster more teamwork among feeding

professionals and give parents a better idea of how their baby's mouth develops. Most breast-feeding problems can be prevented or corrected with better understanding and proper help."
Peg Merrill, BS, IBCLC, International Board Certified Lactation Consultant

"If you find the introduction fascinating—wait till you read the book! Infant feeding and normal development is my specialty, so it's nice to see a book that helps all children achieve good feeding and eating skills. The strategies to assist bottle-feeders are long overdue—since about 1975. There are still some health professionals who think that *books for parents* are 'not for them'—this one will teach everyone something!"
Ailsa Rothenbury, MA, RN, CHN, IBCLC, author of *Breastfeeding Is Not a Spectator Sport: Strategies for the Domestic Coaching Team*

"As both parents and physicians, we were able to appreciate Diane's work and teachings on many different levels. Her book serves as a superb educational tool to both parents and other health professionals interested in feeding. We especially feel that this book should be mandatory reading for every single pediatrician and pediatric gastroenterologist. Feeding is such a complex issue that it requires the collaboration of specialists in several different disciplines—such as speech-language pathologists, occupational therapists, dieticians/ nutritionists, pediatricians, and pediatric gastroenterologists—working together to ascertain the right diagnosis to develop the proper solution and effective treatment. It is Diane's unique insight into this often-difficult matter that brings solutions that can be implemented by parents and professionals alike to promote health and well-being to our children. We believe that Diane accomplishes this through this exquisitely written book. Congratulations, Diane, you did it!"
Inga Polyak, MD, *and Mark Degen*, MD, DDS

"Diane Bahr's new book, *Nobody Ever Told Me (or My Mother) That! Everything from Bottles and Breathing to Healthy Speech Development*, shares all her expertise and is the gold standard for parents to easily understand and assist in their child's development."
Susan Harrison, Parent of a child with special needs

"Full of useful, field-tested advice on your child's feeding, speech, and oral motor development—this gem of a book reaches out to parents across cultures and boundaries."
Christine Tan, Parent Support Coordinator, Ovspring Developmental Clinic, Singapore

"Bahr's new book provides a wealth of information for parents. Her extensive clinical experience and personal knowledge demonstrates her insight into the needs of parents. New parents will find the charts especially helpful in preparing for visits with medical professionals. It is always difficult for a parent to remember all that they want to discuss at a medical visit. This is a resource they can write in to log developmental milestones, identify concerns, carry with them to an appointment, and use as a starting point for discussion with their pediatrician, dentist, etc."
Pat Taylor, MEd COM, CCC/SLP

Reader's Note

This book reflects the ideas and opinions of the author. Its purpose is to give the reader helpful information on the topics covered in the book. It is not meant to provide health, medical, or professional consultation. The reader is advised to consult appropriate health, medical, and other professionals for these processes. The author and publisher do not take responsibility for any personal or other risk, loss, or liability incurred as a direct or indirect consequence of application or use of information found in this book.

Acknowledgments

I would like to acknowledge the many extraordinary people who assisted me in the completion of this book. If I have forgotten anyone, I sincerely apologize.

First, I would like to thank Cris and Anthony Fotia for allowing me to use the photographs of their fabulous son, Anthony, Jr, in this book, and artist Anthony Fotia, Sr, who created original artwork for the book. In addition, I would like to thank the many parents and colleagues who helped to make this the best book possible.

To those who read, reviewed, and made suggestions for the entire book:

Susan Abbott, PhD, CCC-A/SLP, Assistant Professor, Stephen F. Austin State University

Daniela Rodrigues, MA, CCC-SLP, Trilingual Speech-Language Pathologist

Sara Rosenfeld-Johnson, MS, CCC-SLP, Inventor and Entrepreneur

Sheryn Wright, Master-Level English Teacher

Acknowledgments (continued)

To those who read, reviewed, and made suggestions for appropriate sections of the book:

Charlotte Boshart, MA, CCC-SLP

Chris Brown, Parent

Anthony Fotia, Parent

Dee Dee Franke, RN, BSN, IBCLC

Catherine Watson Genna, BS, IBCLC

David Hammer, MA, CCC-SLP

Kathleen A. Harrington, MA, CCC-SLP

Susan Harrison, Parent

Deborah Hayden, MA, CCC-SLP

Christina Johanson, MS, CCC-SLP

Nancy Kaufman, MS, CCC-SLP

Raymond D. Kent, PhD, CCC-SLP

Debbie Lowsky, MS, CCC-SLP

Pamela Marshalla, MA, CCC-SLP

Cindy McCartin, RN, BSN, IBCLC

Peg Merrill, BS, IBCLC, RLC

Suzanne Evans Morris, PhD, SLP

Marla Newmark, RN, BSN, IBCLC

David C. Page, DDS

Brian Palmer, DDS

Donna Ridley, MEd, CCC-SLP

Jaime Sandlin, Reader

Mary Sandlin, Parent

Will Schermerhorn, Parent

Mary Shiavoni, MS, CCC-SLP

Patricia Taylor, MEd, COM/CCC-SLP

Alicia Wopat, Parent

To Christine Tan of OvSpring Developmental Clinic in Singapore, who introduced me to David Brown, JD.

To Polly McGlew, JD, and David Brown, JD, who encouraged me to write this book and worked with its first writing.

To my outstanding editor Heather Babiar, who truly understood the information I was trying to convey and helped me to say it.

To the Gilpins of Future Horizons, my wonderful publisher, originally from my home town of Baltimore. Thank you Jennifer, Wayne, and Kelly.

To the staff at Publication Services, Inc., who made this a beautiful book.

Contents

Foreword

Awareness is the first step toward change. Through the eye of awareness, parents and professionals first gain an understanding of how a process such as the development of feeding skills unfolds. Awareness without judgment enables them to apply general knowledge and observation to specific children and make better decisions.

Infants and young children are highly resilient. Most have the internal sensory and movement abilities to adjust to feeding situations that are less than ideal. They learn to eat and drink in spite of irregular schedules, poor positioning for nursing, spoons that are too large, or food textures that are too challenging for their current experience and skills. They may struggle or protest, but eventually they learn, because taking in enough food and liquid is essential to life and survival.

Some children are born with poorer coordination, a high level of sensitivity to their environment, allergies, or structural difficulties that make eating and drinking exceptionally challenging. Some babies and toddlers, such as those born prematurely, simply need more time and adult guidance to develop these skills. When they are offered eating challenges that are too difficult or experience foods or feeding utensils that don't fit their current needs, they may become discouraged or frustrated; some may even refuse to eat whole categories of food or reject the spoon or cup because they associate it with discomfort or failure.

This is a book that builds awareness. Diane Bahr asks the simple question, "Do children learn more easily when parents understand their needs and the significance of the various stages of development?" Her answer is a clear "yes." Many parents worry that something is wrong with a child when their baby doesn't do things that they remember an older brother or sister doing at the same age. They become fearful that their baby will never be able to chew or drink from a cup. If there are feeding difficulties, someone may tell them that their child will be delayed in speech development. When parents are afraid, their emotions get in the way of their ability to connect lovingly with their child. They may pull back from the relationship in their concerns about the baby's development. Their own stress levels can make it harder for their youngster to move freely into newer skills.

This is a book about babies and young children. It is secondarily about how their mouths and faces develop for feeding and early speech. It is a book about parents and their desire to support their child's natural development. Diane provides guidance that enables parents to understand their baby's development of feeding and to see it in relationship to everything else that the baby is doing. It can assure them that their baby is developing in the same way as other infants, setting his own pace and timing in learning something new. It also offers parents ways to observe and understand when feeding and speech development have become stuck and their baby doesn't seem to be moving to the next level. When feeding and speech are not progressing well, this book offers suggestions that parents can incorporate into their daily life and describes various professionals and other resources that can help them.

Suzanne Evans Morris, PhD

Introduction

As a feeding and speech therapist for almost 30 years, I have seen many children with health and development concerns directly related to problems with feeding and other early mouth experiences. These include sinus and ear problems, allergies, asthma, gastroesophageal reflux, nutritional concerns, sensory processing concerns, late vocal and speech development, and orthodontic issues. Many of these problems could be avoided or reduced if parents and other caregivers had more specific information and training on these topics.

The information in this book comes from my years of experience as a speech-language pathologist while working with children on the development of improved feeding and communication skills. The book also contains the best research I could find on the topics presented. I will tell you the secrets many therapists have learned over the years that the typical parent may never hear, information your child's pediatrician may not know to tell you. I wish I had had this information when I was a young mom more than 30 years ago.

There are many books on breast-feeding, childhood nutrition, and child development, but I have not found any book for parents that outlines the mechanics of feeding, speech, and mouth development. Good feeding techniques and appropriate mouth activities are essential for your child's overall health, well-being, and, ultimately, proper speech development.

Today, parents often do not have the role models of extended families living nearby to demonstrate techniques that were used successfully by previous generations. This information is not innate in our modern world, and feeding can become a tedious pattern of trial and error for parents and their babies if they don't have help.

Just ask some parents:

1. How many bottles they tried before finding one that worked
2. How they finally got their child to keep food in his or her mouth when they began spoon-feeding

There are horror stories about children who refuse to eat an appropriate variety of foods necessary for basic nutrition. Many of these struggles began with incorrect and/or unsuccessful feeding techniques. Speech-language pathologists are also seeing an increase in the number of children with late-developing speech. These are often the same children who had feeding problems.

The ideas presented in this book help parents and other caregivers solve these problems easily and naturally. Giving parents the appropriate tools to feed their baby and stimulate his or her mouth development is crucial for decreasing parent anxiety and frustration, as well as increasing positive interactions between parent and baby. In his book *The Happiest Baby on the Block*, Dr Harvey Karp says that parents who succeed in feeding and calming their babies "feel proud, confident, and on top of the world!"[1] What could be more important than proper nutrition and good communication?

By using the simple, appropriate techniques presented in this book, you will:

1. Help your baby develop good mouth structures that will support overall health

2. Help your child develop appropriate eating and drinking skills that will be used throughout life

3. Help your child develop mouth structures that will support the development of good speech

4. Help your child develop his or her best natural appearance

Just follow these simple, healthy guidelines as you go through your everyday activities with your child. They will make your life easier and eliminate the guesswork. This is a guilt-free, pressure-free, success-oriented approach, so you can have more fun and enjoy watching your child develop these marvelous new skills.

Some special features of this book include:

1. Charts to help you identify important characteristics of mouth development for feeding and speech, so you can decide what may need to change for the improved health and well-being of your child

2. Information repeated as needed (particularly in charts), so you don't have to flip through the book to find it

3. Activities to help you learn techniques quickly, easily, and naturally

4. Pictures of techniques described and discussed

The book contains 10 chapters that are easy to understand and use.

1. Chapter 1 helps you learn about the important differences between your mouth and your newborn baby's mouth.

2. In chapter 2, you learn the most effective techniques for breast- and bottle-feeding, as well as information on nutrition and hydration.

3. In chapter 3, you find out about the importance of breathing through the nose, belly time, and sleeping on the back, as well as information about many health problems.

4. Chapter 4 discusses how your baby's hands and mouth work together. Pacifier use and thumb-sucking guidelines are provided, as well as information on teething and drooling.

5. In chapter 5, you'll discover how to touch and work with your baby's little face and mouth for activities such as maintaining oral hygiene and other important mouth experiences.

6. The most effective methods of spoon-feeding, drinking from a cup and straw, and introducing solid foods are covered in chapter 6. Here, we also talk about picky eaters.

7. Chapter 7 will give you the secrets of good speech development that are often not covered in other resources.

8. In chapter 8, you will learn more about face and mouth development that can affect your child's appearance throughout life. You will also learn how to minimize your child's need for future orthodontic treatment.

9. Chapter 9 discusses ways to work with professionals in your child's life (such as your pediatrician and others).

10. Finally, chapter 10 provides specific information on feeding and mouth development for parents of children with special needs.

1

Let's Learn about Your Newborn Baby's Mouth

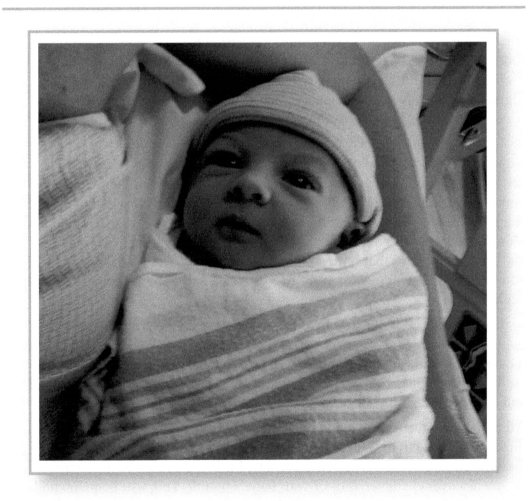

Key Topics in This Chapter

■ Differences between Your Mouth and Your Newborn Baby's Mouth

■ Your Newborn Baby's Mouth Reflexes

Good mouth development is extremely important for the health and well-being of your baby. The mouth is not only the route to good nutrition, but it is an area through which your child will gather information about the world and ultimately learn to express him- or herself through speech.

Birth to 2 years of age is a critical learning period for mouth skills. This is the time when your child will develop the majority of his eating and drinking skills used throughout life. It is also the time when your child will begin to speak. Significant changes in your baby's mouth structure and movement (function) occur at this time. These structure and function changes assist with the many new mouth skills your baby is learning.

Now, you might be wondering why this is important for you to know. Well, getting acquainted with your baby's mouth from the start will help you understand feeding and other aspects of mouth development as your baby grows. If a problem does arise, you will know what to do or where to go for help. I have seen and worked with many frustrated parents whose children had small feeding and speech problems that turned into larger problems over time. My goal is for you to feel successful in your child's feeding and speech development from the beginning.

In this chapter, you will learn the differences between the structure of your mouth and your baby's mouth, as well as how your newborn baby's mouth moves and works from birth. There will be two hands-on activities to guide you with your learning process. These activities will help you become acquainted and comfortable with your baby and his mouth.

All of the activities in this book are simple and easy to do, if you follow the directions. The activities take only a few minutes, and you will learn a lot about your baby's mouth. For each activity, I ask you to date each statement as you discover characteristics of your baby's mouth. This will help you build a record of your baby's development. It will be fun to look at all your baby is accomplishing and to look back on this in the future. Think of it as a type of baby book.

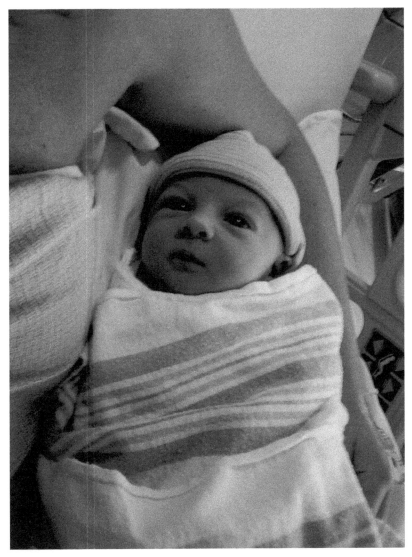

Photo 1.1: Meet our model Anthony as a newborn.

Differences between Your Mouth and Your Newborn Baby's Mouth

Your baby's mouth at birth is very different from your mouth. This is one reason why most babies can drink from the bottle or breast. Just try drinking from a bottle, and see how difficult this really is. It is very difficult for you, because you no longer have the mouth structures and functions most babies have at birth. Figure 1.1 shows the structural differences between your mouth and your newborn's mouth. Activity 1.1 teaches you about these differences.

The directions for completing Activity 1.1 are listed below the Activity 1.1 checklist. Please follow these directions to help you understand the details of the checklist. The checklist, by itself, does not explain what you need to know.

THE MOUTH AND PHARYNX OF THE NEWBORN
(sagittal section)

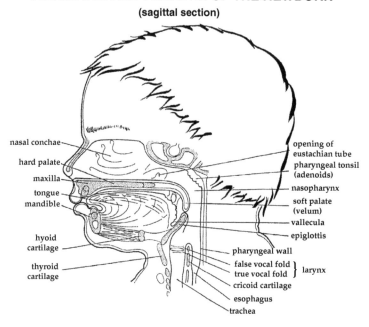

nasal conchae

hard palate

maxilla

tongue

mandible

hyoid cartilage

thyroid cartilage

opening of eustachian tube

pharyngeal tonsil (adenoids)

nasopharynx

soft palate (velum)

vallecula

epiglottis

pharyngeal wall

false vocal fold
true vocal fold } larynx

cricoid cartilage

esophagus

trachea

THE MOUTH AND PHARYNX OF THE ADULT
(sagittal section)

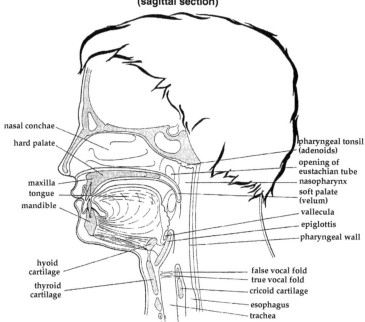

nasal conchae

hard palate

maxilla

tongue

mandible

hyoid cartilage

thyroid cartilage

pharyngeal tonsil (adenoids)

opening of eustachian tube

nasopharynx

soft palate (velum)

vallecula

epiglottis

pharyngeal wall

false vocal fold

true vocal fold

cricoid cartilage

esophagus

trachea

Figure 1.1: Structural differences between the newborn and the adult mouth and pharynx.

Source: Reproduced with permission of Suzanne Evans Morris. Original artwork of artist Betsy True.

You will need to trim your fingernails for the activities in this and other chapters. You may also want to use disposable gloves for these activities. You can buy these at the pharmacy or medical supply store or get them from your dentist. Ask for nonlatex, nonpowdered gloves that are made to go into the mouth. Some other gloves taste bad, smell bad, and are made of latex (a common allergen).

Now, let's have some fun exploring your baby's mouth. This is your newborn baby's "window to the world." You are going to be placing your finger into your baby's mouth to calm him anyway, so you might want to know something about where you are going.

Important Note: If your baby is not in the mood for you to explore his mouth, wait until he is in the mood. Babies usually enjoy this. Your baby will be the leader in the process of mouth exploration. You will watch your baby's facial expressions and body language to see if he is enjoying the process.

Some babies do not enjoy mouth play as much as others. In my work as a therapist, I discovered that many of these babies have belly problems (such as reflux) from birth, which keeps them from enjoying mouth play. This seems to occur because the babies associate the discomfort of belly problems with feeding. We will talk about reflux and other health problems in chapter 3.

ACTIVITY 1.1: YOUR BABY'S MOUTH[2-8]

Items to Check in Your Newborn	Date
1. The open space in your baby's mouth is very small. Your baby seals and compresses the bottle nipple or breast by using the lips, tongue, and gums in the front of the mouth. Your baby then creates a vacuum within the mouth by moving the back of the tongue and jaw downward.	
2. Your baby's bottom jaw is small and pulled slightly back; his top and bottom jaws have a "flat" appearance (approximately 30% of adult size at birth).[9]	
3. The roof of your baby's mouth (the hard palate) may be more than 20–25 mm wide (approximately ¾ to 1 inch) from edge to edge across the middle of the palate (more than 50% of the adult width of 40–50 mm, approximately 1⅝ to 2 inches); ideal shape of the hard palate is a wide "U."	
4. Your baby's hard palate (the roof of the mouth) is composed of several bones that touch one another in the center and toward the back (they're very flexible and easily misshapen in a newborn).	

ACTIVITY 1.1: (cont.)

Items to Check in Your Newborn	Date
5. Your baby's tongue fills his mouth and helps maintain the shape of the mouth's roof (the hard palate) when your baby's mouth is resting.	
6. Your baby's deeply cupped tongue moves from front to back evenly (about 50% forward and 50% back) in a wavelike motion, sealing and unsealing the back third, so that he can extract liquid from the breast or bottle.	
7. Your baby's gums contain some special tissue that swells to help seal the mouth when nursing or bottle-feeding (called *the third lips*).[10]	
8. If your baby was born full-term, he should have sucking pads in the cheek area (balls of fat that keep the cheeks against the gums).	
9. Your baby will breathe through his nose, even when his nose appears to be very close to the breast. You may often hear your baby produce nasal-sounding vowels when he is making vocal sounds.	
10. The structures in your baby's throat (the soft palate, epiglottis, and larynx) are close together to protect him from choking on formula or breast milk.	

DIRECTIONS FOR ACTIVITY 1.1:

1. Look at Figure 1.1 to see the difference between your mouth and your baby's mouth structure. Now you are ready to feel the difference. Place your freshly washed and/or gloved index finger into your newborn's mouth (pad side down, trimmed nail side up). Feel your baby's tongue cup around your finger. You should also feel a good suction within his mouth. This is because of the small amount of open space within your baby's mouth.

DIRECTIONS FOR ACTIVITY 1.1: (continued)

Several mouth structures contribute to making the amount of open space within your newborn's mouth so small. These include the size, shape, and position of the jaws and tongue, the cheek pads, and the relative position of the soft palate to the epiglottis, as seen in Figure 1.1.

The amount of open space in your newborn's mouth is very small so that something called *appropriate intraoral pressure* can occur. This pressure allows liquid to be drawn into the mouth and moved back to the throat for swallowing.

Newborn babies seal and compress the bottle nipple or breast by using the lips, tongue, and gums in the front of the mouth. They create a vacuum within the mouth by moving the back of the tongue downward.[11] Babies who do not have this pressure in the mouth struggle with feeding. The details of this process are discussed thoroughly in chapter 2.

2. Look at your newborn's jaw as he is lying on his back. See how his small bottom jaw is pulled back just a little. This is typical at birth but will begin to change significantly within the first 6 months of your baby's life. Also, if you look at where your baby's lips meet, they will form a fairly straight left-to-right horizontal line. This reflects the normal "flatness" of your baby's jaw. At birth, your baby's jaw is approximately 30% of its adult size.

3. When your baby yawns or cries, take a look at the roof of his mouth. It may be a little more than 20 to 25 millimeters across the center from left to right near the middle of the mouth. Of course, you are only going to look at this visually—don't try to actually measure it! However, you can look at a ruler to see what 20 to 25 millimeters looks like. It is approximately ¾ to 1 inch. Also, the shape of your baby's hard palate (the roof of the mouth) should look like a wide "*U*." Any other shape may indicate a problem.

4. Your baby's hard palate (the roof of the mouth) is composed of several bones that touch one another in the center and toward the back. These bones also touch other bones that create the nasal areas, sinuses, and other parts of the skull. They are very flexible and easily moved out of position in newborns. This entire mouth roof will seem to "harden" as your baby grows.

DIRECTIONS FOR ACTIVITY 1.1: (continued)

When your baby has a closed mouth at rest (that is, when the mouth is not in use), the tongue fills the mouth to help maintain the relatively broad shape of the roof of the mouth or hard palate. The mother's breast during nursing can also help with this process. During proper nursing, the breast is drawn deeply into the child's mouth to help keep the shape of the palate. We will discuss mouth development in detail in chapter 8.

If you touch your baby's hard palate, **you must touch it very gently.** Touching the roof of your baby's mouth can facilitate suckling. This is probably the reason that lactation consultants often teach parents to allow the infant to suckle on the index finger (pad side up, trimmed nail side down). I teach you to turn your finger in the opposite direction (pad side down, trimmed nail side up) when you place it into your baby's mouth for suckling if possible. This will help you avoid placing too much pressure on your baby's very flexible hard palate.

So, why is it important for your child's hard palate or roof of the mouth to remain fairly broad? A high, narrow hard palate will change the shape of the nasal and sinus areas. If this occurs, your child's nasal areas and sinuses may become misshapen, and structures within the sinuses (such as turbinates) may actually block the sinuses.[12]

Children with small or misshapen nasal and sinus areas tend to have more sinus problems. For example, small sinuses are more difficult to clear than typically sized sinuses if your child should develop a cold or upper respiratory infection. This may lead to sinus infection and can contribute to allergies and other upper respiratory illness. Your baby may also have more difficulty breathing through the nose if the nasal and sinus areas are small or misshapen. Nose breathing is important for good health, as it ensures better development of the facial and jaw bones and directs air to the lower lung areas, where more blood is oxygenated.[13] Your baby's brain and body need oxygen for all aspects of life.

5. Look at your baby's mouth at rest (when he is just relaxing or sleeping, not eating or making vocal sounds). Is your baby's mouth closed? If it is, then your baby's tongue is probably resting against the roof of his mouth. Remember, we want this rest position to help keep the shape of the palate. If your baby's mouth is open at rest, there are some techniques in chapter 5 that can help.

6. Again, place your washed and/or gloved index finger into your baby's mouth (pad side down, trimmed nail side up). Focus on your baby's

deeply cupped/grooved tongue around your finger. Can you feel your baby's tongue moving front to back evenly in a wavelike motion (about 50% front and 50% back)? You may also feel the back of your baby's tongue moving up and down at the same time (sealing and unsealing the back third of the tongue), creating a vacuum to extract liquid from the breast or bottle. Isn't this amazing?

If you feel any differences in your baby's mouth (such as the tongue humping—pushing up the middle of the tongue—instead of grooving/cupping, or too much or too little forward movement of the tongue), this will affect the way your baby feeds. These are subtle problems that we frequently see in babies' mouths.

7. You may notice some enlargement of your baby's gums when your finger is placed into your baby's mouth. If you can't feel this, don't worry about it. The slight swelling of the gums that you see or feel helps your baby to seal and compress the bottle nipple or breast when drinking. These are called *the third lips* and will no longer be needed or seen between 3 and 6 months of age.

8. To feel your baby's sucking pads, place the pad of your index finger inside your baby's cheek and your thumb on the outside. Now, move your thumb and index finger up and down, front and back. You can apply some very gentle pressure between your thumb and index finger, but **don't pinch your baby.** You should feel a ball of fat within each cheek. The fat pads may actually make it a little difficult for you to move your index finger inside your baby's mouth. If you don't feel these fat pads, the following may be true:

    a. Your baby may have been born prematurely. Preemies are not born with sucking pads.
    b. Your baby may have been induced or born a little early. Sucking pads develop toward the end of pregnancy, when the rest of the fat is developing on the body.
    c. Your baby may have inherited thin sucking pads.

The presence or absence of sucking pads can make a significant difference in how your baby feeds. As mentioned above, your baby's sucking pads develop toward the end of pregnancy, when the other fat is developing within the body. This is the reason that preemies are born without sucking pads.

DIRECTIONS FOR ACTIVITY 1.1: (continued)

I have worked with many babies with feeding problems who were born close to full-term and did not have adequately developed sucking pads. I often asked the lactation consultants who made the referrals why this might be. One hypothesis was that many babies are induced and may not truly be full-term. An article that appeared in *The Washington Post* on May 20, 2006, stated that 350,000 babies are born "slightly early" (ie, near term) in the United States each year (the average pregnancy is shortened to 39 weeks).[14] Many of these children have been reported to have feeding and other developmental difficulties.

If your baby was born early (either prematurely or even a little early), your baby may not have developed adequate sucking pads. This will affect the way your baby drinks. Sucking pads help to close the mouth space by bringing the cheek areas against the gums, so that your baby has appropriate pressure within the mouth to draw in and swallow liquid.

No matter the cause, there are a number of things you can do to help your baby compensate for thin or nonexistent sucking pads. We will discuss this in detail in chapter 2.

9. Watch how your baby coordinates suckling, swallowing, and breathing. While the breast or bottle is within his mouth, he is still breathing through his nose. If your baby is breast-feeding, his nose will be very close to your breast. When your baby takes a break from feeding and vocalizes, you may hear vowel-like nasal sounds (often a short "*a*," as in the word "at," or a long "*e*," as in the word "eat," depending on whether your baby's jaw is open or closed). The sound may be coming through your baby's nose instead of his mouth. This will change as your baby grows. See chapter 7 for more details on speech sound development.

10. Look again at Figure 1.1, so you can see the structures in your baby's mouth and throat. Notice that the proximity of the structures helps to make the open space within your baby's mouth and throat very small. This helps to naturally protect your baby from choking.

Note: If you are concerned about your baby's mouth structures or functions, talk to your pediatrician. He can refer you to specially trained therapists (eg, feeding therapists) or other professionals who can help you and your baby with these problems.

Your Newborn Baby's Mouth Reflexes

Now, let's see how your baby's mouth moves at birth. Your baby is born with a number of reflexes that assist with feeding until he is mature enough to make these movements on his own. These are listed in Activity 1.2.

Date each reflex as you see it in your newborn. If your baby is a little older, you can still see many of these reflexes. Your baby will not develop control over many of the reflexes for a little while. Reflexes don't really disappear. The motor (or movement) area of your baby's brain actually takes control over time, and your baby no longer needs the reflex to do the activity. So when you see the reflex disappearing, it means that your baby's brain is developing.

It is fun to explore your baby's mouth and see these in action. The directions for completing Activity 1.2 are listed below the chart. Don't forget to trim your fingernails and perhaps wear gloves (nonlatex, nonpowdered gloves meant to be used in the mouth).

Note: If you do not see some of these reflexes in your baby's mouth, ask your pediatrician to check for them. Also, if your baby has reflexes beyond the age when they normally seem to disappear, talk to your pediatrician. Reflexes that remain can indicate a problem with development.

ACTIVITY 1.2: YOUR BABY'S MOUTH REFLEXES[15–21]

Reflex	Date	How You Get Your Baby to Do It	What It Looks Like	Apparent Use	When Your Baby Can Begin to Control It	When the Reflex Seems to Disappear
Rooting		Touch your baby's cheek or lips	Your baby's mouth will move toward your touch	Helps your baby locate the breast for nursing	1 month of age	3 to 6 months of age
Suckling		Place your finger, a bottle nipple, or the breast nipple into your baby's mouth; triggers touch receptors in lips and deep within mouth	Suckling (front to back wavelike movement of your baby's deeply cupped tongue, sealing and unsealing the back third of the tongue to extract liquid from breast or bottle) with lips latched and sucking pads engaged	Allows your baby to breast- and bottle-feed or take a pacifier	2 to 3 months of age	6 to 12 months of age reflexively

Tongue	Touch your baby's lips or tongue	Front to back wavelike tongue movement used in suckling	Helps your baby suckle	Unknown	12 to 18 months of age
Swallowing	Triggered when saliva, liquid, or food reaches your baby's throat	Your baby swallows	Moves saliva, food, and liquid toward your baby's stomach	18 months	Continues as an important reflex throughout our lives
Bite	Press on your baby's gums with "firm but gentle" pressure	Your baby will begin to open and close the jaw, biting up and down	This movement works important jaw muscles (jaw elevators and depressors) that are needed to close the mouth at rest, take bites of food, chew, and make jaw movements for speech	5 to 9 months of age	9 to 12 months of age

ACTIVITY 1.2: (cont.)

Reflex	Date	How You Get Your Baby to Do It	What It Looks Like	Apparent Use	When Your Baby Can Begin to Control It	When the Reflex Seems to Disappear
Transverse Tongue		This occurs when your baby receives touch, food, or taste on either side of the tongue	Your baby moves his tongue sideways toward the touch, food, or taste	Side-to-side tongue movements will eventually be needed for your child to place food for chewing and retrieve food for swallowing	6 to 8 months of age	9 to 24 months of age
Gag		Touch to the back ¾ of your baby's tongue	Your baby's mouth opens wide, head may go back, soft palate rapidly rises, voice box and diaphragm may rise	Protects your baby from swallowing items that are too large to swallow	4 to 6 months of age; at 6–9 months, the reflex moves to the back ⅓ of the tongue[22]	Continues as an important reflex throughout our lives on the back ¼ of the tongue

DIRECTIONS FOR ACTIVITY 1.2:

1. Rooting Reflex: Touch your newborn baby's cheek or lips with your finger, the bottle nipple, or the breast. Your baby's mouth searches for the touch with small side-to-side head movements. This reflex helps your baby find the breast or his own hand for suckling. Your baby will begin to gain some control over this reflex around 1 month of age. Bottle-fed babies quickly develop control over this reflex, because they do not need it to locate the bottle nipple. Bottle nipples are placed directly into a baby's mouth. You will no longer see the reflex beyond 3 to 6 months of age.

2. Suckling Reflex: Place your finger (pad side down, trimmed nail side up), the bottle nipple, or the breast nipple into your newborn baby's mouth. Feel the front-to-back wavelike movement of your baby's tongue while sealing and unsealing the back third of the tongue, so he can extract liquid from the breast or bottle. You felt this in Activity 1.1. The movement is approximately 50% front and 50% back, with the tongue cupped or grooved around your finger.

This reflex helps your baby to suckle liquids from the bottle or breast. It is stimulated by touch receptors in the lips and deep within the mouth. This is why it is important for the mother's breast to be drawn deeply into the infant's mouth. It is also the reason that some nurses, physicians, and therapists give babies longer bottle nipples rather than shorter ones. We will discuss the problems associated with bottle nipples that are "too long" in chapter 2.

Your baby will have the easiest time learning to suckle around the time of birth.[23] This is the reason that babies should be put to the breast or given the bottle as soon as possible after birth. Your baby will begin to gain some control over this reflex by about 2 to 3 months of age. Between 6 and 12 months of age, you will no longer see your baby suckling reflexively. Twelve months of age is also the time when the mature swallowing pattern (tongue-tip touching the ridge behind the top front teeth to begin the swallow) becomes apparent. We will discuss this in chapter 6.

3. Tongue Reflex: Touch your baby's lips or tongue. You will feel the same front-to-back wavelike tongue movement you felt with the suckling reflex. By 12 to 18 months of age, you will no longer see this reflex.

DIRECTIONS FOR ACTIVITY 1.2: (continued)

4. Swallowing Reflex: As you feed your baby, you will see your baby swallow. Your baby develops an increasingly coordinated swallow as he grows and develops. By 18 months of age, your baby will have good control over the swallow. The swallow reflex is one we use many times per day. As an adult, you swallow approximately every 30 seconds when you are awake and use about 26 muscles in the mouth and throat for this process.[24]

5. Bite Reflex: Place your washed and/or gloved finger into your baby's mouth. Apply little (firm but gentle) presses on your baby's gums. Your baby will start to bite repeatedly on your finger in a rhythmic manner. This can be a particularly useful reflex when babies are not born with a complete set of sucking pads. The motion of rhythmic biting at the back of the mouth will help the jaw muscles develop. Jaw and cheek muscles can "take on" the work that the sucking pads were meant to do. See chapter 5 for further information.

The bite reflex can sometimes be a problem for nursing moms. It is not a very good feeling when a baby clamps down on Mom's breast. This can usually be avoided if your baby is breast-feeding properly. See chapter 2 for further details. Babies develop control of the bite reflex between 5 and 9 months of age, when they are learning to take bites and chew foods. The reflex seems to disappear between 9 and 12 months of age, when chewing and taking bites of food are well established.

6. Transverse Tongue Reflex: If you place your washed and/or gloved finger into the side of your baby's mouth, touching the side of his tongue, your baby's tongue will move toward your touch. Your baby begins to develop control over this reflex between 6 and 8 months of age, as he begins to eat soft, solid foods. It seems to disappear between 9 and 24 months of age, when your baby is developing the very sophisticated tongue movements needed to place and collect food within the mouth.

7. Gag Reflex: In your newborn baby, you will see your baby gag if you touch the back three-fourths of his tongue (most of the tongue, toward the back). This may occur during breast- and bottle-feeding and is normal. You **should never** gag your baby on purpose. By 4 to 6 months of age, your baby will begin to develop some control over this reflex, with the gag moving to the back third of the tongue by 6 to 9 months. Again, this is the period of time you are introducing soft, solid foods to your baby.

Through feeding and other important mouth experiences, your baby's gag reflex will eventually move to the back quarter of the tongue. This is a vital process as your baby learns to handle different food textures within the mouth and goes through the critical period of discriminative mouthing. We will talk about discriminative mouthing in chapter 4.

8. Some General Comments about Reflexes: You can feel comfortable stimulating all of the reflexes except the gag. You **do not** want to gag your baby on purpose. In some babies, it may take a little extra time to stimulate their other reflexes. Don't hesitate to keep your finger in place and press or touch the area that stimulates the reflex a little longer. Stimulating reflexes should be fun for you and your baby. If your baby appears uncomfortable, continue this process when your baby is in the mood. We don't want this to be a traumatic experience for you or your baby. In fact, we are beginning this exploration at birth so that things like introducing foods and tooth-brushing will be easier for you and your child later on.

Note: If you are concerned about your baby's mouth structures or functions, talk to your pediatrician. He can refer you to specially trained therapists (such as feeding therapists) or other professionals who can help you and your baby with these problems.

Now that you are acquainted with your baby's mouth, let's go to chapter 2 and learn about breast- and bottle-feeding. Successfully feeding your baby is important for both you and your baby. Of course you know that your baby needs good nutrition to grow properly. However, in his book *The Happiest Baby on the Block*, Dr Harvey Karp also says that parents who succeed in feeding and calming their babies "feel proud, confident, and on top of the world!"[25]

2

Secrets for Better Breast- and Bottle-Feeding

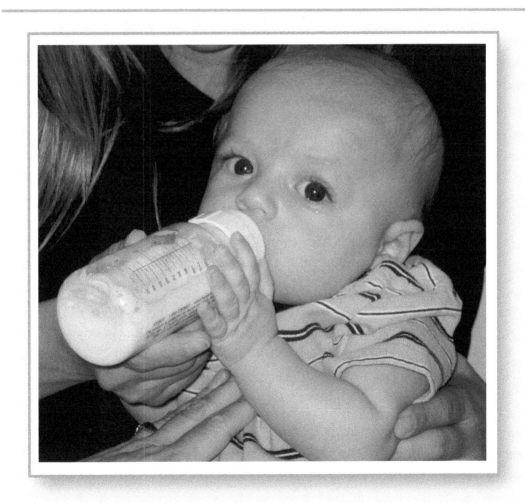

Key Topics in This Chapter

- Important Mouth Characteristics for Feeding
- The Best Positioning for Feeding and Why
- What Breast-Feeding Can Do for Your Baby's Mouth That Bottle-Feeding Cannot
- Help with Nursing/Breast-Feeding
- Finding an Appropriate Bottle Nipple
- What to Do If Your Baby Has Difficulty Maintaining a Latch
- What to Do If Liquid Is Flowing Too Fast or Too Slowly
- Subtle Difficulties That Can Affect Feeding and What to Do About Them
- Nutrition
- Hydration
- Feeding Development: One to 6 Months of Age

P arents often receive very little instruction on ways to feed their children, yet good eating and drinking skills encourage the best mouth development. You are going to feed your child, so why not use appropriate feeding techniques that can support your child's mouth development?

Most of our eating and drinking skills are developed in the first 2 years of life. Every 3 months from birth, your baby will have a growth spurt in this area. You can help with this process by using appropriate feeding techniques from birth.

In this chapter, we are going to address many topics related to nursing and bottle-feeding. You will learn proper breast- and bottle-feeding techniques, as well as what to do if you have a problem with either process. While I prefer that a mom breast-feed when possible, this is not always possible for some families. Therefore, we will also cover the best bottle-feeding practices.

Feeding is like dancing. You and your baby are partners in this dance. The best feeding method for you and your baby may be somewhat different from what someone else may do. As in ballroom dancing, many of the steps are similar, with specific variations that suit you and your child. However, there are some important guidelines that can help you learn the "feeding dance" easily and successfully.

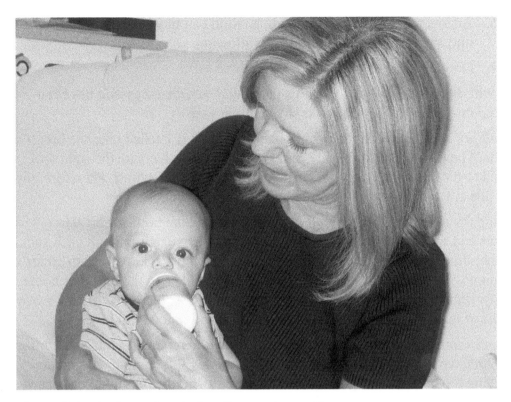

Photo 2.1: Anthony bottle-feeding at 4 months.

Important Mouth Characteristics for Feeding

In chapter 1, you became familiar with your newborn baby's mouth. Now, we are going to see how your baby accomplishes breast- or bottle-feeding successfully. Ideally, your baby should demonstrate the following characteristics, whether you are nursing or bottle-feeding. Most full-term babies are born with the potential for these characteristics. Premature and near-term babies can be assisted in developing most of them.

1. Small jaw movement once latched

2. Tongue cupping/grooving

3. Even, front-to-back wavelike tongue movement (50% front and 50% back), with the back of the tongue moving downward to create a vacuum when drinking (suckling)[26–27]

4. The tongue comes over the lower gum area during front tongue movement, but does not protrude out of the mouth

5. A stable mouth, with the tongue acting as the lower stabilizer, the sucking pads acting as side stabilizers, and the roof of the mouth acting as the top stabilizer

6. Adequate pressure in the mouth, so fluid can move safely and efficiently into and through the mouth for swallowing

7. Good feeding rhythm

We will discuss these characteristics in detail. Each characteristic has been placed into bold italics, so you can locate topics easily.

Small jaw movement should occur once your baby is latched onto the breast or bottle. The tongue, sucking pads, and roof of the mouth create the right space for liquid to move safely, easily, and efficiently through the mouth. Therefore, the jaw doesn't need to move very much.

Your baby's ***tongue needs to cup or groove*** around the bottle or breast nipple and move 50% front to 50% back in a wavelike motion with each suckle. At the same time, the back of your baby's tongue moves downward to create a vacuum within the mouth. This will pump the liquid from the breast or bottle easily. Babies who move their tongues too far front (sometimes called a *tongue thrust* or *exaggerated tongue protrusion*) are working too hard.

Tongue humping (pushing up the middle of the tongue) means that something has gone wrong. Children who hump their tongues and pump the liquid are working too hard and fatigue easily. They usually hump their tongues because they do not have adequate sucking pads, the tongue is tied, and/or their heads and necks are extended back. Tongue humping is an attempt to make the space inside the mouth smaller, which then adjusts the suckling pressure. This is not an efficient method for pressure adjustment within the mouth.

As mentioned previously, your baby should have even, ***front-to-back wavelike tongue movement***. The tongue should come out over the lower gum during the suckle but not thrust. Babies often thrust their tongues because their heads and necks are too far back. These babies are working very hard, and tongue thrusting can become a lifelong pattern that is known to affect the development and shape of the hard palate (the roof of the mouth) and teeth (ie, occlusion). We will discuss this in detail in chapter 8.

Babies whose ***tongues do not come out over the lower gum*** also have a very difficult time nursing and tend to bite down on their mom's nipples (ouch!) or bottle nipples. They do this because the bite reflex is being triggered. They also learn that biting down can help keep the jaw from moving too much.

Some babies are born with a tongue restriction (ie, tongue-tie), which can inhibit proper tongue movements. Small restrictions are often resolved through the use of appropriate feeding techniques. However, some babies have significant restrictions, and the most severe have heart-shaped tongues. The restriction is caused by a structure under the tongue, called the *lingual frenum*. You might hear the medical term *frenulum* when a tongue is restricted in this way. Some pediatricians will recommend clipping the tissue under the tongue if the tongue is so restricted that the baby cannot properly nurse or bottle-feed. See the American Academy of Pediatrics Web site for further information on management of a tongue-tie.[28] Dr Brian Palmer also has information on his Web site regarding tongue-tie at *www.BrianPalmerDDS.com*.

There has been some controversy in the professional literature about whether to clip a tongue-tie or not. Clipping is most important to consider if the tongue is significantly restricted and the baby cannot feed properly. This is sometimes done near the time of birth and is a decision that parents need to make with their physicians, because it is surgery.

In my experience as a feeding therapist, babies who have the clipping at a later date (several weeks after birth or later) usually need some therapy to get their feeding back on track. Babies who feed with a restriction for a period of time develop feeding habits that usually lead to feeding and mouth development problems in the future.

If a baby's tongue is significantly restricted, it is also important to check the baby's lips for restrictions. There is a frenum system, and each lip also has one (a piece of tissue that connects the lip to the gum). These are called the *labial frenums*. If lips are restricted or too tight, the breast or bottle latch can be significantly affected. Lip restrictions can often be resolved with the use of proper feeding and some massage facilitation techniques. Clipping is done occasionally, usually in conjunction with orthodontic work if it has not been done earlier for feeding purposes. Any clipping is surgery and is a decision for parents and their physician to make.

Your baby also needs *a stable mouth* with just enough space inside to effectively nurse or bottle-feed. This stability is provided by the structures with which your baby was born (the roof of the mouth, sucking or fat pads in the cheeks, a cupped tongue, and closeness of the mouth structures). Without this balance in the mouth, your baby will develop patterns that may affect the way she will drink and swallow for the rest of her life.

The roof of the mouth, sucking pads, cupped tongue, and proximity of the structures allow your baby to develop what therapists call *good intraoral pressure*. Just like so many other systems in the body, the mouth is a "pressure system." Without the right pressure in the mouth, the liquid cannot move smoothly and easily to the throat for swallowing. This can cause your baby to work harder than necessary when feeding.

Your baby should also have *a good feeding rhythm*. This means that the entire mouth moves in a rhythmic manner. The nutritive suckle (where your baby takes in breast milk or formula) occurs approximately once per second. As your baby becomes more skilled with the suck-swallow-breathe sequence, she will suckle for longer periods of time without breaks. Nursing or bottle-feeding should occur in a relatively quiet, smooth process. If your baby makes high-pitched sounds, gulping sounds, or other struggling sounds, the liquid may be flowing too quickly from the bottle or breast. Your baby may also be out of position for feeding. We will discuss positioning after Activity 2.1.

ACTIVITY 2.1: WHAT IS YOUR BABY DOING DURING NURSING OR BOTTLE-FEEDING?

Place a date in the column next to the description that matches what your baby is doing.

Date	What You Want My Baby:	Date	Things to Change My Baby:
	Has small, up-down jaw movements once latched		Has wide, awkward-looking up-down jaw movements once latched
	Cups or grooves the tongue to conform to the shape of the bottle nipple or breast		Humps or mounds the tongue to remove liquid from the bottle or breast
	Has even front-to-back wavelike tongue movement (50% front and 50% back), with the back of the tongue moving downward to create a vacuum when drinking		Has greater forward tongue movement than backward tongue movement or a tongue restriction (eg, a heart-shaped tongue)
	Moves the tongue forward "just" over the lower gum when drinking		Cannot get the tongue over the lower gum, is pushing or thrusting the tongue out of the mouth, has a tongue restriction, and/or bites on nipple

Date	What You Want My Baby:	Date	Things to Change My Baby:
	Has a good latch on the breast or bottle		Loses the latch frequently
	Can draw liquid easily into the mouth		Has to work hard to draw in liquid
	Has rhythmic and coordinated suckling, sucking, swallowing, and breathing during feeding		Makes gulping or struggling sounds, gasps for air, and/or does not have a good feeding rhythm

If you have dates to the left of the "Things to Change" column, locate the appropriate section of this chapter that talks about how to address that particular problem.

The Best Positioning for Feeding Your Baby and Why

Positioning can also affect your baby's ability to feed properly. Whether you have chosen to breast-feed or bottle-feed, see if you can follow these guidelines.

1. Keep your baby's head in alignment with her body (keep the head, neck, and body in a straight line).

2. Do not allow your baby's head and neck to extend backward. Hyperextension of the head and neck can cause some irregular patterns to occur in your baby's mouth. These patterns include wide jaw movement, excessive tongue protrusion, tongue humping or mounding, and biting down for stability (ouch for the breast-feeding mom!).

   Note for Breast-Feeding Moms: Your lactation consultant may teach you to have your baby latch by leading with the chin. This will help your baby open the mouth wide. Once your baby is latched, be sure her nose is close to your breast. This allows proper extension in your baby's neck without hyperextension. Your baby may slightly adjust the position so she can breathe, but her nose will be very close to your breast.

3. Keep your baby's ear above the mouth so that fluid will not enter the Eustachian tubes. This means holding your baby when possible at approximately a 45° angle or more. As your child grows, she can be more upright. This is critical for bottle-fed babies. If your bottle-fed baby is positioned at 45° to 90°, then your bottle can be held in such a way that gravity does not make the liquid flow too fast.

This is paced bottle-feeding.[29] *The Breastfeeding Mother's Guide to Making More Milk,* a book by Diana West and Lisa Marasco, contains detailed information on paced bottle-feeding, which is similar to breast-feeding:[30]

a. Stroke the baby's lips with the bottle nipple.

b. Roll the bottle nipple into the baby's mouth when she opens the mouth wide, demonstrating readiness to accept the nipple.

c. Allow the baby a break after four to five suckles by stopping the liquid flow (ie, gentle nipple removal from the mouth or tipping the bottle).

d. Use a slow-flow nipple.

e. Keep the baby more upright and the bottle more horizontal to reduce the effects of gravity.

f. Follow your baby's hunger cues to avoid overfeeding.

Note for Breast-Feeding Moms: If your baby is breast-feeding properly, it is unlikely that fluid will enter the Eustachian tubes, because the pressures within the mouth and nasopharynx are equalized. Breast milk is "living tissue," and macrophage cell activity in breast milk may destroy bacteria in the Eustachian tubes if any milk should enter them.[31] Macrophage cells are the most numerous cells in breast milk. They appear to have antibacterial characteristics to assist the baby in the development of a healthy immune system.[32] When you first breast-feed your baby, the cradle hold or side-lying position may work best for you. Many lactation consultants recommend the cradle hold. However, new information is available on breast-feeding positioning (eg, the DVD *Baby-Led Breastfeeding: The Mother-Baby Dance* from Geddes Productions). Suzanne Colson and colleagues have written several recent articles on the topic of breast-feeding positioning. The articles discuss research and include photos of appropriate breast-feeding positions. Colson and colleagues demonstrate that the newborn may actually be an abdominal feeder, with antigravity reflexes assisting the latch.[33–35] At this point, do not become overly concerned with your baby's ear being above the mouth if you are using a cradle hold or side-lying during breast-feeding. Be sure your baby's head and body are in the best alignment possible (ie, the head, neck, and body are in a straight line with the nose close to the breast). You can move to a football hold when you and your baby become more skilled with the nursing process. This hold will place your baby's ear above the mouth. Breast-feeding has so many health benefits for you and your baby that it is important for the two of you to find a way to successfully breast-feed.

The positioning of your baby while he or she bottle-feeds can be very important. While research is needed, it has long been suspected that babies who are bottle-fed lying down have a higher incidence of ear and sinus infections. This is related to the positioning of the Eustachian tubes, the sinuses, and gravity.

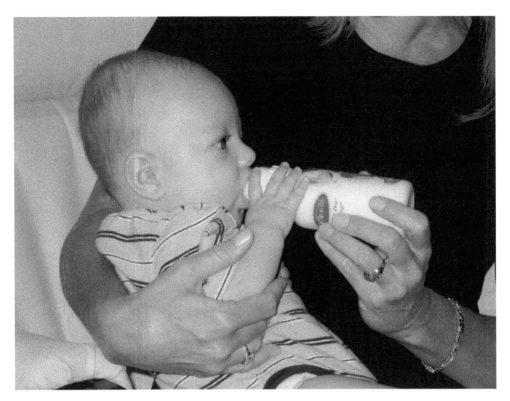

Photo 2.2: Anthony's ear is above his mouth.

The Eustachian tubes are positioned horizontally in the newborn and become more vertical as the child grows. Each Eustachian tube (one in each ear) leads from the back of the nasopharynx (where the nasal area meets the throat) to the middle-ear space. Fluid is more likely to enter the baby's Eustachian tube if the child is lying down because of gravity pulling the liquid downward. Figure 1.1 in chapter 1 shows you the location of the opening of the Eustachian tube.

If fluid from the bottle or the stomach (due to reflux or spit-up) enters the Eustachian tube, it can travel into the middle-ear space behind the eardrum. This space is essentially a sinus, as it is lined with mucus-producing membranes. If a foreign substance enters this area, more mucus is produced in the body's attempt to clear away the foreign substance. This mucus build-up in the middle-ear space can become an ear infection.

When your baby was born, a gelatinous substance[36] filled the middle-ear space. However, this substance is absorbed during the first few weeks of life, leaving an open middle-ear space. The middle ear contains three little bones that help the eardrum communicate sound to the inner ear. If the middle-ear space is filled with fluid or infected mucus, your child may have a significant hearing loss (eg, a 30-decibel loss; conversational speech is approximately 65 decibels).[37-38]

Having a healthy middle ear is important for your child's hearing and speech-language development.

Fluid in the middle ear can distort the way your child hears sounds. It may be most similar to when you hold your fingers in your ears or hear sound from under water. Children are learning to discriminate the sounds of their own language from birth.[39] Discriminating the different sounds of speech allows the child to learn language and speech. Therefore, your child's middle ear needs to be kept clear from fluid or infection.

Sinus infections can also be caused by foreign matter, such as reflux (commonly known as spit-up), entering the nasal sinus areas. Despite the cause, sinus infections or congestion make it very difficult for your baby to feed. This is the reason that most parents use a hand-held suctioning bulb to clear the baby's nose of mucus.

When babies feed, they coordinate suckling, swallowing, and breathing in a sophisticated manner. A stuffy nose may cause your baby to struggle with this process and possibly to compensate by taking more breaths through the mouth. Long-term mouth breathing is unhealthy and makes it almost impossible to adequately coordinate suckling, swallowing, and breathing. By bottle-feeding your baby at a 45° to 90° angle (with the ear above the mouth) with the head and body in alignment, you can help your child avoid ear and sinus problems.

ACTIVITY 2.2: WHAT IS YOUR BABY'S POSITION DURING NURSING OR BOTTLE-FEEDING?

Place a date in the column next to the description that matches what your baby is doing.

Date	What You Want My Baby's:	Date	Things to Change My Baby's:
	Head, neck, and body are aligned during feeding		Head and neck are turned or tipped back
	Ear is at least slightly above the mouth during bottle-feeding (body and head at approximately a 45° angle or more to the earth)		Ear is not above the mouth, because my baby is lying flat or at less than 45°

Date	What You Want My Baby's:	Date	Things to Change My Baby's:
	Body is in a correct cradle (belly-to-belly), side-lying, or football-hold position during nursing		Head and neck are turned or tipped back
	Nose is very close to the breast during nursing		Head and neck are tipped back

If you have dated items in the "Things to Change" column, review the chapter for the appropriate section on addressing these items.

What Breast-Feeding Can Do for Your Baby's Mouth That Bottle-Feeding Cannot[40-42]

Nursing has made a comeback as the preferred feeding method for many reasons. First of all, breast-feeding is biologically normal. Babies who are nursed tend to have fewer allergies, better immune systems, and better mouth development than those who are bottle-fed. A popular resource on breast-feeding is *The Nursing Mother's Companion,* by Kathleen Huggins.[43] *Breastfeeding Made Simple,* by Nancy Mohrbacher and Kathleen Kendall Tackett, is a newer, research-based book. If you are breast-feeding, I suggest that you purchase a book for your reference.

I would like to see all mothers breast-feed their babies. However, I know that this is not realistic for some. Therefore, I want you to know the benefits of breast-feeding, whether you are breast- or bottle-feeding. If you are bottle-feeding, you can help counteract some of the negatives of bottle-feeding by understanding what breast-feeding does for mouth development.

1. When your baby breast-feeds, the breast is drawn deeply into the mouth. This helps to maintain the shape of the hard palate (the roof of the mouth). A bottle-fed baby may develop a high, narrow hard palate due to the forces involved in bottle-feeding. If you are bottle-feeding, I will teach you an exercise in chapter 5 to help keep your baby's hard palate in shape.

2. A breast-feeding mom feeds her baby on alternate breasts. This provides stimulation and exercise to both sides of the infant's face, head, and body.[44]

3. Mouth structures move in a more sophisticated manner during breast-feeding than during bottle-feeding. This leads to better mouth development.

4. Development of the face,[45] jaw, dental arches, palates (hard and soft), teeth,[46-47] and speech[48-49] is better in breast-fed infants than bottle-fed infants. Bottle-feeding may result in underdeveloped jaws and subsequent orthodontic problems.[50] We will discuss this further in chapter 8.

5. Breast-feeding supports sophisticated suck-swallow-breathe synchronization, allowing the structures of the mouth, throat, and respiratory system to move together as a unified oral-motor organ.[51]

According to Dr David C. Page, considered a pioneer in functional jaw orthopedics, breast-feeding is the best way to ensure proper jaw growth. The jaw is the keystone for the development of the other structures around it (ie, "the gateway to the human airway"[52]). Dr Page recommends "exclusive" breast-feeding for the first 3 to 6 months, with continued breast-feeding until 12 months. This is similar to the recommendations of the American Academy of Pediatrics. Dr Page says that the movements of breast-feeding assist jaw growth, which is most rapid during the first year of life.

Dr Page does not recommend bottle-feeding. He says that "bottle, pacifier, and digit sucking create backward destructive forces on both upper and lower jaws."[53] These forces can narrow the dental arches and hard palate and ultimately cause malocclusion.[54-56] Some of these malocclusions include cross-bite,[57] crooked teeth, and other jaw problems. These difficulties and what to do about them will be discussed in chapter 8.

According to Dr Page, research shows that bottle-fed infants are generally sicker than successfully breast-fed infants.[58] This makes sense if you think about a high, narrow hard palate making the nasal and sinus areas smaller. A number of studies have shown that breast-fed babies are less likely to develop allergies, ear[59] and other respiratory[60] infections, insulin-dependent diabetes,[61] and gastrointestinal problems.[62] They are also less likely to be overweight and to die from sudden infant death syndrome.[63-65] Dr. Page has a website at *www .smilepage.com*.

Dr Brian Palmer also has a Web site containing important breast-feeding information at *www.BrianPalmerDDS.com*. He discusses topics such as the importance of breast-feeding to total health, breast-feeding and frenulums, SIDS, otitis media (ie, middle-ear problems), and obligate nose breathing. Dr Palmer is the author of the journal article, "The Influence of Breastfeeding on the Development of the Oral Cavity: A Commentary."[66]

Dr Ashley Montagu, a social scientist, presents significant research on breast-feeding in the book *Touching: The Human Significance of the Skin.*[67] In my opinion, every mother- and father-to-be should read the chapter on breast-feeding in this book. It will help parents make a more informed decision on how to feed their newborn, because it is based on research from many different fields of study and cultures.

Dr Montagu discusses one study of 173 children followed from birth to 10 years of age. Babies who were breast-fed had four times fewer respiratory infections, 20 times fewer bouts of diarrhea, 22 times fewer infections of other kinds, eight times fewer cases of eczema, 21 times fewer cases of asthma, and 27 times fewer cases of hay fever.[68] Another study of 383 children indicated that bottle-fed children were nutritionally poorer, more susceptible to childhood diseases, and slower to learn walking and talking than breast-fed children.[69] Both Drs Page and Montagu comment that the research suggests higher intelligence and better physical health in breast-fed children.[70–71]

The superior physical health of breast-fed children seems to be related to airway development. Breast-feeding supports proper airway development. The airway consists of your baby's nose, mouth, throat, windpipe, and voice box, leading to the lungs. Airway development is dependent upon appropriate face and jaw growth, and vise versa.[72] Airway obstruction can cause mouth breathing and change face and jaw development.[73] There is a connection between airway obstruction, allergies, asthma, ear problems, sinus problems, reflux, and stress.[74] Obstructive sleep disorders, blood pressure concerns, and heart problems can be added to this list.[75] Proper airway development is crucial for your baby's health.

As you can see, there is a substantial amount of research to support the value of breast-feeding for good and appropriate mouth and airway development. However, I do not want parents who choose to bottle-feed their babies to become overly concerned. There are activities in chapter 5 to help you counteract some of the possible negative effects of bottle-feeding. Actually, the activities and exercises in chapter 5 are "good" for all babies, whether they are breast- or bottle-feeding. I have frequently assigned these activities to moms and dads whose babies were having difficulty breast-feeding.

While nursing may be a preferred method for many, this book is an equal-opportunity manual that values whatever choice you make as a parent. You, as a parent, will make the best choice possible for your child and family situation. I respect your decision and want to help you with your child's feeding and mouth development, whether you breast- or bottle-feed.

Help with Nursing/Breast-Feeding

Nursing moms often have the advantage of working with a lactation consultant. If you are a nursing mom or plan to nurse, try to find a lactation consultant with whom you feel comfortable before giving birth. Many hospitals have these specialists. Lactation consultants are usually nurses who are specifically trained in this area. There are also some other professionals (such as speech-language pathologists and occupational therapists) who have received this training and certification. A nursing mom should look for a breast-feeding professional who is an International Board Certified Lactation Consultant (IBCLC). These are some of the most qualified breast-feeding professionals.

Lactation consultants have access to important tools and techniques that can make nursing easier and more effective. Medela is one company that specializes in products for nursing mothers, and lactation consultants have access to these products. Some Medela products are sold at stores such as Target and Babies R Us. Lactation consultants can also help parents to supplement their children's intake with other feeding methods until the mom and baby can work out any difficulties with the nursing process.

If you are having problems with breast-feeding, refer to Activities 2.1 and 2.2 in this chapter. Chapter 5 has some activities and exercises to improve awareness in and movement of your baby's mouth.

Finding an Appropriate Bottle Nipple

Feeding is a nurturing and bonding process. Parents choose to bottle-feed exclusively or part-time for many reasons. This allows Dad and others to take part in feeding the baby. It can give Mom a much-needed break and allow others to connect and bond with the baby. Also, if Mom needs to be away from the baby for an extended period of time, the baby can continue to be fed on demand or on schedule. If you bottle-feed your baby, review the information on paced bottle-feeding discussed earlier in this chapter.

Choosing an appropriate bottle for your baby can be confusing, because there are many products on the market. Basically, you want a bottle nipple that fits your baby's mouth. If your baby has a small mouth, you will need a short, small nipple. A child with a larger mouth may be able to handle a longer nipple. In my opinion, it is better to give your child a nipple that is a little too short than one that is too long.

A nipple that is too long may encourage your baby to use incorrect movements that may negatively affect mouth development (such as tongue thrust or exaggerated tongue protrusion). If your baby has difficulty maintaining a good latch on the nipple, the nipple may be too long. If the bottle nipple is too long, it will often move in and out of your baby's mouth while your baby is drinking. This makes feeding inefficient and can tire your child.

There is a simple test to determine if nipple length is the problem or if your baby is having trouble getting enough pressure at the lips and inside the mouth to maintain the latch. Support your baby's cheeks during bottle drinking (see information on "maintaining a latch" in the next section of this chapter). If the nipple stops moving in and out of your baby's mouth while the cheeks are supported, nipple length is not the problem. You will need to provide your baby with cheek support until she learns to use the muscles of the jaw, cheeks, and lips to keep the latch.

However, if the bottle nipple continues to move in and out of your baby's mouth when you give your baby cheek support, you need to find a nipple that fits your baby's mouth. Product labeling can be misleading. Your child may require a nipple that is labeled differently than you would expect. For example, some nipples are labeled preemie, newborn, or mini but may be a perfect nipple size for your child. This does not say anything about your baby's development, except that she may require a certain nipple to appropriately fit her mouth. Like the saying goes, "There is a key for every lock." Finding the right key is important.

Nipple shape can be another consideration when choosing a bottle for your baby. Many nipples are rounded so the tongue can cup around them. I prefer these, because they encourage tongue cupping. This is particularly important for the newborn baby, who uses a deeply cupped tongue while drinking. However, some babies drink better from what may be identified as an orthodontic nipple. These nipples may encourage up-down front tongue movement, which is typically seen as babies mature. See the discussion of three-dimensional sucking that develops by 4 months of age in the Feeding Development Checklist at the end of this chapter.

A good latch on the bottle means that your baby's lips maintain a hold on the "latch area" of the bottle nipple. The "latch area" is the part of the nipple that flares out from the nipple itself. A wide latch area may encourage better mouth development. However, more research is needed in the area of bottle-feeding and mouth development.

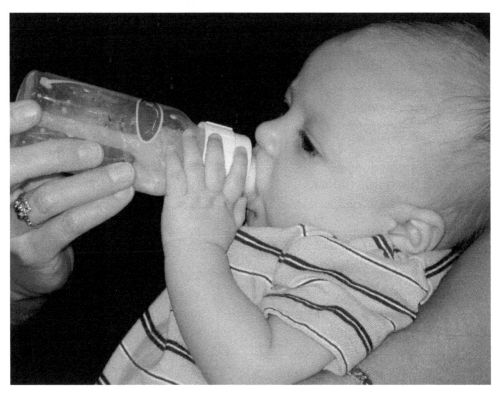

Photo 2.3: Anthony has a balanced lip latch even when sleepy.

If your baby is using an appropriately sized nipple and still has difficulty maintaining a latch, your baby may have a jaw weakness or some other difficulty that you may not be able to determine on your own. As mentioned previously, providing your baby with cheek support can help your baby appropriately compensate for a weak latch until the difficulty is resolved. Activity 2.3 can help you avoid some of the problems parents encounter with bottle nipples.

However, if you still have questions or concerns about the right nipple for your baby or your baby's latch on the nipple, work with a professional. Appropriately trained occupational therapists, speech-language pathologists, lactation consultants, nurse practitioners, and pediatricians can help you with this process. Check with the hospital where you delivered your baby or hospitals that specialize in feeding to find professionals who can help you. The International Lactation Consultant Association *(www.ilca.org)*, the American Speech-Language-Hearing Association *(www.asha.org),* and the American Occupational Therapy Association *(www.aota.org)* are other sources for finding feeding professionals.

ACTIVITY 2.3: CHOOSING THE "RIGHT" BOTTLE NIPPLE FOR YOUR BABY

Circle the problem you are seeing, and place a date in the column next to what you want to try. Be sure that you have completed Activities 2.1 and 2.2 prior to doing this activity.

Problem	Date	Things to Try
My baby's tongue does not cup around the bottle nipple		Choose a rounded nipple rather than an orthodontic-type nipple
The bottle nipple moves in and out of my baby's mouth		Provide cheek support
The bottle nipple moves in and out of my baby's mouth when I give cheek support		Try a shorter nipple, even if the packaging is labeled for a younger baby

If you have dates next to the "Things to Try" column, review the chapter for the appropriate section on addressing these items.

What to Do If Your Baby Has Difficulty Maintaining a Latch

Maintaining a good latch on the bottle or breast is a common problem. As mentioned previously, it is important to check nipple size and shape if you are bottle-feeding. Also pay attention to your baby's positioning. If your baby's head and body are out of alignment (head, shoulders, and hips not in a fairly straight line), this can significantly affect the latch.

You may need to provide your baby with some cheek support if your child is still having difficulty maintaining a latch. This can be a temporary measure to assist your baby in maintaining the lateral, or side, stability needed in the mouth and bringing the lips forward to suckle properly. Cheek support can help your baby create an appropriate amount of interior mouth pressure to draw in liquid from the bottle or breast easily and efficiently.

To provide cheek support, place your thumb on one of your baby's cheeks and your index or middle finger on the other. Press gently but firmly inward toward your baby's gums while pulling your fingers slightly forward toward your baby's lips. Do not slide your fingers over your baby's skin in any direction. You will

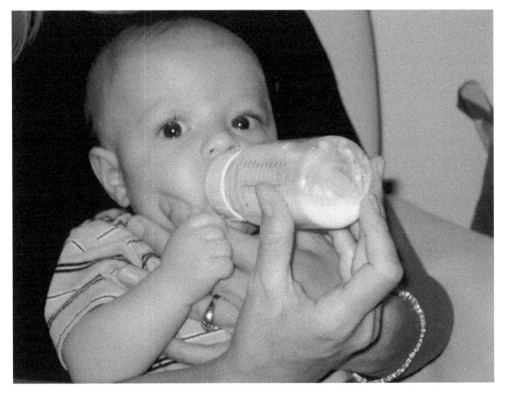

Photo 2.4: Anthony demonstrates cheek support with therapist Diane.

see your baby's lips flare, because the muscles of the cheeks help to move the lips. You may also see your baby's tongue cup, because you are now providing the lateral stability your child needs to suckle properly.

For many years, lactation consultants have taught moms the "Dancer" hand position (ie, Mom supports the baby's cheeks and chin with her free hand while baby is nursing) to support babies' cheeks and jaws while they nursed. Some moms have found this hold difficult to maintain, particularly when using a cradle (ie, cross-over) position.

However, modified cheek support can be used with the cradle hold. Gravity is often the culprit in this situation, as gravity pulls the lower cheek toward the ground. Therefore, the lower cheek does not remain against your baby's gum surface during nursing. Appropriate pressure in the mouth is lost. Nursing moms using a cradle hold can apply gentle but firm pressure on the baby's lower cheek surface to help the baby compensate for this difficulty.

You can also give your baby a little jaw support along with cheek support, if needed. This can be done by placing the area between your thumb and index finger under your baby's chin while you provide cheek support. However, it is essential that you do not stop your baby's jaw from moving or force the jaw to move in an unnatural direction. Providing jaw support is like dancing smoothly with a partner and will be discussed in detail in chapter 6.

See Activity 2.4 below if your baby is having difficulty latching. Cheek and jaw support can help your baby to latch. However, these are usually temporary measures. Your baby may have a subtle difficulty in the mouth that is causing the latching concern. Subtle concerns are often problematic because they can be difficult to identify. These are discussed later in this chapter.

ACTIVITY 2.4: HELPING YOUR BABY LATCH ONTO THE BREAST OR BOTTLE

Circle the problem you are seeing, and place a date in the column next to what you want to try. Be sure that you have completed Activities 2.1 and 2.2 prior to doing this activity if you are breast-feeding. If you are bottle-feeding, complete Activities 2.1, 2.2, and 2.3 prior to completing this activity.

Problem	Date	Things to Try
Your baby is not latching properly on the bottle (lips are not latched to the flared part of the nipple)		Provide cheek support with your thumb and index or middle finger; check nipple length if this does not work

Problem	Date	Things to Try
Your baby is not latching properly on the breast (the breast should be drawn deeply into the mouth with your baby's lips latched)		1. When using a cradle hold or side-lying position, provide cheek support to the lower cheek; provide jaw support if needed; or try the "Dancer" hand position if working with a professional who can demonstrate it for you 2. When using a football hold, provide cheek support with your thumb and index or middle finger; you will have to switch hands so that the hand on the side you are feeding is free to provide support

If you have dates next to the "Things to Try" column, review the chapter for the appropriate section on addressing these items.

What to Do If Liquid Is Flowing Too Fast or Too Slowly

The best way to tell if liquid is flowing too fast from the breast or bottle is to listen for the sounds your baby makes while drinking. Mom's breast milk can let down very quickly, or fluid can flow through the bottle nipple too fast. When this occurs, your baby may make little high-pitched gulping sounds. Your baby's vocal cords are making the high-pitched sound while closing to keep liquid from going into the airway. You may also hear little struggling sounds like your baby is trying to clear her throat. This means that your baby is working too hard and may be aspirating fluid. If your baby is gasping for breath, there is definitely a problem.

If you hear any of these sounds, find a way to slow the flow. For quick let-down while breast-feeding, position your baby in a more upright position to limit the effects of gravity.[76] Your lactation consultant can help you with this. For bottle-fed babies, flow can be controlled to match your baby's suckling by choosing the correct bottle nipple. Some nipples flow more slowly than others.

There are variable-flow nipples available (such as the Haberman), where the flow can be adjusted according to your baby's suckling ability. I prefer the Haberman nipple, because it is very easy to control. Variable-flow nipples allow liquid to flow more slowly if your baby is gasping, gulping, or struggling in any way. They also permit liquid to flow faster as your baby develops more skill. If your baby has a weak suckle, the variable-flow nipple will allow your baby an easier flow until her suckle is stronger. You can actually assist your baby in developing a stronger suckle by having her work a "little harder" (but not to the point of fatigue) as you change the flow of the nipple over time.

Paced bottle-feeding, where the bottle is held even with the horizon, can also keep the liquid from flowing too fast. *The Breastfeeding Mother's Guide to Making More Milk,* a book by Diana West and Lisa Marasco, contains detailed information on paced bottle-feeding. See the description of paced bottle-feeding in the positioning section of this chapter.

Important Note for Parents Who Are Bottle-Feeding: Please do not attempt to modify or change the bottle nipple your baby uses. Some parents have enlarged the hole of a nipple for a faster flow. Nipples that flow too fast can cause significant mouth development problems. Some parents have cut the nipple so that formula mixed with cereal can come through the bottle nipple. Cereal is best presented from a spoon or an open cup when the time is right. If your baby has trouble drinking from a nipple, try some different nipples. However, there are so many on the market you may need an appropriately trained professional (such as a lactation consultant, pediatrician, nurse practitioner, occupational therapist, or speech therapist) to help you with this process.

I like the story of "The Three Bears" when we talk about liquid flow. We want liquid flow from the breast or bottle to be "just right" for your baby. If liquid flows too fast, it can cause your baby to cough or choke. Some babies learn to pull their tongues back to protect the airway from the fast-flowing liquid. This is a hard habit to break. If liquid flows too slowly, your baby may hump or thrust the tongue to apply more pressure. The greatest concern about inappropriate liquid flow is that your baby can develop incorrect feeding habits that can affect swallowing for a lifetime. See Activity 2.5 if your baby is having problems with liquid flow.

ACTIVITY 2.5: LIQUID FLOW FROM THE BREAST OR BOTTLE

Circle the problem you are seeing, and place a date in the column next to what you want to try. Be sure that you have completed Activities 2.1, 2.2, and 2.4 prior to doing this activity if you are breast-feeding. If you are bottle-feeding, complete Activities 2.1, 2.2, 2.3, and 2.4 prior to completing this activity.

Problem	Date	Things to Try or Do
Breast-feeding: Milk let-down is too fast		Feed your baby in a more upright position; work with your lactation consultant

Problem	Date	Things to Try or Do
Bottle nipple flow is too fast		Change nipple to a slower-flow nipple; consider a variable-flow nipple or paced bottle-feeding
Bottle nipple flow is too slow		Change nipple to a faster-flow nipple; consider a variable-flow nipple
It's difficult to find the correct nipple flow		Consult a professional for help

If you have dates next to a "Things to Try or Do" column, review the chapter for the appropriate section on addressing these items.

Subtle Difficulties That Can Affect Feeding and What to Do about Them

During my work as a feeding and speech therapist for almost 30 years, I have had the opportunity to work closely with very skilled lactation consultants. However, certain babies had difficulty nursing, despite all of the wonderful techniques recommended. These babies were often referred to my private practice and had problems related to subtle structural or movement difficulties in the mouth, which we will discuss here.

Some babies are more successful with bottle-feeding than breast-feeding. Many nursing moms assume that they (the moms) are having the difficulties, not the babies. However, there may be some small but significant differences with mouth development that can affect your baby's ability to nurse or bottle-feed. Professional evaluation can help. Some lactation consultants, occupational therapists, and speech-language pathologists are specifically trained to evaluate these subtle concerns.

So, what are the small difficulties that can affect your baby's feeding? One problem I have seen is mild jaw weakness. The muscles on one or both sides of the jaw may not be doing their jobs. Often parents will report that they also had some difficulties with feeding as babies (particularly nursing). Since mouth structures are inherited, one of the parents will often have a similar pattern in the jaw.

Another problem that some babies have is underdeveloped sucking pads (the fat pads in the cheeks that your baby develops during the last month of pregnancy). Premature babies do not have a chance to develop these, and babies do not develop them after birth. Some reportedly full-term babies have only partial sucking pads. We do not know for sure why some babies are born with only partially developed sucking pads. Some babies may be born a little early (ie, near term) because of scheduled delivery dates. Underdeveloped sucking pads may also be an inherited trait.

As we discussed in chapter 1, the sucking pads are important stabilizers for your baby's mouth during feeding. They assist the mouth in obtaining appropriate internal pressure, so formula or breast milk can be efficiently managed and swallowed. You can feel your baby's sucking pads by placing your index finger inside your baby's cheek and your thumb outside. A fully developed sucking pad feels like a "ball" of flesh in each cheek. If your newborn baby has well-developed sucking pads, it may be difficult for you to place your finger inside her cheek.

If your child does not have fully developed sucking pads or has a mild jaw weakness, you can help. There are a number of things you can do to assist feeding and other aspects of mouth development. These are activities you can do as you play and interact with your baby on a daily basis. See chapter 5 for further information on this topic.

Activity 2.6 helps you identify problems that can occur within the larger feeding picture. It brings together the different aspects of feeding that tend to cause feeding problems. If you can identify how these fit together, you can usually see how the problems can be solved easily and quickly.

ACTIVITY 2.6: THINGS TO DO OR TRY IF YOUR BABY IS HAVING DIFFICULTY FEEDING

Circle the problem you are seeing, and place a date in the column next to what you want to try.

Problem	Date	Things to Do or Try
Baby changes color while feeding (blue, gray, pink, or red)		**Call your pediatrician;** work with your pediatrician or a feeding specialist on suck-swallow-breathe coordination
Very wide jaw movement, tongue humping and/or thrusting, or biting on nipple occurs		Be sure your baby's head and neck are in line with her body and there is no hyperextension of the neck (backward tilting of the head)

Problem	Date	Things to Do or Try
Baby has a significant tongue or lip restriction or a heart-shaped tongue		Talk to your pediatrician or other appropriate physician about whether or not a clipping procedure is needed; get therapy if needed (often needed if the child is older than newborn)
Baby can't maintain lip latch		Provide cheek and/or jaw support; check nipple length
Bottle nipple moves in and out of mouth		Provide cheek and/or jaw support; try a smaller, shorter nipple if cheek support does not help
Reduced pressure in the mouth results in a shallow or poor latch on the breast or bottle		Check head, neck, body, and nose positioning; try cheek and/or jaw support
Problems do not resolve and may be related to subtle differences in your baby's mouth		See chapter 5 on "Face, Jaw, and Mouth Massage with 'Jaws-ercise'"

If you have dates next to the "Things to Do or Try" column, review the chapter for the appropriate section on addressing these items.

Nutrition

There are many good books on nutrition. This book is not meant to replace them. In fact, I recommend books on nutrition by Ellyn Satter to the parents with whom I work. These are:

1. *Child of Mine: Feeding with Love and Good Sense*[77]
2. *How to Get Your Kid to Eat . . . But Not Too Much*[78]

Good nutrition is difficult to attain if your baby's mouth and digestive system are not working well. You now know a lot about how your baby's mouth works. Let's talk about some basics of nutrition.

Appropriate weight gain is crucial. This means that your baby should not be overweight or underweight. Breast-fed infants are seldom overweight, because they stop eating when they are full. Sometimes they eat bigger meals, and sometimes they snack.[79] Breast-feeding usually takes 15 minutes or less per breast, beginning about every 2 hours with a newborn. The mother's breast milk production adjusts to the infant's nutritional needs when breast-feeding is going well. Therefore, Mom's nutrition and hydration are important to the baby's nutrition and hydration.

It is a little trickier to judge whether a bottle-fed baby is getting appropriate nutrition. I believe this is one reason some bottle-fed babies may be overfed. As a therapist, I have worked with babies who continue drinking from or suckling at a bottle for apparent comfort after their nutritional needs are apparently met.

In my experience, bottle-fed babies tend to have more problems with excessive spit-up, technically called *gastroesophageal reflux*. Breast-fed babies do not seem to have this problem as often. This is probably because Mom's milk supply adjusts to her baby's nutritional needs.

A baby's stomach is very small (about the size of her fist). If a baby overfills her stomach by even one-half ounce, this can contribute to gastroesophageal reflux (spit-up) and discomfort. You know how it feels to overeat. If you suffer from reflux, you know that you are more likely to experience reflux if you overfill your stomach.

Both breast-fed and bottle-fed babies need to self-regulate the amount they eat according to their own needs. It is crucial to allow your baby to decide how much and how often to eat, unless she is demonstrating signs of poor growth and/or dehydration.

Your baby will also go through some growth spurts, so some days she will be hungrier than others. According to Ellyn Satter, some predictable growth spurts appear to occur at 7 to 10 days, 5 to 6 weeks, and 3 months of age.[80]

The best way to track your baby's growth is through frequent weight and measurement checks. Most hospitals with lactation consultants and most pediatricians' offices have scales and measurement equipment available. You can also rent a scale if you need to track your baby's weight between office visits.

Your pediatrician and/or lactation consultant will have growth charts to help you follow increases in your baby's weight, head circumference, and length. Many books on nutrition (such as Ellyn Satter's books) contain these charts, as well. Ask your pediatrician to use growth charts developed by the World Health Organization *(www.who.int)* if you are breast-feeding, because many other growth charts are based on data obtained in formula-fed babies.[81] Formula-fed and breast-fed babies grow somewhat differently.

Also, many parents are anxious about their child's nutrition. This can cause some parents to err on the side of overfeeding. While I think this concern is perfectly normal, it may cause problems with weight and feeding later on. If you are nervous about how much your baby is eating, your baby can sense your feelings. This makes feeding stressful for you and for your baby. I want you to be relaxed and confident when you feed your baby. Get good information on nutrition and how your child is growing. Work with your pediatrician and/or lactation consultant on this.

Children tend to eat what they need and self-limit the amount of food they take. Parents need to learn their baby's body language and communication signals to know when their baby is full. In the following activity, you will find information from Ellyn Satter on the body language of babies to help you with this process.[82]

ACTIVITY 2.7: WHAT MY BABY'S BODY IS TELLING ME	
Place a date in the column next to the description that matches what your baby is doing.	
Ready to Eat	**Date**
Eyes open wider than usual	
Face looks bright	
Arms and legs curl over belly	
Touch around mouth stimulates a rooting reflex and/or mouthing	
Baby may suck on hands	
Fussing is a last resort	
Ready to Take a Break	
May pause to rest	
May pause to look at you and/or socialize	
How to Tell When Baby Is Full, or Something Does Not Feel Right	
Sucking or suckling slows down	

ACTIVITY 2.7: (cont.)	
How to Tell When Baby Is Full, or Something Does Not Feel Right	
Baby lets go of nipple	
Baby will turn away	
Baby will begin to kick, squirm, arch back, get fussy if you don't pay attention to the signals listed above	

Remember that the amount your baby eats is individual and is based on her own metabolism and stomach size. Age, growth rate, and activity level[83] will also factor into this equation.

If you are bottle-feeding, here are some of Ellyn Satter's guidelines on formula amounts.[84] These are only guidelines. They are given per day, not per feeding. It is also better to feed your baby more frequently throughout the day than to overfeed your baby at any one meal. See previous discussion about gastroesophageal reflux.

- Birth to 1 month: 14–28 ounces per day
- 1 to 2 months: 23–34 ounces per day
- 2 to 3 months: 25–40 ounces per day
- 3 to 4 months: 27–39 ounces per day
- 4 to 5 months: 29–46 ounces per day
- 5 to 6 months: 32–48 ounces per day
- Once you introduce solid foods to your baby's diet (between 4 and 6 months of age), these requirements change significantly.

There are iron-fortified formulas for babies. Have your pediatrician check to see if your baby needs extra iron. Also, if you are using a powdered formula that you mix with water, have your water tested for lead and other contaminants. It is best to boil the water you use for 3 minutes during your baby's first 6 months of life.[85] Check with your pediatrician on the safety of using powdered formula, as there have been a number of recalls on powdered formula.[86] See the American Academy of Pediatrics Web site *(www.aap.org)* for further information.

Hydration

Your child may act hungry but actually be thirsty. Seventy-five percent of the body and 85% of the brain is water.[87–88] Your baby's body and brain need water. Breast milk and formula contain water, so you usually don't need to give your baby extra water until she begins to experiment with drinking from an open cup around 4 to 6 months of age. Talk to your pediatrician about this. According to Suzanne Evans Morris and Marsha Dunn Klein, authors of *Pre-Feeding Skills: A Comprehensive Resource for Mealtime Development*, infants require 1½ oz of fluid per pound of body weight each day.[89]

Water "regulates all functions of the body."[90] It helps to keep body chemistry in balance by carrying hormones, nutrients, and other important substances to the cells of the body. Water also removes waste from these cells. Your child should drink two-thirds of her body weight in ounces each day (eg, a 36-lb child needs 24 oz of water per day).[91–92] Breast milk and formula contain water. Baby foods also contain water. Work with your child's pediatrician to determine how much water your baby needs.

Adequate hydration is connected to immune system function. Dehydration leads to disease. Some signs and symptoms of dehydration can include chronic drowsiness, chronic pain, constipation, belly pain, head pain, stress, depression, chronic upper respiratory illness, asthma, allergies, excessive body weight, diabetes, and problems with sleep.[93]

The following may lead to or indicate poor growth and dehydration in your baby:[94]

- Decrease in "pees and poops"
- Few feedings
- Decrease in number of feedings
- Overly sleepy
- Weak sucking ability
- Little interest in feeding.

Here are some signs of significant dehydration. Please **contact your baby's physician** if you see any of these signs: [95]

- Dry mouth and decreased "pees"
- Sunken eyes with few tears when crying
- Sunken soft spot
- Tight, dry skin
- Fast pulse and breathing
- Skin unusually blue
- Cold hands and/or feet
- Listlessness, drowsiness, or unconsciousness

Feeding Development: One to 6 Months of Age

Here is a feeding development checklist, so you can look at your baby's progress in feeding during the first 6 months. It will also help you prepare for all of the new feeding activities you and your baby will be doing around 5 to 6 months of age.

Feeding Development Checklist: One to 6 Months of Age[96-104]

Place a date next to the skills your baby is accomplishing. Circle the items your baby needs to accomplish. Know that these checklists are approximate, and not absolute. Every baby has her own unique developmental sequence. These checklists should be used as a guide to let you know if your baby is basically on track or not. If your baby is not showing you some of the skills listed in these checklists or you do not understand the item, review the chapter for further information. Always talk to your pediatrician or another knowledgeable professional if you have questions regarding your baby's development.

Date	Age: 1 Month
	Control of rooting reflex developing
	Easily locates nipple with mouth
	Suckles or sucks thin liquid from bottle or breast, sequencing two or more sucks

By 1 month of age, your baby can locate the breast or bottle nipple easily with her mouth. The rooting reflex is coming under control. You will see the rooting reflex more often in breast-fed babies than in bottle-fed babies. Breast-fed babies use the rooting reflex to find Mom's nipple. Bottle-fed babies have the nipple placed into their mouths and don't really use the reflex. Your baby can now suckle or suck breast milk or formula, sequencing two or (usually) more sucks at a time with good suck-swallow-breathe coordination.

Date	Age: 2–3 Months
	Control of the suckling reflex is developing
	The mouth is beginning to change shape, and the tongue is beginning to move more within the mouth

Date	Age: 2–3 Months
	Longer suckling or sucking occurs without a pause on the bottle or breast
	Baby brings her hands together

By 2 to 3 months of age, your baby is developing control of the suckling reflex. She will suckle or suck for longer periods of time without pausing. The mouth is beginning to change shape, and the tongue is beginning to move more within the mouth. You will see your baby bring her hands together when feeding. She may rest them on the breast or bottle. Babies that have difficulty with breast- or bottle-feeding often improve significantly by 6–8 weeks of age, as suck-swallow-breathe coordination increases.

Date	Age: 3–4 Months
	Suck-swallow-breathe coordination improves
	More space develops between the structures in the throat (the soft palate, epiglottis, and larynx)
	The tongue seal toward the front third of the tongue leads to three-dimensional sucking by 4 months (the tip of the tongue and sides come up with the lips puckered, the fat pads shrink, and the cheek and jaw muscles develop)
	A sequence of 20+ suckles or sucks occurs without a pause
	Coughing or choking occurs only occasionally
	Baby recognizes the bottle when she sees it
	Baby pats the bottle or breast with her hand(s)

At 3 to 4 months of age, your baby now recognizes the bottle or breast when she sees it. She will pat the bottle or breast with her hand(s). Your baby's suck-swallow-breathe coordination is increasing substantially. You will hear only occasional coughing if your baby loses control of this coordination. Your baby is adapting to the increasing space between the structures in the mouth and throat. She will suck or suckle 20 or more times without a pause from the breast or bottle. Your baby is developing a mature, three-dimensional suck, where the tongue seals toward the front third of the mouth, the tip of the tongue and sides move up, the lips pucker, and the cheek muscles replace the work of the sucking pads. The sucking pads are getting smaller.

The mature, three-dimensional suck is different from the suckle your baby used previously. Remember that the suckle involved front-to-back wavelike tongue movement, with significant tongue cupping and little open space inside the mouth. Now, there is more space within the mouth, and the tongue is beginning to do what therapists call *dissociate*. This means that one part (ie, the front) of the tongue is learning to move independently of the rest of the tongue. Dissociation is a very important process for higher-level eating and drinking skills.

Date	Age: 3–6 Months
	Rooting reflex is seen less and less; seems to be disappearing; baby locates breast nipple frequently without use of rooting reflex (3–6 months)
	Third lips disappear (3–6 months)
	Gag reflex comes under control (4–6 months)
	Space between mouth and nasal area increases (4–6 months)
	Open space in mouth continues to increase through jaw growth and shrinking of the sucking pads (4–6 months)
	The tongue seal toward the front third of the tongue leads to three-dimensional sucking by 4 months (the tip of the tongue and sides come up with the lips puckered, the fat pads shrink, and the cheek and jaw muscles develop)
	Baby develops increased lip control and movement (4–6 months)
	Baby begins to learn to use jaw, lip, and tongue muscles separately

Date	Age: 3–6 Months
	Appropriate intraoral air pressure is maintained through the valving of structures (ie, appropriate mouth structures coming together and moving apart, like the closing and opening of a valve)
	Teeth begin to come in, with increased chewing and biting experiences (5–6 months)
	Baby places hands on bottle (4½ months); holds bottle with hand or hands (5½ months)
	Mouth and digestive system are getting ready for cereals and pureed foods (4–6 months)
	Baby is ready to experiment with drinking from an open cup, with the cup held by the parent or care provider (4–6 months); drinks from an open cup held by the parent (6 months)
	Baby's mouth is ready for a soft baby cookie, thicker puree or cereal, and foods with very small, soft lumps (5–6 months)
	Baby bites and chews on a soft cookie with a rhythmic bite reflex (5–6 months)
	Baby may use a diagonal rotary chewing pattern if food is placed on the sides of the gum surfaces (5–6 months)
	Baby suckles or sucks to swallow food and liquid (5–6 months)

A lot of changes are happening in your baby's feeding abilities between 3 and 6 months of age. You will see your baby's rooting reflex less and less—it seems to be disappearing. Reflexes do not really disappear; the motor (movement) area of your baby's brain is developing and taking control, so the reflex is not needed. The third lips (the slight gum swelling during feeding) will also seem to disappear.

Between 4 and 6 months, the gag will be stimulated farther back on the tongue. New mouthing and feeding experiences allow this to occur. Breast-fed babies have a particular advantage—Mom's breast is drawn deeply into the mouth, which helps to integrate the gag reflex. As your baby gains more control over mouth space and movement, the gag reflex does not need to occur as far forward on the tongue. However, it will still help protect your baby from items that are too large to swallow. We will discuss this topic further in chapters 4 and 5.

By 4 to 6 months, the space between your baby's mouth and nasal area (nose) increases. Your baby's hard palate and nasal and sinus areas are developing. There is more open space in your baby's mouth, because her jaw is growing and the sucking pads are getting smaller. By 4 months, your baby's tongue seals toward the front third of the mouth in a three-dimensional suck. You will begin to see your baby have more lip control and movement.

Your baby's mouth structures are beginning to move independently of one another over time (eg, the tongue and lips move independently of the jaw). As mentioned previously, therapists call this *dissociation*. This allows valving within the mouth (ie, appropriate mouth structures coming together and moving apart, like the closing and opening of a valve). Through this valving, your baby will learn to control the pressure changes within the mouth. Therapists call this intraoral pressure. The mouth, throat, esophagus, voice box, and respiratory system are really systems of valves and pressure changes. The processes of dissociation and pressure valving allow the development of mature eating, drinking, and speaking skills.

Your baby puts her hands on the bottle around 4½ months and holds the bottle around 5½ months of age. Her mouth and digestive system are getting ready for cereals and pureed foods between 4 and 6 months. Formula-fed babies may need to begin cereals and pureed foods earlier than breast-fed babies. Breast milk is said to be a complete food, while formula is not.[105] Check with your baby's pediatrician about when to begin these foods. There are also iron-fortified baby cereals. Have your pediatrician check to see if your baby needs extra iron.

By 6 months of age, your baby is usually sitting up. This places her in a good position for eating from a spoon and drinking from an open cup. Baby cereals and other pureed foods can be given with a spoon or an open cup when your baby is ready to learn these skills. We will discuss spoon-feeding and drinking from an open cup extensively in chapter 6. At 5 to 6 months, your baby will still suck or suckle to swallow. The mature, adultlike swallowing pattern (where the tip of the tongue touches the ridge behind the top front teeth to start the swallow) will not appear until around 12 months.

Between 5 and 6 months of age, your baby's teeth will begin to come in. The processes of chewing and taking bites help develop the jaw muscles and assist in the appearance of teeth. In my experience, babies who don't chew and bite on toys and foods are often late in tooth development and have more problems with jaw development.

With an increase in biting and chewing activities at 5 to 6 months of age, your baby is ready to bite on a soft baby cookie (such as an arrowroot cookie). She will use the rhythmic bite reflex to bite on the cookie. If a small piece of cookie or a soft, small lump of food is placed on your baby's side gums, you may see some diagonal rotary chewing. This means that the jaw is moving sideways and diagonally and then back to center to chew the food. Circular rotary chewing (when the jaw moves in a circle) is the way we chew our food as adults. Your baby will develop this by 2 years of age. Even though you have just started giving your baby solid foods at 5 to 6 months of age, she is quickly ready to begin foods with small, soft lumps, as well as thicker purees and cereals. Details will be provided for you in chapter 6.

Now, let's proceed to chapter 3 to learn some more about your baby's development. In chapter 3, we are going to talk about breathing, belly time, common health problems, and my opinion on vaccines.

3

Breathing through the Nose, Belly Time, Allergies, Spit-Up, SIDS, and Vaccines

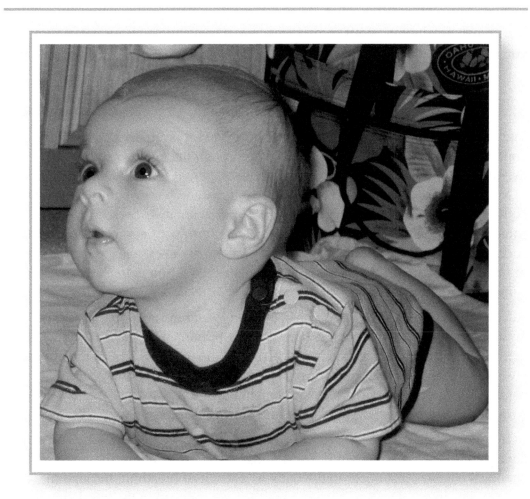

Key Topics in This Chapter

■ The Importance of Breathing through the Nose for Health

■ The Importance of Belly Time When Your Baby Is Awake

■ Health Problems and Possible Treatments

■ Let's Talk about Allergies and Sensitivities

■ Reflux, SIDS, and Sleeping on the Back

■ What about Vaccines?

In this chapter, we will cover a number of topics related to your baby's health and development. We will discuss breathing through the nose, belly time, health problems and possible treatments, allergies, sudden infant death syndrome, or SIDS, and vaccines. These are all important topics for you as a parent.

The Importance of Breathing through the Nose for Health

The importance of breathing through the nose cannot be stressed enough for your baby and all human beings. Breathing through the nose is crucial for overall health. It helps your baby's jaw and facial areas develop. It directs air to lower lung areas, where more blood is oxygenated.[106] Your baby's brain and body need oxygen for all life processes. Newborns are nose breathers, unless some problem exists. However, some babies are born with nasal obstruction.[107] A constantly stuffy nose, feeding difficulty, or "sticky eyes" can be symptoms of nasal obstruction.[108] Speak with your pediatrician if you notice any of these symptoms.

According to Dr David C. Page, considered a pioneer in functional jaw orthopedics, "your jaws form the gateway to your human airway and influence your life, for life."[109] Remember that the roof of the mouth is part of the upper jaw. We talked a lot about the roof of the mouth in chapters 1 and 2. The hard palate, or roof of the mouth, needs to remain fairly broad so that your baby's nasal and sinus areas are adequate for breathing through the nose.

In his book, *Your Jaws—Your Life*, Dr Page says that people with small airways have a tendency toward breathing problems.[110] He also explains the important chemical changes that occur in the body as a result of breathing through the nose. According to Dr Page, nitric oxide[111–112] is produced in the nasal sinuses, secreted into the nasal passages, and inhaled through the nose. It is found in healthy newborns during the first hour of life.[113]

Nitric oxide prevents bacterial growth and can kill some viruses.[114] This chemical helps dilate blood vessels, including those in the lungs, and has an antiinflammatory effect.[115–116] It also helps oxygen to be absorbed by the lungs and transported throughout the body. Babies who breathe through their mouths may have lower levels of blood oxygen and higher levels of carbon dioxide than those who breathe through their noses, because they are not inhaling nitric oxide.[117]

Physician Christine Northrup also discusses the importance of breathing through the nose in several of her books. She says that breathing through the mouth causes a stress response and releases stress hormones within the body. Deep breathing through the nose, into the chest, and into the lower abdomen reduces the production of stress hormones and brings about relaxation.[118] You can watch your baby's abdomen rise and fall as he breathes deeply when relaxed or sleeping. Breathing through the nose is also the first step to good immune system function, because the nose warms and filters the air being inhaled.

Breathing through the nose can be encouraged through appropriate feeding techniques that keep the mouth "in shape." We discussed these in chapter 2. Here are some of the other benefits of breathing through the nose:[119]

- Overall body movement becomes easier for your baby, because he is breathing more deeply.

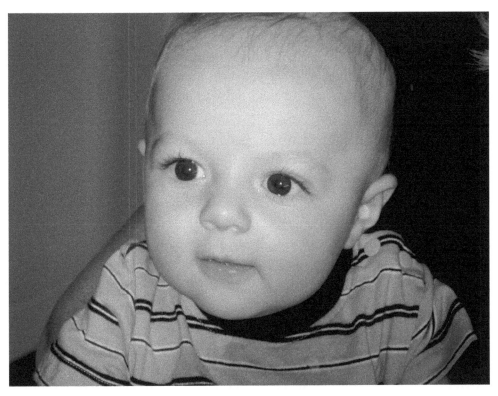

Photo 3.1: Anthony breathes through his nose with his mouth closed.

- The vagus nerve in the upper abdomen is stimulated, allowing your baby to move more vigorously with a lower heart rate as he develops.

- It maintains rib cage flexibility, so your baby's lung capacity is at its best; this way, oxygen can be carried to the body and brain effectively (the rib cage is active by 7 to 8 months of age).[120]

- The chances of developing colds, sinus infections, ear infections, croup, and asthma are reduced, because the air is being warmed and filtered by the nose.

- Metabolism improves, because better oxygen consumption in the body allows better metabolism of food. This is very important for babies.

The Importance of Belly Time When Your Baby Is Awake

Belly time (placing your baby in a face-down, or prone, position) provides the foundation for the development of breathing, postural control (eg, sitting and standing), and movement (eg, rolling, crawling, walking, eating, drinking, and talking). The muscles in your baby's head, neck, upper spine, shoulder girdle, chest, and abdomen develop through belly time and movement. Children who do not have a sufficient amount of belly time often have difficulties with postural development, breathing, feeding, and speech. Unfortunately, therapists are seeing far more of these problems than we would like.

Today, babies are not getting the changes in position and the body movements that babies tended to receive in the past. As a result, we are seeing more developmental problems related to our babies' sedentary lifestyles. Some of this has to do with our mobile lifestyles. We tend to keep our babies in car and infant seats for longer periods of time as we transport them from place to place. This is why it is extremely important for your baby to have belly time each day when your baby is awake.

The amount of belly time in which your baby engages can increase as your baby is awake for longer periods of time during the day. It is very important to place your baby on her back when sleeping, unless you are using a SIDS monitor. Having belly time when your baby is awake is critical for your child's postural, respiratory, and motor development.

Your baby has spent 9 months in your belly, in a position called *flexion*. Baby seats and swings also place your baby into flexion. Since your baby needs to develop muscles on both sides of the body (front and back), your baby will need different movement and positioning experiences to do this. One way to give your baby this experience is to place your baby on the belly for a period of time each day when your baby is awake.

This will help your baby develop the muscles of the neck, back, chest, abdomen, and shoulder girdle, to name a few. These muscles will ultimately assist your baby in developing motor skills, such as controlling head and neck movements, rolling,

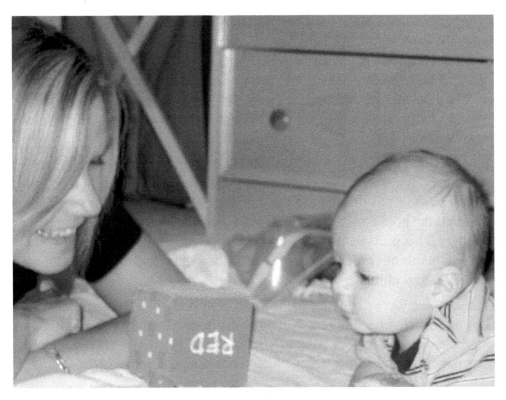

Photo 3.2: Anthony participates in belly time.

sitting, crawling, standing, walking, breathing, and speaking. To develop these skills, there needs to be good co-contraction and coordination of muscle groups in the body—namely, flexors and extensors. Flexors are generally the muscles that bring an area of the body together (such as those needed to bend at the waist or bend the elbow). Extensors generally straighten an area of the body (such as those used to stand up tall or straighten the elbow).

Some parents hear about the importance of placing their baby on her back during sleep and mistakenly think that the baby should be on her back all or most of the time. Currently, therapists, nurses, physicians, and educators have noticed that many children do not seem to be developing motor skills (eg, controlling head and neck movements, rolling, feeding, crawling, walking, talking, and handwriting) on time.

Many speech-language pathologists have noticed a recent increase in the number of children with delayed feeding and speech development. Many occupational therapists have noticed an increase in the number of children with delays in handwriting development and other hand skills. Many physical therapists have noticed an increase in fittings for special headgear to help babies overcome "flat heads." We, as therapists, are wondering whether these delays and differences in development are related to the decreased amount of belly time that babies are getting when awake.

How long should you place your baby on her belly when awake? This changes as your baby grows. As your baby spends more time awake, you will have more opportunities for belly time. There is no "time schedule" for this. However, you will want to make some time for this activity each day. You want your baby to experience a balance of different body positions, so that muscle groups can learn to respond in different ways to support activities that your baby will perform throughout life.

Place your baby in different positions, including lying on the back (supine), lying on the belly (prone), and lying on the side. Your baby should have time in each of these positions throughout the day. Baby seats allow you to move your baby around the house with you, so you can interact with your child as you do other things. This is certainly appropriate at times when you need to use your hands for other things (such as cooking and doing laundry) and still want to interact with your child.

You can also carry your baby on the front of your body in a baby carrier while you do certain activities that require you to use your hands. In my opinion, this is preferable to carrying your baby around in a seat, because it encourages your baby to make postural adjustments, change position, and move.

When your newborn baby comes home from the hospital, you can give your baby some quality belly time by having your baby lie on your chest area as you

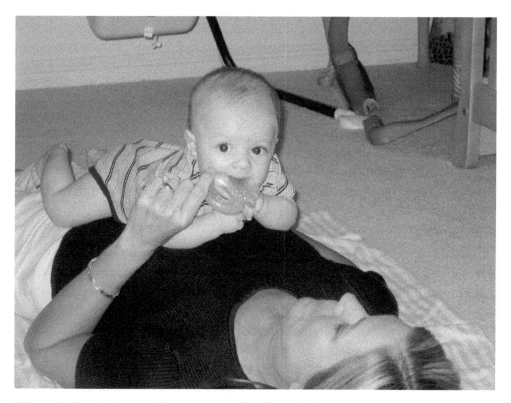

Photo 3.3: Anthony demonstrates belly-to-belly position with Diane.

recline. This gives dads a wonderful opportunity to bond with newborns. If your baby should catnap in this position, you can monitor your baby's breathing, because you will be awake. As your baby grows, he will begin to lift his head, and you can have some fleeting eye contact with your baby. Over time, you and your baby will share increasing eye contact as your baby's head and neck become stronger.

You can also place your baby in a prone position (on his belly) on a large bed prior to your baby learning to roll. You must be with your baby, because babies do wiggle even before they roll. Once your baby learns to roll, the bed is **not** a safe location for belly time. After your baby has learned to roll, the floor or other safe play areas may be good locations. You can place a clean baby blanket or sheet on the floor as long as the sheet or blanket is safely spread and cannot stop your baby from breathing by getting bunched up. Again, your baby must be where you can see him when you do this. You can also interact with your baby in this position by getting down on the floor on your belly, facing your baby. You can place some toys around your baby for him to see.

It is fun to play and vocalize with your baby in this position. You can make eye contact, eventually have your baby look at and reach for toys, and play reciprocal vocal games (you make vocal sounds, and your baby responds with vocal sounds). This can include cooing, babbling, and talking in a conversational manner with your baby and waiting for your baby to make a vocal response. Belly time helps to strengthen the respiratory system, which is used for vocalization and, eventually, speech. Adults often need some strengthening in the prone position, so it will be good for both you and your baby to lie on your bellies while you interact.

Remember, baby seats and swings all have their uses in your life and your baby's life. However, they should not be used to the exclusion of other positioning and movement activities for your baby. They place your baby in generally one position (flexion). Your baby was in this position for 9 months prior to birth and needs a number of other positioning and movement experiences for his body to develop well.

Health Problems and Possible Treatments

Hopefully you will not need the charts in this section very often. However, if you see any of these health problems in your infant or toddler, please keep track of them. Seeing these occasionally is one thing; seeing these chronically is another. Date each occurrence of any of these symptoms. I have divided the health problems into three groups:

- Group 1: Possible Allergy-related Problems
- Group 2: Upper Respiratory Problems
- Group 3: Other Respiratory Problems

GROUP 1: POSSIBLE ALLERGY-RELATED PROBLEMS

Problem	Date	Person(s) to See	Possible Treatments
Excessive spit-up (reflux)		Pediatrician, pediatric gastroenterologist, pediatric allergist, pediatric dietitian, or others as appropriate	Change of diet, change in positioning or movement, infant massage to relax and calm baby, medication
Excessive diarrhea		Pediatrician, pediatric gastroenterologist, pediatric allergist, pediatric dietitian, or others as appropriate	Change of diet, infant massage to relax and calm baby, medication
Possible food sensitivity or allergy		Pediatrician, pediatric gastroenterologist, pediatric allergist, pediatric dietitian, or others as appropriate	Change of diet, rotation diet, activities to boost baby's immune system (eg, infant massage)
Rashes or eczema		Pediatrician, pediatric allergist, pediatric dietitian, or others as appropriate	Evaluation for food or environmental allergies or sensitivities, activities to calm and boost baby's immune system (eg, infant massage), medication

Problem	Date	Person(s) to See	Possible Treatments
Hay fever and other environmental allergies or sensitivities		Pediatrician; pediatric ear, nose, and throat specialist; pediatric allergist; or others as appropriate	Evaluation for food or environmental allergies or sensitivities, activities to calm and boost baby's immune system (eg, infant massage), medication
Feeding problems		Pediatrician, lactation consultant, occupational therapist, speech-language pathologist, pediatric dietitian, feeding team, or others as appropriate	Regular sessions with someone who works with babies' feeding problems; find a professional who can help you learn techniques to resolve your baby's feeding problem

Excessive spit-up. If your baby has excessive spit-up, this could be caused by food allergies or sensitivities, a weak lower esophageal sphincter, or ingesting too much milk too fast.[121] The lower esophageal sphincter is the area at the bottom of the esophagus that keeps food from leaving the stomach. We will discuss allergies in the next section and reflux (spit-up) later in this chapter. If your child has this problem, your pediatrician is the first person who can help you. She will often begin by recommending a change in diet for breast-feeding moms or a change in formula.

You can also introduce changes in your baby's body positioning (eg, more belly time when awake) and other techniques (eg, infant massage) to help your baby's digestive process. See the section in this chapter on reflux and chapter 5 on infant massage for further details. If your pediatrician cannot help you, she will often refer you to another professional, such as a pediatric gastroenterologist (often referred to as a "GI doctor"). The pediatric gastroenterologist may refer you to a pediatric allergist if needed, who may refer you to a pediatric dietitian.

The roles of these professionals are discussed in chapter 9. Medication may be prescribed by your baby's physician to address reflux.

Excessive diarrhea. Excessive diarrhea could also be caused by food allergies or sensitivities. It is important to remember that breast-fed babies have looser stools than bottle-fed babies, and this is normal. However, excessive diarrhea may require a change in Mom's diet if breast-feeding or a change in formula if bottle-feeding. For the breast-feeding mom, an elimination diet and then a rotation diet may be tried. An elimination diet means that Mom removes foods likely to cause an allergic reaction from her diet. She later reintroduces these foods into her diet in a systematic manner to see if her baby has a reaction. A rotation diet means that Mom eats foods possibly causing the reaction only every 4 days. See the next section on allergies and sensitivities for more detail on foods that tend to cause them.

Infant massage and other activities to relieve stress and boost immune system function may also be useful. If excessive diarrhea is a problem, the same list of professionals may be required as those you would consult for excessive reflux. Medication may be prescribed by your baby's physician.

Rashes, eczema, hay fever, and airborne environmental allergies and sensitivities. Rashes and eczema can also be related to food or environmental allergies or sensitivities. As you know, changes in the breast-feeding mom's diet or a change in formula can be used to treat food allergies or sensitivities. Environmental allergies or sensitivities are usually observed and noted as you make or see changes in the environment. Rashes can be related to something as simple as the detergent you are using to wash your clothing. Hay fever and airborne environmental allergens (such as pollen, dust, pet dander, mold, pollutants, and chemicals) can cause sneezing and sinus congestion.

If your baby is suspected of having allergies or sensitivities, it is important to keep a log and/or food diary to help identify the cause (see the sample log sheet and food diary I've provided). Infant massage and other activities to relieve stress and boost immune system function may also help. There are some topical medications (those placed directly on a rash) that your pediatrician may prescribe or suggest. A pediatric ear, nose, and throat specialist or pediatric allergist may have some suggestions for treating hay fever and other airborne environmental allergies or sensitivities.

Feeding problems. Feeding problems experienced by infants and toddlers can be related to allergies, sensitivities, reflux, or other belly problems. It is important that you consult someone for help with your child's feeding problems. These may include your child's pediatrician, your lactation consultant, an occupational therapist, a speech-language pathologist, a pediatric dietitian, and/or a feeding team. You can often locate these specialists through your pediatrician or local children's hospital. See chapter 9 for more information on how these specialists can help you.

The reason I advise getting help for feeding problems early is because they can quickly escalate into behavior problems, even though behavior is not usually the cause. If a feeding problem is not handled well, the entire feeding process can become extremely frustrating for you and your child. See chapter 6 for more information on feeding problems.

ACTIVITY 3.1: FOOD DIARY

Date	Symptom Seen	What Mother Ate/ Drank (Breast-Feeding) or What Your Baby Ate/ Drank	What Change Are You Making?

EXAMPLE OF FOOD DIARY ENTRY

Date	Symptom Seen	What You Ate/ Drank (Breast-Feeding) or What Your Baby Ate/Drank	What Change Are You Making?
8/31/??	Excessive spit-up (breast-fed baby)	Breakfast: Cottage cheese and fruit with orange juice Lunch: Turkey sandwich on wheat bread with mayo; water Dinner: Roast beef, potatoes with gravy, broccoli; water Snacks: Soy protein bar	Replacing foods over time that typically cause allergies or sensitivities, beginning with soy; working with my physician

In this example, Mom's diet consists of the items listed. If the foods eaten by Mom are being considered as a possible cause of her baby's excessive spit-up, she might consider the removal of dairy, wheat, soy, and citrus from her diet (ie, foods that typically cause allergies and sensitivities). She could add foods back into and rotate foods through her diet over time to see if her baby has a reaction. She should work with her pediatrician and/or other appropriate medical professional on this.

ACTIVITY 3.2: LOG SHEET TO TRACK POSSIBLE ALLERGENS

Date	Symptom Seen	Change Made	Did You See Improvement?

Date	Symptom Seen	Change Made	Did You See Improvement?

EXAMPLE OF LOG SHEET ENTRY

Date	Symptom Seen	What You Did	Did You See a Change?
8/31/??	Rash on back	Changed laundry detergent	Yes

In this example, Mom and Dad noticed that their baby had a rash on her back, but not in the diaper area. They switched to a laundry detergent that was said to be more gentle and natural. The rash disappeared.

GROUP 2: UPPER RESPIRATORY PROBLEMS

Problem	Date	Person(s) to See	Possible Treatments
Stuffy or runny nose, sinus concerns		Pediatrician; pediatric ear, nose, and throat specialist; pediatric dentist; pediatric allergist; others as appropriate	Mucus suctioned, use of saline solution (prepared specifically for babies); evaluation of bony structure, swelling, or reflux; imaging examination (eg, MRI or x-ray); facilitaion to improve structure and function; medication
Snoring		Pediatrician; pediatric ear, nose, and throat specialist; pediatric allergist; pediatric dentist; pediatric orofacial-myofunctional or craniosacral therapist; others as appropriate	Evaluation of bony structure, swelling, or reflux; facilitation to improve structure and function; functional jaw orthopedics; craniosacral or orofacial-myofunctional therapy; medication
Frequent colds		Pediatrician; pediatric ear, nose, and throat specialist; pediatric dentist; pediatric allergist; others as appropriate	Evaluation for allergies and sensitivities, activities to boost the immune system (eg, infant massage), medication
Breathing through the mouth		Pediatrician; pediatric ear, nose, and throat specialist, pediatric allergist; pediatric dentist; pediatric orofacial-myofunctional or craniosacral therapist; others as appropriate	Evaluation of bony structure, swelling, or reflux; facilitation to improve structure and function; functional jaw orthopedics; craniosacral or orofacial-myofunctional therapy

Problem	Date	Person(s) to See	Possible Treatments
Pulling or grabbing the ear(s), excessive head shaking, fever, fatigue, irritability		Pediatrician; pediatric ear, nose, and throat specialist; pediatric allergist; pediatric audiologist (after consult with pediatrician); others as appropriate	Evaluation for ear problems, reflux, and food or environmental allergies or sensitivities; feedings administered in an upright position; craniosacral or orofacial-myofunctional treatment; medication

There are a number of upper respiratory problems that babies can have. These could be related to food or environmental allergies or sensitivities. They could also be related to reflux or structural problems of the mouth, nose, and face. If reflux is suspected, a pediatric gastroenterologist may be the person to see. Reflux has recently been connected with sinus, middle ear, and other respiratory problems.

If your baby has a stuffy or runny nose or any problem breathing through the nose (such as snoring or frequent colds), your pediatrician or nurse practitioner can teach you to suction excess mucus by using a bulb purchased at your local pharmacy. Your pediatrician or nurse practitioner can also suggest either homemade or commercially available saline solution that can help keep your baby's nose and sinus area clear. It is important that you use a saline solution that is safe for your baby. There are saline solutions prepared specifically for babies. You already know that problems breathing through the nose often lead to the unhealthy practice of mouth breathing.

It is also important for your pediatrician to check the structure of your baby's face, nose, and mouth if your baby cannot breathe easily through the nose. If your pediatrician needs help with this, he can refer you to another professional who can do this, such as a pediatric ear, nose, and throat specialist or a pediatric dentist. This may require an x-ray or another form of imaging. Your baby's physician may prescribe medication, if needed. There are some pediatric dentists (such as those who provide functional jaw orthopedics) and specially trained pediatric therapists (such as craniosacral and orofacial-myofunctional therapists) who know how to gently manipulate your baby's pliable bony face, nose, and mouth structures to help the structures move into place. This is called *facilitation* and can save your child a lifetime of upper respiratory illnesses and other problems related to the upper respiratory system.

Now let's discuss middle-ear problems. We have already talked about the best positioning for breast- and bottle-feeding in chapter 2. Positioning your baby with his ear above his mouth during feeding will help to keep liquid out of your baby's Eustachian tubes, which lead to the middle ear. Remember, the middle ear is the space behind the eardrum that is lined with mucus-producing membranes. This space has three little bones that communicate with the inner ear, which transmits sound to the brain. It is important that your baby's Eustachian tubes be in good working order, so that any fluid that may accumulate in the middle ear can drain into the throat.

Allergies or sensitivities can cause fluid to build in the middle ear, because mucous membranes tend to swell and secrete mucus when people have allergies or sensitivities. Reflux can also get into the Eustachian tube and middle ear because of the pressure changes that occur during reflux. Therefore, it may be important to keep your baby fairly upright immediately after feeding if he has excessive spit-up. Some parents elevate the head of their baby's bed—you can speak with your baby's physician about this. You may also want to implement other strategies to boost your baby's immune system (such as infant massage or other calming strategies) if your child is having ear or other upper respiratory problems.

Your child's pediatrician may prescribe medication if your child develops a middle-ear infection. However, there are other middle-ear problems that can lead to fluctuating hearing loss. These include retracted ear drums and fluid retention in the middle-ear spaces, which is related to Eustachian tube malfunction. Fluctuating hearing loss can be devastating to young children learning speech and language, because they are not hearing speech sounds accurately as their hearing changes or fluctuates. Your baby is learning the sounds of his language from birth. Many pediatricians have tympanometers in their offices to check middle-ear function in children. There are also pediatric audiologists who can provide this and other tests for your baby or toddler.

GROUP 3: OTHER RESPIRATORY PROBLEMS

Problem	Date	Person(s) to See	Possible Treatments
Wheezing or asthma		Pediatrician; pediatric ear, nose, and throat specialist; pediatric allergist; pediatric pulmonologist; others as appropriate	Evaluation for reflux, allergies, sensitivities, and swallowing problems; treatment for swallowing problem if present; respiratory therapy; activities to calm and boost baby's immune system (eg, infant massage); medication

Problem	Date	Person(s) to See	Possible Treatments
Hoarse or wet-sounding vocal quality		Pediatrician; pediatric ear, nose, and throat specialist; pediatric allergist; others as appropriate	Evaluation for reflux, allergies, sensitivities, and swallowing problems; treatment for swallowing problem if present; activities to calm and boost baby's immune system (eg, infant massage); medication
Persistent croupy-sounding cough		Pediatrician; pediatric ear, nose, and throat specialist; pediatric allergist; pediatric pulmonologist; others as appropriate	Evaluation for reflux, allergies, sensitivities, and swallowing problems; treatment for swallowing problem if present; respiratory therapy; activities to calm and boost baby's immune system (eg, infant massage); medication
Frequent pneumonia		Pediatrician; pediatric ear, nose, and throat specialist; pediatric pulmonologist; others as appropriate	Evaluation for swallowing problems; treatment for swallowing problem if present; respiratory therapy; medication

Some other respiratory problems that babies can have include wheezing, asthma, a hoarse or wet-sounding voice, a persistent croupy-sounding cough, or frequent pneumonia. These can be related to reflux, allergies, sensitivities, and swallowing problems, because something is getting into or irritating your child's airway (sometimes referred to as the "windpipe"). Reflux can easily get into the airway, because it happens so quickly. It spills into the area of the voice box that protects the windpipe and lungs from fluid entering (the voice box is the gateway to the lower airway going to the lungs). You know how this feels if you have ever started coughing immediately after you experienced some reflux. Allergies or sensitivities can also cause swelling and mucus production in the airway. Hopefully you already know that severe allergic reactions can be life threatening and cause the airway to close.

If your child has a problem with suck-swallow-breathe coordination, saliva and other fluid can also enter the lower airway. If you have ever "swallowed the wrong way," then you know what this feels like. This is called *aspiration*—we all aspirate a small amount of fluid at times. However, too much of a foreign substance in the lower airway (the voice box, windpipe, and lungs) can lead to chronic respiratory conditions, such as asthma, wheezing, and persistent croupy cough. It can also result in other respiratory conditions, such as pneumonia. If your child has any of these problems chronically, your pediatrician may refer you to a pediatric pulmonologist.

A hoarse-sounding voice can result from too much crying or acid reflux burning the vocal cords of the voice box. A wet-sounding voice can result from saliva, reflux, or other liquid entering the voice box. Your baby's pediatrician will send you and your baby to an appropriate specialist if he cannot resolve these problems. Some of the specialists who work with respiratory concerns include a pediatric ear, nose, and throat specialist; a pediatric allergist; a pediatric pulmonologist; and others. Don't forget that once you have taken care of the respiratory problem medically, you can work on boosting your child's immune system function through infant massage and other stress-reducing experiences.

ACTIVITY 3.4: SAMPLE LOG SHEET TO TRACK HEALTH CONCERNS

Here is a sample log sheet for you to track your baby's health problems. This can help you and your pediatrician figure out what may be causing your baby's health problem.

Health Problem Seen	Date	Change Made	Did It Work?

Health Problem Seen	Date	Change Made	Did It Work?

Let's Talk about Allergies and Sensitivities

As we know, allergies and sensitivities can be environmental or food related. (The term *sensitivity* is most often used to describe potential allergies in children.) We are also seeing many more people with allergies and sensitivities today than 20 or 30 years ago. The book *Is This Your Child? Discovering and Treating Unrecognized Allergies in Children and Adults* by Dr Doris Rapp has chapters on infant and toddler allergies.[122] Her work is summarized in the following charts. This is very important material for parents to understand, because of the apparent overall increase in allergies and sensitivities in the general population. There has also been an increase in children identified with autism and attention problems who have allergies and sensitivities.

POSSIBLE ALLERGY OR SENSITIVITY SYMPTOMS IN INFANTS AND TODDLERS[123]	
Date	**Things Mom Might Notice Before Birth** **My Baby:**
	Is excessively active
	Hiccups for long periods of time
	Kicks excessively, to the point of Mom's ribs being bruised

Allergies and sensitivities often run in families, and a mom might notice some symptoms in her baby even before he is born. According to Dr Rapp, these might include excessive activity, hiccupping, or kicking, with the mother's ribs becoming bruised[124] from the inside. If you notice this, you might want to keep a food diary and/or log sheet to make note of what foods or other factors seem to cause your baby to become overly active. See the previous section of this chapter for a food diary. Then you can eliminate or modify your intake of the potentially offending foods, if foods indeed seem to be the problem. You can also modify your exposure to certain environmental factors (such as second-hand smoke).

Both Dr Doris Rapp and Dr William Crook have written about elimination and rotation diets.[125–126] An elimination diet means that you take the foods out of your diet that may cause your baby to exhibit the patterns listed previously. Once you have done this, you can then reintroduce those foods once every 4 days, which becomes a rotation diet. Your baby may be able to handle exposure to a food once every 4 days. Be sure that you work with your obstetrician if you are trying an elimination or rotation diet. It is critical that you have excellent, well-balanced nutrition while you are pregnant. Now, let's look at allergy and/or sensitivity symptoms seen in infants.

Date	Possible Infant Allergy and/or Sensitivity Symptoms[127] My Baby:
	Has had colic for a prolonged period of time, with excessive screaming and crying
	Has excessive reflux (spit-up) or frequent vomiting
	Has diarrhea
	Has constipation
	Has nose or chest congestion
	Drools and/or perspires excessively
	Has frequent ear infections

Date	Possible Infant Allergy and/or Sensitivity Symptoms[127]
	My Baby:
	Has bronchiolitis, coughing, or asthma
	Has itchy rashes, eczema, or bright-red buttocks
	Has a fast pulse
	Has extreme restlessness or activity
	Resists cuddling
	Will only calm when walked, bounced, or moved rhythmically
	Rocks his crib or bangs his head excessively
	Has problems sleeping
	Is walking early (by 7–10 months)
	Touches his or her genitals frequently
	Does not like to remain dressed
	Demands frequent or constant attention

According to Dr Harvey Karp, there is a "rule of threes" that can be used to determine if a baby has colic. A baby with colic would cry for at least 3 hours each day, 3 days per week, for 3 consecutive weeks.[128] Dr Karp says that most babies move past this period of fussiness by 3 months of age. Therefore, prolonged colic would last longer than the first 3 months of your baby's life.

Now, you are not going to want to wait that long to know if your baby is showing signs of allergies or sensitivities. Therefore, you will look at the other signs listed. These include excessive reflux, diarrhea, nose and chest congestion, asthma, eczema, rashes, and ear infections. However, there are other physical and behavioral indicators of allergy you can look for.

Other physical indicators of allergy and sensitivity may include constipation, coughing, bronchiolitis, bright-red buttocks, excessive drooling and perspiration, and/ or a fast pulse.[129] Behavioral indicators include resistance to cuddling, need for movement to calm down, excessive rocking or head banging in the crib, sleeping difficulties, early walking, genital touching, dislike for wearing clothes, and demand for frequent or constant attention.

You would have to agree that taking care of a baby with these characteristics could be very challenging and frustrating for the parents. If your baby demonstrates some or many of these characteristics, you may want to explore the possibility of allergies or sensitivities with your pediatrician and/or pediatric allergist. For a bottle-fed infant, you should look at the ingredients in the formula that may be causing an allergy or sensitivity. I have provided a list of foods that commonly cause allergies and sensitivities later in this section. A change of formula is often the remedy of choice.

If a mom is nursing, she can change her diet by using the elimination and rotation strategies discussed earlier. She will need to work with the baby's pediatrician and possibly a nutritionist or dietitian to be sure that she is eating a balanced diet.

If you have changed your baby's diet and you still see many allergy or sensitivity symptoms, your baby may suffer from environmental allergies or sensitivities. These can include pollen, mold, pet dander, chemicals used for cleaning or other purposes in the house, and environmental pollutants. Now, let's look at allergy or sensitivity symptoms we see in toddlers.

Date	Possible Toddler Allergy Symptoms[130]
	My Toddler Has:
	Recurring sinus, ear, and/or chest infections
	Red cheeks and/or earlobes
	Dark circles, bags, and/or wrinkles under his eyes
	Glassy eyes and/or a "spaced-out" look

Date	Possible Toddler Allergy Symptoms[130] My Toddler Has:
	Stuffy or runny nose
	Nose picking, rubbing, and/or wiggling
	Wheezing and/or coughing
	Headaches
	Gagging, belching, vomiting, retching, and/or nausea
	Constipation, diarrhea, rectal gas, and/or abdominal pain
	Bad breath
	Restless legs and/or leg aches
	Whining, clinging, screaming, and/or temper tantrums
	Excessive activity
	Aggressive behavior (eg, hitting, pinching, biting, spitting, and/or kicking)
	A tendency to talk nonstop and/or senselessly or repeat a desire for a craved food
	An apparent reluctance to smile, significant fatigue, apparent depression
	A dislike of cuddling or touch
	A refusal to remain dressed
	A tendency to hide in dark corners or under furniture

A toddler with allergies or sensitivities may be very challenging for parents. Once your child is walking, some of the behavioral concerns that accompany allergies and sensitivities may exhaust you. These can include extreme levels of activity, frequent tantrums with screaming, aggression toward others, whining and clinging, nonstop talking, constant repetition of thoughts and ideas, refusal to keep clothes on, and hiding. Children with these problems are difficult to calm, because they often do not like to be touched or cuddled and are frequently tired. Their moods are often "hard to read," because they do not smile very often and may become depressed.

Physically, these children can be difficult to be around, because they may have bad breath (possibly due to reflux or sinus infection), belching, gagging, vomiting, rectal gas, diarrhea, and runny noses. Other physical symptoms of allergy and sensitivity in toddlers include frequently recurring sinus, ear, and/or chest infections (at times indicated by red cheeks and earlobes); wheezing and/or coughing; dark circles, bags, and/or wrinkles under the eyes (often called *allergic shiners*); glassy eyes and/or a "spaced out" look; stuffy or runny nose with nose picking, rubbing, and/or wiggling; headaches and leg aches; wiggly, restless legs; and bloating, constipation, belly pain, and nausea.[131]

If your toddler has these symptoms, see your pediatrician. You might also want to ask for a referral to a pediatric allergist. There are so many things that may cause your child to suffer from allergies or sensitivities. As you know, some children are allergic or sensitive to foods, some may have environmental sensitivities or allergies, and others may have both food and environmental sensitivities or allergies. Environmental allergies or sensitivities can include pollen, mold, pet dander, chemicals used for cleaning or other purposes in the house, and environmental pollutants.

There are currently many books and resources on the topic of allergies, immune system function, and other related information. Dr William Sears and his family of medical professionals have a Web site *(www.askdrsears.com),* with good advice regarding many topics for parents. The site addresses breast-feeding, the introduction of solid foods, allergies and sensitivities, and many other topics.[132] Here is a summary from this site of the foods that cause the most and the least problems. It is interesting to note that, as a population, we seem most allergic to the foods to which we are constantly exposed. This is the idea upon which elimination diets are based.

Most Common Food Allergies and Sensitivities	Most-Allergenic and Sensitizing Foods	Least-Allergenic and Sensitizing Foods
Dairy Products*	Berries	Apples
Egg Whites*	Buckwheat	Apricots
Peanuts†	Chocolate†	Asparagus
Shellfish†	Cinnamon	Avocados
Soy	Citrus Fruits	Barley
Tree Nuts†	Coconut	Beets
Wheat*	Corn	Broccoli
	Dairy Products*	Carrots
	Egg Whites*	Cauliflower
	Mustard	Chicken
	Nuts†	Cranberries
	Peanut Butter†	Dates
	Peas	Grapes
	Pork	Raw honey (not given before 12 months – botulism risk)§
	Shellfish†	Lamb

Most Common Food Allergies and Sensitivities	Most-Allergenic and Sensitizing Foods	Least-Allergenic and Sensitizing Foods
	Soy	Lettuce
	Sugar	Mangoes
	Tomatoes	Oats
	Wheat*	Papayas
	Yeast	Peaches
		Pears
		Poi
		Raisins†
		Rice
		Rye
		Safflower Oil
		Salmon
		Squash
		Sunflower Oil
		Sweet Potatoes

Most Common Food Allergies and Sensitivities	Most-Allergenic and Sensitizing Foods	Least-Allergenic and Sensitizing Foods
		Turkey
		Veal

*These foods are introduced as your baby's digestive system matures (see guidelines for introducing foods in chapter 6).

†These foods are often given later. Nuts and raisins may be a choking hazard if given too early. Peanuts, peanut butter, tree nuts, and shellfish need to be introduced carefully into the diet, because they are included on the list of most common food allergies and sensitivities. Chocolate contains caffeine.

§Raw honey has been known to cause botulism in children under 12 months of age.

There are a number of common foods listed in the first two columns. You see an overlap between columns 1 and 2. There is a large list of most-allergenic foods, and the most common food allergies and sensitivities are also on that list. However, you can see that you have a wide variety of foods from each food group in the "Least-Allergenic Foods" column that you can safely feed your child. See chapter 6 for information on introducing foods and how much to feed your child.

Reflux, SIDS, and Sleeping on the Back

We have more information on gastroesophageal reflux in infants and children than ever before. Many babies experience reflux, although some babies have silent reflux or "wet-sounding burps" without exhibiting overt signs of spit-up. In other words, you don't always see it. Reflux can result from a weakness in the muscles that keep food in the stomach (the lower esophageal sphincter). This may be an inherited trait, or perhaps the area has not developed adequate strength. This is a good reason to provide your baby with daily belly time when he is awake, as it helps the abdominal and many other areas of the body to develop.

Reflux can also result from your baby being overfed, even slightly. A common rule of thumb for stomach size is that the baby's stomach is the size of his or her fist. Your baby's fist is very small, which means your baby's stomach is very small. Therefore, overfeeding your baby by even half an ounce can be too much. This is the reason why many pediatricians recommend smaller, more frequent feedings for babies throughout the day when a baby has reflux.

Reflux has also been connected to a variety of other health concerns, particularly respiratory issues. If reflux travels into the middle-ear spaces (via the Eustachian tubes) or the nasal and sinus areas, your baby can develop ear or sinus problems. If reflux flows over into the airway, your child could eventually develop asthma.

The potential connection between reflux and sudden infant death syndrome, or SIDS, may be one reason why the idea of placing your baby on her back to sleep has become a standard practice recommended by most pediatricians. Not only has this sleeping position been reported to significantly reduce the number of deaths from SIDS, but it also decreases the chance of reflux spilling over into the airway. In fact, reflux may be a major contributor to SIDS.

If your baby is sleeping on her stomach and reflux occurs, there is a greater chance that the reflux will spill over into the airway than if your baby is sleeping on her back (due to gravity pulling the spit-up downward into the airway). As a natural protective mechanism, the baby may cough and clear the airway. However, if the baby cannot do this, then the vocal cords may spasm or contract in a closed position. This could happen if the baby's young vocal mechanism is overwhelmed by the reflux while the baby is asleep.

If your baby is sleeping on her back and reflux occurs, she is likely to wake up because of the startle reflux. The reflux can also be ejected from the mouth, if your baby's head is turned even slightly. Less reflux is likely to spill over into the airway when she is sleeping on her back, and your baby can cough to clear it out.

Your baby is very experienced with swallowing through feeding but may be less experienced with clearing the airway via coughing. If you hear your baby coughing frequently when awake or asleep, please mention this to your pediatrician. Coughing is a sign that something has gotten into the airway or windpipe. It may be a sign that your baby has reflux or a swallowing incoordination.

Babies who sleep on their backs also tend to not sleep as deeply as babies who sleep on their stomachs. This is believed to be the result of the Moro or startle reflex. If your baby spits up, he is likely to startle and wake up if sleeping on his back. For information on calming your baby and getting him to sleep well on his back, refer to Dr Harvey Karp's book, *The Happiest Baby on the Block*.[133]

There are exceptions to every rule, however. For some cases of reflux, your pediatrician or other appropriate professional may recommend that your baby sleep on his belly with a SIDS monitor. This is because the occurrences of reflux seem to decrease while a child is sleeping on the stomach.[134–136] The SIDS monitor is very important to use if your baby is in the age group most affected by SIDS (ie, birth to 1 year with a peak at 2 to 4 months of age)[137] or if your baby has immature development.

Placing babies with reflux on their bellies (ie, in the prone position) on a wedge or raised mattress has been used in hospitals and by parents for many years. In some hospitals, the professionals working with the babies pin a cloth diaper (not the baby's diaper) to the mattress in a certain way to keep the baby in place. A SIDS monitor is used.

The prone position allows the baby's digestive system to elongate and can place a small amount of pressure on the lower esophageal sphincter, assisting it with keeping food in the stomach. Elevation of the baby's head can also allow gravity to keep the food in the stomach. However, it is important to remember that little babies who sleep on their bellies will need a SIDS monitor.

Some professionals have recommended that parents allow a baby with reflux to sleep upright in a baby seat or car seat after a meal. This is usually recommended because gravity can help keep food and/or fluid in the stomach. However, many parents have noticed greater reflux or fussiness with this position. Little babies have a lot of natural flexion in their bodies. This means that they tend to sit "slouched" in these seats. This position would place the digestive system in a less-than-ideal position for effective digestion, because everything in this area is pushed together or crowded. The next time you have finished eating a full meal, try sitting in a slouched position and see what you think.

If you have a baby who experiences excessive, uncontrollable reflux, you need to work with your pediatrician and possibly others (such as a pediatric gastroenterologist, lactation consultant, occupational therapist, or speech-language pathologist). A pediatrician may change the diet of breast-feeding moms, the formula being used, or the baby's feeding schedule. A pediatric gastroenterologist may be needed if you and your pediatrician cannot resolve the problem. Other professionals, such as lactation consultants, occupational therapists, and speech-language pathologists who work with feeding on a regular basis may be able to work with you and your pediatrician on other ideas to resolve the issue.

Uncontrolled reflux can lead to poor nutrition for obvious reasons. Depending on the age of the child, your pediatrician many recommend that cereal (often rice) be added to your baby's diet to add weight to the breast milk or formula. The added weight is believed to help the food or liquid remain in the stomach, although this has not been proven. However, it may actually just add calories to a smaller volume of milk or formula. Babies can be spoon-fed or fed from a very small open cup from a young age. See chapter 6 for information on spoon-feeding and drinking from an open cup. It is generally not a good idea to enlarge the hole in the bottle nipple if you are feeding cereal to your baby. This may change the way the manufacturer meant the bottle to function.

Giving a young baby cereal before the digestive system is ready may compromise the immune system and increase the potential for the development of allergies and sensitivities. Here is where you and your pediatrician need to weigh your options. It is important to have your baby well fed while the structure that keeps food in the stomach (the lower esophageal sphincter) is developing. Many babies seem to outgrow this difficulty over time. However, many adults have reflux. Therefore, we need to examine whether some babies ever really "outgrow" this problem.

There are some other factors aside from reflux and sleeping on the belly that appear to be related to SIDS. These include loose bedding and soft sleep surfaces (don't use these), overheating (make sure your baby is not too hot), maternal smoking during pregnancy, bed sharing, preterm birth, and low birth weight.[138]

Pacifier use has also been suggested in the prevention of SIDS.[139-142] This may be related to the fact that children who use pacifiers get extra practice in the suck-swallow-breathe sequence. Also, a baby is less likely to reflux if he has the swallowing process engaged and the wavelike motion of the esophagus is moving saliva toward the stomach. This may be why some gastroenterologists recommend that adults chew gum to reduce episodes of reflux. We will discuss appropriate pacifier use in chapter 4.

SIDS is most common between 2 and 4 months of age,[143] when significant changes are occurring in your baby's mouth and swallowing structures. SIDS is a concern until approximately 1 year of age,[144] when your baby's breathing is more mature.

What about Vaccines?

We have certainly seen that the use of vaccines in children has come into question in the past 20 years with the increase in children being identified with autism. I want you as a parent to be as informed as possible when vaccinating your child. Here are three books that I believe can help you. I suggest you purchase the one that appeals to you. Dr Tenpenny's book is well researched, Dr Cave's book has long been a favorite of parents, and Dr Sears' book helps parents sort through often-conflicting information and make informed decisions when vaccinating their children. All have received high ratings from parents on *Amazon.com*.

- *Vaccines: The Risks, the Benefits, the Choices, a Resource Guide for Parents* by Dr Sherri J. Tenpenny[145]

- *What Your Doctor May Not Tell You about Children's Vaccinations* by Dr Stephanie Cave[146]

- *The Vaccine Book: Making the Right Decision for Your Child* by Dr Robert W. Sears[147]

Now, here is my opinion, as a therapist who has treated many individuals with autism (including the children of several pediatricians) for almost 30 years, and as the sister of two individuals on the spectrum. I believe that the vaccines alone are not the culprit. However, if you stress an already stressed immune system with a vaccine, the vaccine may contribute to or possibly trigger autism. This does not mean we should not vaccinate our children. It may, instead, be helpful to reevaluate the schedule of childhood vaccinations.

We currently give babies more vaccines than ever before, beginning with hepatitis B at birth. We have a food supply and an environment that contain more chemicals and toxins than ever before. We are also seeing more allergies and sensitivities than ever before. Some vaccines (such as measles-mumps-rubella, or MMR, and the flu vaccine) are grown on the skin cells of baby chickens and can place an egg- or chicken-sensitive child at risk for a reaction.[148] We know that autism tends to run in families and that people with a certain genetic "make-up" are at greater risk for autism. It is difficult to control genetics or the environment. You, however, do have some control over the food you and your baby eat and the way you vaccinate your child. Please read books such as those listed previously, and make an informed decision with your child's pediatrician.

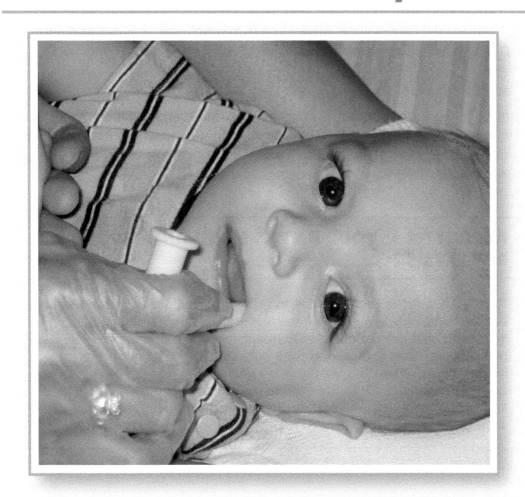

4

The Hand-Mouth Connection: Helping Your Baby Have Mouthing Experiences That Promote Good Development

Key Topics in This Chapter

■ The Hand-Mouth Connection

■ The Importance of Good Mouth Experiences

■ Appropriate Pacifier Use and Thumb- and/or Finger-Sucking

■ Teething and Drooling

■ What to Do about Too Much Drooling

Your baby's exploration of the world will depend on her ability to process and organize sensation in the body. According to Suzanne Evans Morris and Marsha Dunn Klein, the mouth and hand have the most sensory receptors per square inch in the human body.[149] It seems that we, as humans, are prewired to use our hands and mouths together for exploration, feeding, speech, and more. Once you are aware of this idea, you will see the hand-mouth connection in yourself and in your child during everyday experiences. Now, let's talk about the hand-mouth connection.

The Hand-Mouth Connection

Human beings have a hand-mouth connection. This means that our hands and our mouths work together. We will discuss many examples of this connection throughout the book. There are three reflexes that demonstrate this connection from birth: the palmomental, Babkin, and grasp reflexes.

ACTIVITY 4.1: YOUR BABY'S HAND AND MOUTH REFLEXES[150–152]

Place a date next to each reflex as you see your newborn do these. If your baby is a little older, you can still see these reflexes until a certain age. Remember that reflexes don't really disappear—the motor area of your baby's brain actually takes control over time, so your baby no longer needs the reflex for the activity. When you see the reflex going away, it means that your baby's brain is developing. It is fun to explore your baby's hand-mouth connection and look at these reflexes in action. The directions for completing this activity are listed below the chart.

Reflex	Date	How You Get Your Baby to Do It	What It Looks Like	Apparent Use	When the Reflex Seems to Disappear
Palmomental		Touch your baby's palm	Your baby's mentalis muscle under the lower lip will wrinkle	The mentalis muscle everts (turns out) the lower lip for latching onto the bottle or breast	Can be seen into adulthood in some individuals
Babkin		Gently press the base of your baby's palm	Your baby's mouth opens, eyes close, and head moves forward	This reflex helps your baby prepare to feed	3–4 months
Grasp		Gently press your finger into your baby's palm	Your baby will grasp your finger tightly	Your baby's grasp tightens as she sucks, and your baby can hold on to the feeder's clothing	8 months

DIRECTIONS FOR THIS ACTIVITY:

1. Palmomental Reflex: When you touch your newborn's palm, the small mentalis muscle beneath your baby's lower lip contracts, or wrinkles. The mentalis muscle allows us to evert (or protrude) the lower lip (make a "pouty" lip).

You can experience the movement of this muscle. Touch right below the pink part of your bottom lip in the center. Make the "er" sound, as in the word "mother" or "father." Can you feel your lower lip protruding a little? If not, make a "pouty" lip and feel the mentalis evert (or protrude) your lower lip.

DIRECTIONS FOR THIS ACTIVITY: (continued)

The mentalis muscle is important for maintaining a lip latch on the bottle or breast. Some parents have actually assisted their baby's lip latch by touching the baby's palm to assist the mentalis in contracting. The palmomental reflex can be seen into adulthood in some individuals.

2. Babkin Reflex: This is another reflex that is present at birth. When you gently press the base of your baby's palm, the mouth opens, the eyes close, and the head moves forward. You can easily see how this response helps your baby get ready to feed. The reflex will seem to disappear around 3 to 4 months of age as it becomes integrated by the brain into the motor system. Many parents elicit the palmomental, Babkin, and grasp responses naturally by touching the palms of their babies' hands when they feed.

3. Grasp Reflex: This is the hand reflex with which most parents are familiar. However, many people do not realize that it is also related to mouth movement. As your baby sucks, her grasp gets tighter. This reflex is believed to be important in cultures where babies are carried around all day in slings on the front of the mother's body. Many of these babies nurse at will. The grasp reflex seems to disappear around 8 months of age and may be a precursor for self-feeding.

The hand-mouth connection is also seen when your baby brings her hands together at the center or midline of her body during feeding. This becomes more apparent around 2 to 3 months of age. At 3 to 4 months of age, your baby may pat the bottle or Mom's breast with her hand(s) as she feeds. Around 4½ months of age, your baby places her hands on the bottle. Around 5½ months, your baby can hold her bottle.

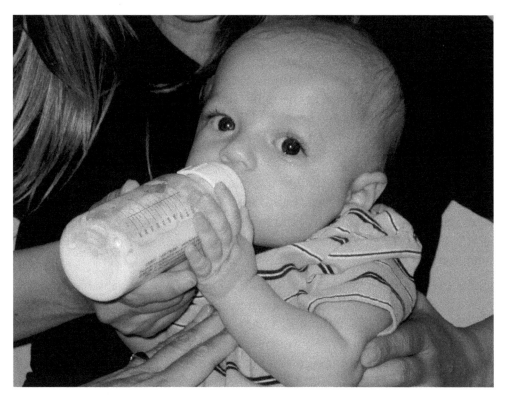

Photo 4.1: Anthony's hands are at midline on his bottle.

ACTIVITY 4.2: YOUR BABY'S HANDS AT MIDLINE DURING FEEDING[153–154]

Place a date next to when your baby brings her hands to midline while feeding. It is really fun to observe your baby's development. Aren't you a proud parent?

Date	Age	What You Want to See My Baby
	2–3 Months	Brings her hands together at the center of her body during feeding
	3–4 Months	Pats the bottle or breast with her hand(s)
	4½ Months	Places her hands on the bottle
	5½ Months	Can hold her bottle

It is important to allow your baby to bring her hands toward one another while feeding and at other times. Some well-meaning individuals try to move the baby's hands out of the way during feeding by placing the baby's arm away from the midline or center of her body. This can elicit an asymmetric tonic neck reflex in the baby and can make feeding more difficult. When the baby's arm is moved to the side, her face naturally follows. This takes the baby's head and mouth out of position for efficient and effective feeding.

Bringing the hands to midline and to the mouth is another hand-mouth activity that can be very calming for your baby. Your baby needs to explore her hands with her mouth. She will also explore her feet with her mouth, beginning around 6 months of age. We will discuss the specifics of mouthing in the next section of this chapter.

As adults, we can relate to the hand-mouth connection your baby has from birth. We use a hand-to-mouth pattern when eating and drinking. We cannot feed ourselves effectively without it. There is also a hand-mouth connection during speech production. When we try to speak without using our hands and other body language to communicate, it can become very difficult. The use of

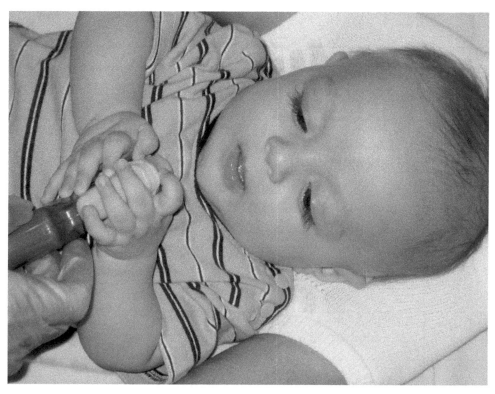

Photo 4.2: Anthony's hands are at midline as he prepares to mouth this toy.

our hands when speaking is a natural part of our expression as human beings. Another example can be seen when people become anxious. Some people use a hand-to-mouth pattern to calm themselves (such as biting or chewing on food, fingernails, or another item, or taking sips of a liquid). As you can see, the hand-mouth connection is still apparent in adults, even though we may not always recognize it.

The Importance of Good Mouth Experiences

Remember that your baby's mouth is her window to the world. The developmental process of mouthing and mouth play is outlined for you here. We will discuss the critical learning periods of generalized mouthing, discriminative mouthing, and mouth play. Mouthing is important for mouth development. As a therapist, I am always concerned when parents tell me that their child did not go through these stages. Mouthing is a means for exploration, as well as a means for calming.

Your baby will mouth her fingers, fists, and/or thumbs to calm herself. You may see this shortly after birth. In fact, some babies suck their thumbs before they are born (in utero). Over the first 6 months, you will see less suckling (wavelike front-to-back tongue movement used at birth) and more sucking, biting, chewing, and exploration. Your baby will do this with the hands, feet, and appropriate mouth toys.

The trick is to find appropriate and safe objects and toys for your baby to mouth. Look for safe toys that you can help your baby hold with her hands and explore with her mouth. The objects need to be large enough that they are not a choking hazard. They need to be safe for oral use by a baby (ie, made of materials that have been approved for babies' mouths). They also need to be small enough for your baby to explore safely in the front, middle, and back of the mouth.

It is difficult to find safe and appropriate items for your baby to mouth on her own. Many currently available mouth toys found in stores can only be effectively explored near the front of the mouth. This leads to a lot of sucking or suckling and nothing else. Some safe and appropriate mouth toys, along with information on where to purchase them, are listed here and in chapter 5. I recommend Chewy Tubes, Grabbers (made by ARK Therapeutics, Inc), and Debra Beckman's Tri-Chews (by ARK). Chewy Tubes are nontoxic, latex free, and lead free; do not contain polyvinyl chloride, or PVC, or phthalates; and colors are approved by the U.S. Food and Drug Administration, or FDA. ARK products are manufactured in the United States with FDA-approved materials, scents, and colors, and made without latex or phthalates. Here is a list of some of the companies that carry these products.

COMPANIES THAT CARRY PRODUCTS FOR CHILDREN THAT CANNOT BE FOUND IN MOST STORES

Company	Phone Number	Web Site
ARK Therapeutic Services, Inc	(803) 438-9779	www.arktherapeutic.com
New Visions	(800) 606-7112	www.new-vis.com
The Speech Bin	(800) 850-8602	www.speechbin.com
SuperDuper Publications	(800) 277-8737	www.superduperinc.com
TalkTools	(888) 529-2879	www.talktools.net
Therapro	(800) 257-5376	www.theraproducts.com

Parents sometimes express concerns about giving babies items to chew if they have no teeth. Let me put your mind at ease. Chewing and biting on mouth toys, beginning around 3 months of age, will help your baby's teeth to emerge. Three months of age is when the swelling of the gums disappears during your baby's latch (ie, the third lips).[155] Your baby is then ready to do something with the gums (to work on getting teeth). Even though teeth do not usually begin to erupt until 5 to 6 months of age, your baby begins to work on this process at 3 months. Babies who have limited biting and chewing experiences seem to develop teeth later than babies who are provided with appropriate chewing and biting experiences.

ACTIVITY 4.3: MOUTHING AND MOUTH PLAY DEVELOPMENT CHECKLIST (ONE TO 24 MONTHS)[156–169]

This checklist is presented in a manner that will help you encourage your baby's best mouth development through appropriate mouthing and mouth play. Place a date in the appropriate column as your child develops these skills. Suggested mouth toys are listed after each age group.

GENERALIZED MOUTHING PERIOD (BIRTH TO 4–5 MONTHS)

Date	Age: 1 Month
	Control of rooting reflex developing
	Decreased rooting noted when hands or items are brought to the mouth
	Locates and suckles or sucks on fist near the front of the mouth

As your baby develops control over the rooting reflex, you will see a decrease in rooting as items touch your baby's mouth. Your baby is in a period called *generalized mouthing*. This means that your baby will suck on items that come in contact with the mouth (such as your finger, a pacifier, or your baby's own hand). Remember, sucking is calming. Your baby is also learning about general sensations (such as softness, hardness, and firmness) through mouthing experiences.[170] You may often see her suckle or suck on her fist near the front of the mouth.

Date	Age: 2–3 Months*
	Control of suckling reflex is developing
	The mouth begins to change shape, and the tongue begins to move more within the mouth
	Baby brings hands to her mouth while on her back and belly (2 months)
	Baby brings a toy placed in her hand to her mouth (3 months)
	Baby suckles or sucks on fist and/or fingers with increased control
	You may see some biting motion if the bite reflex is stimulated

*Suggested mouth toys: ARK's Baby Grabber and Debra Beckman's Tri-Chews by ARK (used with a parent's help and supervision)

The 2- to 3-month period is a time when your baby's mouth is beginning to grow and change shape. There is now more space within your baby's mouth, so she can move the tongue more. Your baby is still within the period of generalized mouthing. However, you will begin to see your baby suck on her fist or fingers with increased control.

Around 2 months of age, your baby can bring her hands to her mouth while lying on her back or belly. If you put a small, safe mouth toy in your 3-month-old baby's hand, she will bring it to her mouth. You might see some biting on the toy if your baby's bite reflex is stimulated. Some recommended toys are ARK's Baby Grabber and Debra Beckman's Tri-Chews by ARK, to be used with your help and supervision.

Date	Age: 3–4 Months*
	Suck-swallow-breathe coordination improves
	Baby's swallow adapts to the increased space developing between structures in the throat (soft palate, epiglottis, and larynx)
	The tongue seals toward the front third, leading to three-dimensional suck by 4 months (tip of the tongue and sides come up, lips pucker, fat pads get smaller, cheek and jaw muscles develop)
	Begins to reach for and grasp objects
	Sucks longer on hand, toy, pacifier, or thumb
	Bites on mouth toy or fingers when bite reflex is stimulated

*Suggested mouth toys: ARK's Baby Grabber and Debra Beckman's Tri-Chews by ARK (used with a parent's help and supervision)

By 3 to 4 months of age, your baby has improved her suck-swallow-breathe coordination. This allows more consecutive swallows during feeding and mouthing. The increase in this coordination is needed, because your baby now has even more space between the structures in the mouth and throat. Your baby is now using a more mature, three-dimensional sucking pattern.

The three-dimensional sucking pattern will be used on everything that goes into your baby's mouth (such as mouth toys, a thumb, and a pacifier). Your baby will reach for and grasp objects. You will notice her sucking on and mouthing her

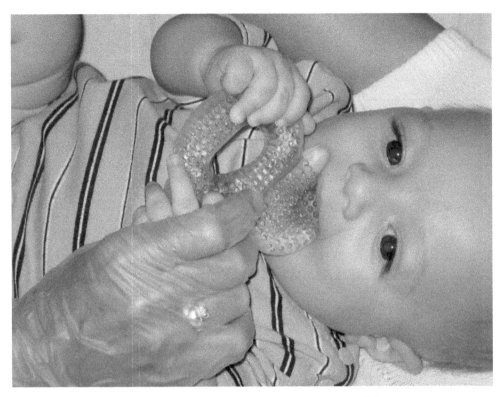

Photo 4.3: Anthony participates in generalized mouthing.

hand, pacifier, toy, or thumb for longer periods of time. Your baby will also bite on toys or fingers. You can help your baby hold ARK's Baby Grabber or Debra Beckman's Tri-Chews by ARK for biting and chewing. These movements work the muscles that open and close the jaw. Your baby will suck and bite on mouth toys for exploration, exercise, and calming. Have your baby use mouth toys with your help and supervision.

Date	Age: 3–6 Months*
	Rooting reflex is seen less and less; seems to be disappearing (3–6 months)
	Baby locates toy, hand, or other item with mouth, without use of rooting reflex (3–6 months)
	Gag reflex comes under control (4–6 months)
	Mouthing of toys increases (4–6 months)

The Hand-Mouth Connection

Date	Age: 3–6 Months*
	Space between mouth and nasal area increases (4–6 months)
	Open space within mouth continues to increase through jaw growth and sucking pads getting smaller (4–6 months)
	Tongue moves up and down and front to back with a little less cupping (4–6 months)
	Lip control and movement increases (4–6 months)
	Baby begins to learn to use jaw, lip, and tongue muscles independently of one another
	Discriminative mouthing begins (5–6 months)
	It is important for baby to have appropriate toys for biting, chewing, and discriminative mouthing (5–6 months)
	Teeth begin to come in with increased chewing and biting experiences (5–6 months)
	Chewing and taking sips from an open cup begin to replace sucking and suckling for calming (5–6 months)

*Suggested mouth toys: ARK's Baby Grabber, Debra Beckman's Tri-Chews by ARK, Yellow Chewy Tube, ARK's Grabber (soft and purple), and other appropriately sized mouth toys approved for use with babies (used with a parent's help and supervision)

You have to admit, the changes you are seeing in your baby's mouth are pretty amazing. Just look at all the things that are happening in the 3- to 6-month period. Your baby's rooting reflex is seen less and less. It seems to be disappearing, because your baby now has more sophisticated mouth movement to replace it. Your baby can now locate a toy, her hand(s), and other items with her mouth, without rooting to find them.

Between 4 and 6 months of age, your baby's gag reflex is coming under control. This means that your baby can explore her hands and mouth toys without

The Hand-Mouth Connection

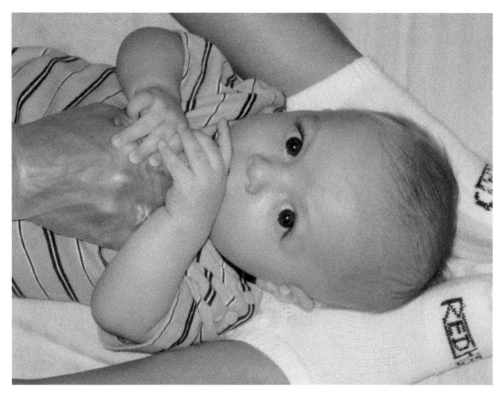

Photo 4.4: Anthony controls mouthing of adult's finger with his hands.

gagging. You will see an increase in your baby's mouthing of toys during this period of time. Your baby's exploration of hands, fingers, and mouth toys helps the gag response move toward the back of the tongue.

During the 4- to 6-month period, you will also see the space between your baby's mouth and nasal area increasing. There will be more open space in your baby's mouth, because the jaw is growing and the sucking pads are getting smaller. Your baby's tongue can now move up and down, as well as front to back with a little less cupping. Your baby's lips will also start to move more. You can see your baby beginning to use the jaw, lips, and tongue independently of one another.

The very important period of discriminative mouthing begins around 5 to 6 months of age. During this process, your baby will move items around within the mouth to explore them. She will use the mouth to learn about textures, shapes, temperatures, and sizes of toys, food, liquid, and fingers. It is vital that your child has safe and appropriate toys to mouth during this critical learning period (to use with your help and supervision). In my experience, children who don't discriminatively mouth are often late in speech development.

In addition to moving the items around within the mouth for exploration, your baby will bite and chew on toys, fingers, and foods. This is part of the

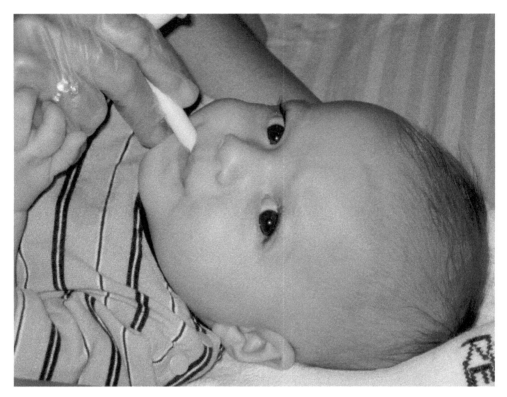

Photo 4.5: Anthony can chew on a yellow Chewy Tube at 4 months with assistance.

teething process. It also prepares your baby for new feeding skills. Between 5 and 6 months of age, your baby's teeth will begin to come in. The processes of chewing and taking bites help develop the jaw muscles and help teeth to emerge. In my experience, babies who don't chew and bite on toys and foods often seem to be late in tooth development.

Now, let's talk about mouthing for calming. Up to this point, your baby may have used a pacifier for calming. You will begin to wean your baby from the pacifier beginning at 5 to 6 months of age. I will give you pacifier guidelines in another section of this chapter. As an adult, you hopefully don't suck on your thumb or a pacifier to calm yourself. You do other things for calming (such as chew gum, crunch on ice, and take sips of water). During the 5- to 6-month period, you will give your baby appropriate mouth toys and soft, solid foods for biting and chewing. You will also begin to give your child sips of liquid from an open cup. These new activities can be just as calming as suckling or sucking on the bottle or pacifier.

THE DISCRIMINITIVE MOUTHING PERIOD (BEGINNING AT 5–6 MONTHS)

Date	Age: 5–9 Months*
	The most pronounced period of discriminative mouthing occurs (5–7 months)
	The gag reflex is found on the back third of the tongue (6–9 months)[171]
	A greater variety of movements are noted during mouth play (eg, biting and chewing on toys and fingers, exploring toys in different parts of the mouth, bringing the feet to the mouth)
	Baby bites and chews on appropriate toys or fingers, so the teeth can come in
	The bottom two front teeth (central incisors) come in (5–9 months)
	The top two front teeth (central incisors) come in (6–10 months)
	The bottom side teeth (lateral incisors) come in (7–20 months)
	The top side teeth (lateral incisors) come in (8–10 months)
	Control over the bite reflex develops; more diagonal rotary jaw movement is seen
	Control over the transverse tongue reflex develops (6–8 months)
	Around 7 months, the tongue moves toward a toy or fingers placed on the side of the gums with a rolling, shifting motion
	The involuntary suckling reflex is seen less and less; it seems to be disappearing (6–12 months)

THE DISCRIMINITIVE MOUTHING PERIOD (BEGINNING AT 5–6 MONTHS) (cont.)

Date	Age: 5–9 Months*
	Control of air coming through the throat, mouth, and nose develops
	Vocalization with mouth play increases
	Chewing on appropriate items and taking sips from an open cup or straw can replace sucking and suckling for calming
	It is time to begin weaning from pacifier, thumb, and/or finger-sucking

*Suggested mouth toys: ARK's Baby Grabber, Debra Beckman's Tri-Chews by ARK, Yellow Chewy Tube, ARK's Grabber (soft and purple), and other appropriately sized mouth toys approved for use by babies (with a parent's supervision)

Your baby has now entered the period of discriminative mouthing. Between 5 and 7 months, you will see a marked increase in the quality and amount of your baby's mouthing. Your baby's gag reflex will move to the back third of the tongue between 6 and 9 months of age. You will see a greater variety of movements during your baby's mouth play. Your baby will explore toys throughout the mouth (front, middle, back, and side). Around 6 months of age, it is typical for a baby to bring his feet to his mouth as part of this exploration.

The increase in biting and chewing on safe toys and safe foods with your supervision helps your baby's teeth to erupt. Look at all the teeth that emerge during this period of time. Your baby is now developing control over his bite reflex. With safe foods, you will see an increasing amount of diagonal rotary chewing. With safe mouth toys, you will see mostly up and down chewing movements. When your baby places mouth toys or fingers on his side gums, you may see the tongue move toward the area with a rolling, shifting motion. This occurs because your baby is developing control over the transverse tongue reflex between 6 and 8 months of age.

Your baby also has increased control over the flow of air from the lungs through the throat, mouth, and nose. You will now hear more vocal play with mouth play. It is time to begin weaning your baby from the pacifier or thumb if your baby sucks on these. You will do this by encouraging your baby to bite, chew, and

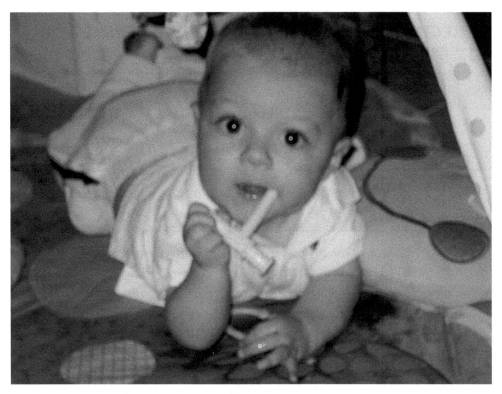

Photo 4.6: Anthony discriminatively mouths and chews on a Chewy Tube at 6 months with supervision.

mouth safe toys for calming, as well as for exploration and mouth exercise. See the discussion on calming in the previous 3- to 6-month section.

THE BEGINNING OF TRUE MOUTH PLAY PERIOD (9–12 MONTHS)

Date	Age: 9–12 Months*
	Bottom first molars come in (10–12 months)
	Bite reflex is seen less and less; seems to be disappearing
	Diagonal rotary jaw movement increases when chewing food
	Baby develops increasingly sophisticated biting, chewing, and manipulation of toys within the mouth

THE BEGINNING OF TRUE MOUTH PLAY PERIOD (9–12 MONTHS) (cont.)

Date	Age: 9–12 Months*
	Chewing and taking sips from an open cup or straw continues to replace sucking and suckling for calming
	From 9–24 months, the transverse tongue reflex is seen less and less; seems to be disappearing
	The tongue moves toward or away from items placed in the mouth, as appropriate
	Mouthing of toys lessens, and baby develops a greater interest in using the mouth appropriately with toys (eg, begins to show interest in blowing horns and bubbles)

*Suggested mouth toys: Yellow and red Chewy Tubes, P's and Q's; ARK's Grabbers, and other appropriately sized mouth toys approved for use with babies (with a parent's supervision); baby horns and bubbles (with a parent's activation and demonstration)

I am calling the 9- to 12-month period "the beginning of true mouth play." Your baby's mouth play between 9 and 12 months will mature. You will see increasingly sophisticated biting, chewing, and manipulation of toys within the mouth. By this time, many children move from the critical learning period of discriminative mouthing to more sophisticated mouth activities. You will begin to see an interest in horn- and bubble-blowing activities, as you show your child how they are used. In my experience, children who skip discriminative mouthing seem to have greater difficulty feeding, developing speech, and participating in new mouth activities, such as blowing horns and bubbles.

Your child will hopefully chew and take sips of liquid to calm himself now, instead of using less mature sucking and suckling. He will hopefully be weaned from a pacifier and/or thumb- and finger-sucking by this time. See the section on pacifier use and thumb- and finger-sucking for further information.

Between 9 and 12 months of age, you will see less and less of your baby's bite reflex. It will seem to disappear like so many other reflexes we have discussed. You will see more diagonal rotary chewing during feeding. Jaw movement will match the shape and size of food or toys placed in the mouth. You will usually see diagonal rotary chewing with food and up-and-down jaw movement with a toy. This shows that your child already knows different ways to use his jaw for different activities.[172] Isn't that amazing?

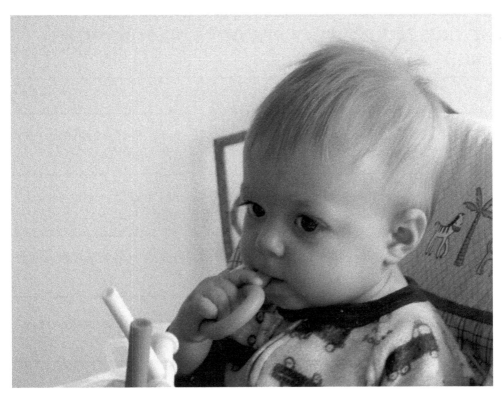

Photo 4.7: Anthony bites and chews on "P's" and "Q's" at 12 months.

Between 10 and 12 months, your baby's bottom first molars will erupt as he chews on foods and appropriate toys. Between 9 and 24 months, the transverse tongue reflex will also seem to disappear. You will see your baby develop much more skill with his tongue. The tongue will move easily toward toys placed into his mouth.

THE TRUE MOUTH PLAY PERIOD (12–24+ MONTHS)	
Date	Age: 12–18 Months*
	Respiration is maturing
	Rapid lip growth occurs (12–24 months)
	Baby continues experimenting with many mouth activities (eg, bubbles and horns)
	Baby may bite on a horn mouthpiece or a straw to obtain jaw stability

THE TRUE MOUTH PLAY PERIOD (12–24+ MONTHS) (cont.)

Date	Age: 12–18 Months*
	Baby uses lips and cheeks together to shape lips for drinking from a straw or some beginning horn or bubble activities
	Increasingly sophisticated biting, chewing, and manipulation of appropriate items occurs within the mouth
	The tongue reflex is seen less and less; seems to be disappearing (12–18 months)
	The transverse tongue reflex is seen less and less; seems to be disappearing (9–24 months)
	The jaw, lips, and tongue continue to learn to move independently of one another
	The different parts of each structure continue to learn to move separately (eg, the tip of the tongue moves independently of the rest of the tongue, and each lip corner contracts independently of the rest of the lips)
	Top first molars come in (14–16 months)
	Bottom cuspids come in (16–18 months)
	Chewing and taking sips from open cups and straws replace sucking and suckling for calming

*Suggested mouth toys: Yellow and red Chewy Tubes, P's and Q's, and ARK's Grabbers (with a parent's supervision); baby horns and bubbles (with a parent's activation, demonstration, and presentation to the child)

I am calling 15 to 24 months the "true mouth play" period. However, mouth play will continue beyond 24 months. Your baby's breathing patterns continue to mature. Your child's jaw has grown rapidly between birth and 12 months. Her lips are growing rapidly between 12 and 24 months. These changes lend themselves to the fun of more sophisticated mouth activities like horn blowing,

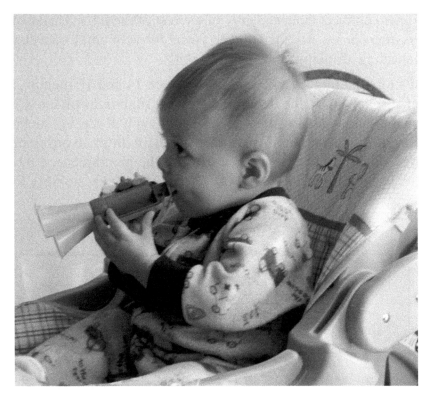

Photo 4.8: Anthony begins horn play at 12 months.

bubble play, and drinking from a straw. There are horns that can be activated if your child sucks on the mouthpiece like a straw. These can be good first horns, because you may have begun teaching your child how to drink from a straw as early as 6 months of age.

Blowing horns and bubbles and sucking on straws require your child to use her lips and cheeks together. Your child's cheeks not only help move her lips, they help your child to maintain the right amount of pressure within the mouth. We talked about the need for the right amount of pressure within your child's mouth for breast- or bottle-feeding. This pressure is also required for blowing bubbles and horns, as well as drinking from straws. Maintaining "just the right pressure" within the mouth is called *appropriate intraoral pressure*. We will discuss the importance of appropriate intraoral pressure in the mouth again when we talk about speech in chapter 7.

During the 12- to 18-month period, your child will continue to develop increasingly sophisticated biting, chewing, and manipulation skills within the mouth. Her tongue reflex will be seen less and less between 12 and 18 months. Her transverse tongue reflex will be seen less and less between 9 and 24 months of age. The jaw, lips, and tongue continue to learn to move independently of one another. The different parts of these structures also continue to move separately (eg, the tip of the tongue moves independently of the rest of the tongue, and each lip corner contracts independently of the rest of the lips). Therapists call this process *dissociation*. Dissociation is crucial for your child's development of higher-level eating, drinking, and speaking skills.

Your child's top first molars will come in between 14 and 16 months, and her bottom cuspids will come in between 16 and 18 months of age. Chewing activities and taking sips from an open cup or straw will replace sucking and suckling for calming. Jaw stability develops along with tooth development. You may see your child bite down on a straw or the mouthpiece of a horn to stabilize the jaw during this time period. Discussion of jaw stability follows.

Date	Age: 18–24 Months*
	Respiration is maturing
	Baby develops good control of swallowing by 18 months
	Rapid lip growth occurs (12–24 months)
	Experimentation with many mouth activities continues (eg, bubbles and horns)
	Baby uses lips and cheeks together to shape the lips for drinking from a straw or for horn and/or bubble activities
	Baby develops increasingly sophisticated biting, chewing, and manipulation of appropriate items with the mouth
	The tongue reflex is seen less and less; seems to be disappearing (12–18 months)
	The transverse tongue reflex is seen less and less; seems to be disappearing (9–24 months)
	The jaw, lips, and tongue continue to learn to move independently of one another

Date	Age: 18–24 Months*
	Different parts of each structure continue to learn to move separately (eg, the tip of the tongue moves independently of the rest of the tongue, and each lip corner contracts independently of the rest of the lips)
	Top cuspids come in (18–20 months)
	Bottom second molars come in (20–24 months)
	Top second molars come in (24–30 months)
	All first and primary teeth come in by 24–30 months
	Jaw stability increases substantially (16–24 months)
	Baby may bite on a mouthpiece or straw when trying to blow into a horn or suck from a straw until around 18 months
	Chewing, taking sips from an open cup or straw, and blowing activities have replaced sucking and suckling for calming

*Suggested mouth toys: Horns and bubbles (with parents and others), yellow and red Chewy Tubes, P's and Q's, and ARK's Grabbers (with a parent's supervision)

During the 18- to 24-month period, your child is developing increasingly sophisticated mouth movements for eating, drinking, mouth play, and speaking. Your child will get better and better at these mouth activities.

You will see improved grading, dissociation, and direction of movement. Grading means that your child moves the mouth just far enough with just enough strength to accomplish the movement. For example, you will see your child open her mouth just enough to place a horn on her lips. Dissociation of movement means that your child is now moving one mouth structure or part of a mouth structure separately from another. For example, your child will just place her lips on the horn and will no longer bite on it to stabilize it with the jaw around 18 months. You will also see direction of movement. For example, your child's lips will come forward and round to blow bubbles. More examples of grading, dissociation, and direction of movement will be provided in chapter 5.

There is always going to be some overlap between age ranges as mouth development occurs. These are ongoing processes. However, here are some changes that happen specifically between 16 and 24 months. Your child will have increasingly mature swallowing control by 18 months. Prior to 16–18 months, you might see your child biting down on a horn mouthpiece or a straw to obtain jaw stability. However, you will see a marked increase in your child's ability to stabilize the jaw between 16 and 24 months. This means that your child can easily move the jaw into any variety of positions, keeping the jaw still when needed and in good alignment while moving the lips and tongue independently of the jaw. Good alignment means that top and bottom jaws are "lined up" during mouth activities, such as biting on toys or talking. You will see something different when your child is chewing food (ie, rotary jaw movement). See chapter 6 for more detail.

The improvement in jaw stability seems to be related to the remaining primary teeth coming in. All primary teeth erupt by 24–30 months. The top cuspids come in between 18 and 20 months. The bottom second molars come in between 20 and 24 months. The top second molars come in between 24 and 30 months.

Appropriate Pacifier Use and Thumb- and Finger-Sucking

Pacifier use has often been considered controversial. Some parents and professionals feel that it is better for your baby to use a pacifier than to suck on her thumb. Some think the opposite. Some feel that pacifier use and thumb- and finger-sucking are bad habits that should not be allowed. The reality is that babies primarily use suckling and sucking to calm themselves during the first 5 to 6 months of life. In some cultures, young babies are allowed to suckle at the breast as needed throughout the day.[173] Some babies need more suckling and sucking than others. Pacifier use during sleep has been recommended to avoid SIDS.[174–175]

When your baby was born, she had few ways to calm herself. Suckling was one way. Some babies have been seen to suckle on their thumbs in the womb on ultrasound images. It was easy for your baby to suckle on the thumb in utero because she was in a flexed or rounded position, and the thumb was easy to get to. Babies have somewhat less control over this process after birth, because they are moving in relation to gravity.

Pacifier use will be a decision that you make as a parent. Whether your child uses a pacifier or suckles on the thumb, it is most important that these activities occur appropriately. You can assist your baby in bringing the thumb or fingers to the mouth to calm herself. As discussed previously, hand-to-mouth play is very important for your child. This can begin with suckling and move toward various types of hand-to-mouth play (such as exploring appropriate toys with the mouth) as your baby is ready for these. See the previous section on the importance and development of good mouthing experiences.

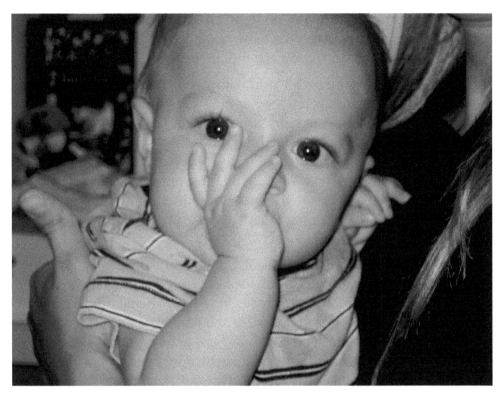

Photo 4.9: Thumb-sucking is still appropriate at 4 months.

Many lactation consultants will recommend that the pacifier not be introduced until breast-feeding is well established. Dr Harvey Karp[176] recommends avoiding both bottles and pacifiers for the first 2 to 3 weeks of life to avoid breast-feeding problems. Breast-feeding has been shown to reduce the risk of middle-ear problems,[177] while prolonged pacifier use is correlated with middle-ear concerns, oral candida, cavities, and malocclusion (eg, overbite, open bite, and cross-bite).[178]

Middle-ear problems (commonly resulting in ear infections) have been connected with pacifier use beyond 10 months of age.[179] They are usually treated with antibiotics. Excessive use of antibiotics is a worldwide concern, because it promotes the development of new strains of bacteria that are resistant to antibiotics. Persistent middle-ear problems affect a child's ability to learn speech, language, and, ultimately, related academic skills (such as reading). It is believed that pacifier use changes the pressure balance between the middle ear and the nasopharynx and therefore affects Eustachian tube function.[180]

Aside from middle-ear concerns, there are good developmental reasons to follow the guidelines for pacifier use presented in this chapter. We want your baby to develop her feeding and speech skills on time. Excessive, long-term pacifier use can keep your child from developing mature food manipulation and swallowing patterns. It can also keep your child from developing mature mouth movements needed for speech. Remember, the suckling pattern used with the pacifier is a movement your baby needed at birth. See chapters 7 and 8 for further information on speech and mouth development.

If you choose to use a pacifier with your baby, the pacifier needs to fit your baby's mouth. If the pacifier is too long, it may gag your baby or move in and out of the mouth when your baby suckles or sucks on it. Don't be fooled by packaging. If your baby has a small mouth, she will need a small pacifier. For example, don't be concerned about using a pacifier that was originally developed for a preemie (eg, the Wee Soothie) if your child is a newborn. As your child grows, the pacifier you use may not reflect your child's age. Do not worry about this. Get a pacifier that fits your baby's mouth. People have different mouth sizes, just as they have different shoe, clothing, and hat sizes.

If you are having difficulty finding a pacifier to fit your baby's mouth, see Activity 2.3 in chapter 2. You will check the fit of the pacifier nipple in the same way you checked the fit of the bottle nipple. Your baby should have a good lip latch on the pacifier, and your baby's tongue should move in an even, front-to-back wavelike motion during the suckle (newborn to 3 or 4 months of age). Since your baby is doing what therapists call nonnutritive suckling, you will probably see your baby suckle two times per second. This is different than the nutritive suckle you see on the bottle or breast (ie, usually one time per second). You also want your baby's tongue to be cupped (not humped) when suckling on a pacifier. This should be an easy, relaxed movement, with little jaw movement. The tongue is the primary actor, but you may not see it if the lips are latched properly.

If your baby has difficulty keeping the pacifier in the mouth after you have checked for a fit, you can assist your baby by providing cheek support. See the section on What to Do If Your Baby Has Difficulty Maintaining a Latch in chapter 2. Dr Harvey Karp[181] also recommends that you play a gentle tug of war game with the pacifier. By gently tugging on the pacifier when your baby starts to suck, you can teach your baby to keep the pacifier in the mouth.

I often recommend a pacifier with a rounded nipple, such as the Soothie or the Wee Soothie, because the tongue can cup around the nipple. However, your baby may prefer a different type of pacifier nipple. Some pacifiers are called *orthodontic* and may encourage the three-dimensional suck that develops by 4 months of age. However, no pacifier has been shown to benefit mouth development in the same way as the mother's breast.[182-184] The mother's breast is drawn deeply into the baby's mouth and can help to maintain the shape of the hard palate (the roof of the mouth) if the baby is nursing properly. There does not seem to be any pacifier that works like the mother's breast for shaping the mouth.

Some guidelines for pacifier use and thumb- and finger-sucking are listed as follows. These are based on studies of pacifier use[185-187] and knowledge of mouth development.

ACTIVITY 4.4: PACIFIER USE AND WEANING

Place a date by each skill as your child accomplishes it. Review the chapter to address relevant "Things to Change." Date the changes you made.

Date	What You Want	Date	Things to Change
	Birth to 5–6 months: Takes pacifier only for calming		Keeps pacifier in the mouth much of the time while awake
	6–10 months: Weaning from pacifier begins—takes pacifier only to sleep; participates in higher-level mouth activities (eg, mouthing safe, appropriate toys)		Relies on pacifier to calm self throughout the day
	10 months: Proper eating, drinking, and true mouth play; no longer uses a pacifier		Still uses pacifier

Here are pacifier and thumb- and finger-sucking guidelines, based on current research:

- Between birth and 6 months of age, give your baby the pacifier for calming purposes. When your baby is asleep or calm, remove the pacifier when possible. (**Note:** Authors of studies on SIDS[188–189] recommend pacifier use during sleep; studies on middle-ear problems[190] recommend pacifier use as your baby is falling asleep). Babies who have difficulty calming may need the pacifier for longer periods of time. However, there is generally no reason to place the pacifier back into your baby's mouth once she is calm. Thumb-sucking and finger-sucking are appropriate at this age if you are not using a pacifier. (**Note:** Dr Harvey Karp recommends that parents discontinue pacifier use at 4 to 5 months of age.)[191]

- Between 6 and 10 months of age, begin to wean your baby from the pacifier by providing the pacifier only when your baby is most cranky and needs to sleep.

- At 6 months of age, you can give your baby appropriate items to chew or mouth for calming in place of the pacifier, thumb-sucking, or finger-sucking (eg, toys that can be safely chewed and mouthed). Six-month-old babies can sit up, hold objects in their hands, and bring toys to their mouths. This is also a critical time for oral exploration, called *discriminative mouthing*. Good discrimination in the mouth is important for feeding and speech development. (See the previous section for discussion of discriminative mouthing).

- By 10 months, your baby can be weaned completely from the pacifier, because she has learned to use the mouth in other appropriate ways (such as chewing, taking bites, taking sips, and babbling). It may be a little more difficult to wean your child from thumb- or finger-sucking, because they are part of your child's body.

- Keep in mind that these are guidelines and not rigid timelines. You and your child will negotiate your way through this process. You will praise your baby as she uses her mouth for more sophisticated movements, such as chewing and interacting with appropriate mouth toys, which begins by 6 months of age. It is important that neither you nor your child feels pressure as you work your way through this stage of development. There are many beliefs and wives' tales about pacifier use and thumb- and finger-sucking. You may use the information gained here to help you navigate the process easily with your child.

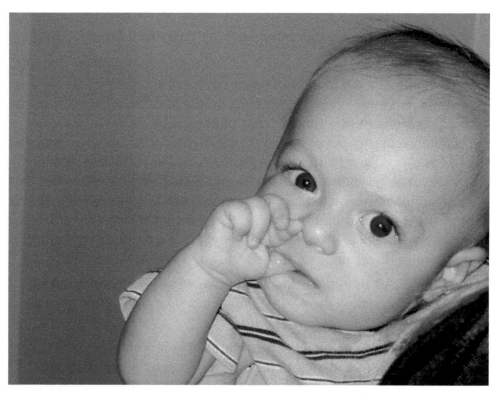

Photo 4.10: Thumb sucking may change to thumb and finger chewing as part of jaw development.

Here is a summary of ideas to help you with the pacifier, thumb-, and finger-sucking weaning process at the ages recommended previously. These ideas can also be used with older children who are still using pacifiers.

Weaning Summary:

1. Replace pacifier use, thumb-sucking, or other sucking habits with an appropriate mouth behavior (such as chewing on Chewy Tubes, ARK's Grabbers, and other appropriate mouth toys, and taking sips of water).

2. Gently offer the replacement when your child asks for the pacifier or starts sucking on her thumb or fingers.

3. If your child will not accept the replacement right away, keep the replacement where your child can chew on it as she chooses.

4. You can change your child's pacifier into a type of replacement by poking holes into it or cutting it. This way your child's pacifier no longer works like a pacifier. **See the drawbacks and warning below**.

5. Give your child attention and praise when she is using an appropriate replacement for the pacifier or other sucking habit.

6. Give your child attention and praise at other times throughout the day when she is using her mouth appropriately (such as babbling, smiling, talking, eating, and drinking).

7. Ignore thumb-, finger-, and other sucking behaviors when your child engages in them, but **do not** ignore your child. Just act like the behavior is not occurring.

8. If your child is older, consider reasoning with her and coming up with a plan to give away or get rid of the pacifier or other sucking habit.

Most young children welcome new and novel mouth experiences (such as chewing on Chewy Tubes and ARK's Grabbers). However, if your child insists upon using the pacifier, you can change your child's pacifier by poking holes into it or cutting it as mentioned previously.[192] This way, your child's pacifier no longer works like a pacifier.

The **major drawbacks** of using this method are:

1. The pacifier is no longer safe for your child to use independently.

2. Dirt can collect in areas that were modified.

3. You will need to throw the modified pacifier away after one use.[193]

If you use this method to show your child that the pacifier no longer works, you may need to buy several of your child's pacifiers for this process, as they will need to be discarded after a single use. Children will often throw away their own pacifiers when they don't work and then look for something else to mouth.

Some people have tried punishment to wean a child from a pacifier or from a thumb- or finger-sucking habit. I personally don't like to use punishment (eg, use of bad-tasting substances painted on the thumb or nagging the child) during the weaning process. Punishment is known only to have temporary results and can be traumatic. Children (and adults, for that matter) respond better to praise.

The best way to get rid of any behavior is to ignore the behavior (when possible), and praise the behavior you want. For example, you can praise your child when he or she is not sucking on the pacifier, thumb, or fingers, by saying something like, "Emily, your mouth looks so pretty right now." Remember that pacifier, thumb, and finger-sucking are habits your child has established. Habits are changed over time by replacing them with new, more appropriate behaviors. Anyone who has quit smoking or has lost weight on a systematic program can understand this.

So, what should you do if you feel caught in the pacifier or thumb- and finger-sucking trap? For example, what if you have an older child who continues to suck on a pacifier, thumb, fingers, or blanket? It is important to understand why your child may want to suck on the pacifier, thumb, fingers, or blanket. Is your child doing this when upset or tired? Is there another reason? Many children use sucking to help improve attention, focus, and concentration. You now know that chewing activities and taking sips of water can be calming. You will

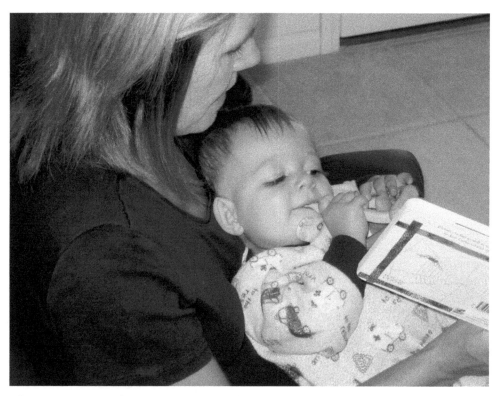

Photo 4.11: Anthony attends to a book while chewing on a Grabber.

systematically help your child replace one behavior with another more effective one over time by using the previous weaning suggestions.

Another way to work through this process with an older child is to reason with him. Create a plan for stopping use of the pacifier with your child, making him part of the process. Plan to give the pacifier away to the new baby down the street. Wrap it up like a present. This is a pretend activity, and it is helpful to have the other mom on board with the plan. One mom told me her child wanted to bury her pacifiers in the back yard as a way of separating from their use. When you plan together, you are partners in the process. Pam Marshalla's book, *How to STOP Thumbsucking and Other Oral Habits,* is a resource for parents on this topic.[194] There is also a book entitled *David Decides about Thumbsucking: A Story for Children; A Guide for Parents,* by Susan Heitler.[195] This book has a story for the older child, as well as information for parents.

Teething and Drooling

Teething and drooling are related to the hand-mouth connection. This section will help you to decide if your child's teething and drooling are appropriate. Many people think that a lot of drooling is normal for a baby or toddler. It never is. This is what you can expect to see.

ACTIVITY 4.5: TEETHING AND DROOLING CHECKLIST[196–200]

Place a check mark and a date in the column below as your child accomplishes these milestones. If your child is doing some of the things you don't want to see, review the chapter for guidance on how to address it.

Date	Age	What You Want to See	What You Don't Want to See
	1 month	Rare drooling	A lot of drooling
	2–4 months	May see some drooling between 2 and 4 months when mouthing objects[201]	A lot of drooling
	3–6 months	May see some drooling around 5–6 months with teething and mouthing	A lot of drooling

ACTIVITY 4.5: TEETHING AND DROOLING CHECKLIST (cont.)[196–200]

Date	Age	What You Want to See	What You Don't Want to See
	3–6 months	Teeth begin to erupt with increased chewing and biting experiences (5–6 months)	No sign of teeth (5–9 months)
	5–9 months	Some drooling may occur while on back or belly or while sitting and babbling or using hands; with teething; during or after feeding; with certain foods	A lot of drooling
	5–9 months	Bottom two front teeth (central incisors) erupt (5–9 months)	No teeth; teeth erupting late or in an irregular sequence
	5–9 months	Top two front teeth (central incisors) erupt (6–10 months)	No teeth; teeth erupting late or in an irregular sequence
	5–9 months	Bottom lateral incisors erupt (7–20 months)	No teeth; teeth erupting late or in an irregular sequence
	5–9 months	Top lateral incisors erupt (8–10 months)	No teeth; teeth erupting late or in an irregular sequence
	9–12 months	No drooling with movements such as rolling or crawling	Drooling during these movements

Date	Age	What You Want to See	What You Don't Want to See
	9–12 months	Some drooling while teething	A lot of drooling
	9–12 months	Bottom first molars erupt (10–12 months)	Teeth erupting late or in an irregular sequence
	12–15 months	No drooling with previously learned body movements	Drooling during these movements
	12–15 months	Some drooling while teething	A lot of drooling
	12–15 months	Top first molars erupt (14–16 months)	Teeth erupting late or in an irregular sequence
	15–18 months	No drooling with previously learned movements, such as walking and running	Drooling during these movements
	15–18 months	Some drooling while getting teeth	A lot of drooling
	15–18 months	Bottom cuspids erupt (16–18 months)	Teeth erupting late or in an irregular sequence
	18–21 months	No drooling with previously learned hand movements (eg, feeding self, handling toys)	Drooling during these movements

ACTIVITY 4.5: TEETHING AND DROOLING CHECKLIST (cont.)[196-200]

Date	Age	What You Want to See	What You Don't Want to See
	18–21 months	Some drooling while getting teeth	A lot of drooling
	18–21 months	Top cuspids erupt (18–20 months)	Teeth erupting late or in an irregular sequence
	21–24 months	No drooling with more advanced hand and mouth movements (eg, coloring, finger plays, speech)	Drooling during these movements
	21–24 months	Bottom second molars erupt (20–24 months)	Teeth erupting late or in an irregular sequence
	21–24 months	Top second molars erupt (24–30 months)	Teeth erupting late or in an irregular sequence

Drooling is seen with the development of motor skills and teething. It is rare in a 1-month-old baby, because little saliva is produced.[202] Between 2 and 4 months of age, you may see some drooling when your baby is mouthing a toy. Between 3 and 6 months of age, your baby may drool when mouthing and teething. Drooling, mouthing, and teething accompany one another. Appropriate mouthing, biting, and chewing help teeth to erupt. Your child will probably get her first teeth around 5 or 6 months of age. See Figure 8.3 for a diagram of the deciduous (primary) teeth.

Between 5 and 9 months of age, your baby may drool while on his back or belly or while sitting and simultaneously using his hands or babbling. You may also notice some drooling with teething, during or after feeding, or with certain foods. The bottom two front teeth (central incisors) usually erupt between 5 and

9 months. The top two front teeth (central incisors) usually erupt between 6 and 10 months. The bottom lateral incisors usually erupt between 7 and 20 months. The top lateral incisors usually erupt between 8 and 10 months.

If your child is not getting teeth at these times or his teeth are emerging in an irregular or different sequence, look at what he is doing with his mouth. An increase in appropriate mouth play and feeding activities to include biting and chewing activities can help with this process.

As your child gains control over whole-body movements, you will see drooling disappear during these activities. For example, between 9 and 12 months of age, you will no longer see drooling during whole-body movements such as rolling or crawling. However, you may continue to see some drooling with teething. In addition to the teeth listed in the previous paragraph, your child's bottom first molars usually erupt between 10 and 12 months. A lot of teeth are emerging during this time.

Your 12- to 15-month-old child will no longer drool with previously learned whole-body movements, such as crawling. Again, you may see your child drooling when teething, as well as when using her hands (one type of fine motor activity). Your child's top first molars usually erupt between 14 and 16 months of age. Between 15 and 18 months, you no longer see drooling with previously learned whole-body movements such as walking or running. Some drooling may be seen with teething and hand movements. Your child's bottom cuspids usually erupt between 16 and 18 months of age.

By 18 to 21 months of age, you will no longer see drooling with previously learned hand movements (such as feeding himself and handling toys). Your child has gained control over these movements. You may see some drooling with more advanced hand and mouth movements, such as coloring, speech, and finger games (eg, "Itsy Bitsy Spider," "Where Is Thumbkin?"). Drooling may still occur with teething. The top cuspids usually erupt between 18 and 20 months of age.

Between 21 and 24 months of age, you will no longer see drooling with more advanced hand and mouth movements. The bottom second molars usually erupt between 20 and 24 months of age, and the top second molars usually erupt between 24 and 30 months of age.

Again, the ages at which your child develops teeth are approximate. You should see your child develop the teeth around the developmental age listed. If you do not see this occurring or your child is developing teeth in an irregular manner (such as irregular sequence, tooth shape, or tooth structure), review the chapter for pertinent information and consult your child's dentist. If you see a large amount of drooling at any time or your child continues to drool beyond the age of 2 years, review the next section of the chapter for guidance on how to address it.

What to Do about Too Much Drooling

Excessive drooling can be frustrating for both you and your child. There are four things you need to think about if your child is drooling "too much." Activity 4.6 can help you to figure out what to do. Place a date in the column next to the description that matches "What You Want" or "Things to Change."

ACTIVITY 4.6: CHECKLIST TO DETERMINE IF YOUR CHILD IS DROOLING TOO MUCH

Date	What You Want	Date	Things to Change
	Clear sinuses, easy breathing through the nose		Stuffy nose, mouth breathing
	Good sensation in the mouth		Child does not seem to feel things in the mouth like you do
	Closed mouth at rest		Mouth hangs open at rest or other times
	Swallowing approximately every 30 seconds		Infrequent swallowing

In chapter 3, we talked about the importance of breathing through the nose for good health. Throughout the book, we discuss the problems that can occur if your child's hard palate is high and narrow. If the roof of your child's mouth is high and narrow, this affects the shape and function of the nasal and sinus areas. It is more difficult to breathe with small or misshapen nasal areas and/or sinuses. These are more difficult to clear if any sinus swelling or congestion occurs. You will need to consult with your child's pediatrician and/or ear, nose, and throat specialist to take care of nasal and sinus problems. See the section on Health Problems and Possible Treatments in chapter 3.

It is also important that your child have good sensation in the mouth. In this chapter, we have already talked about the importance of discriminative mouthing. A child who has a chronically open mouth usually experiences differences in mouth sensation. See what happens when you breathe through your mouth for a few minutes. Does the inside of your mouth feel different? Most people notice the dryness. Dryness changes the way you feel things within the mouth.

Some children have less sensation in the mouth than others. This may be an inherited characteristic. People with decreased muscle tone in their bodies tend to have less acute sensation. If your child does not have good sensation in the mouth, she may not feel the presence of saliva. We will discuss some more ways to improve sensation in the mouth in chapter 5.

You want your child to have a closed mouth when she is not eating, drinking, or speaking. If you see your child's mouth hanging open at rest, when she is using her hands, or at other times, your child may need some jaw exercise, or "jaws-ercise." As you already know, sometimes people keep their mouths open so they can breathe. At other times, the mouth is open because of jaw weakness. The jawbone is very heavy, and gravity is constantly pulling down on it. Jaw muscles need adequate strength to keep the mouth closed. See chapter 5 for "jaws-ercise."

Swallowing is the other thing to consider if your child is drooling too much. Remember that the mature swallow is developing in the first 2 years of life. When we are awake, we swallow about every 30 seconds. This clears the saliva from our mouths. You need good sensation within the mouth to know that saliva is there. Time your child's swallow. If your child does not swallow approximately every 30 seconds (when not eating or drinking), you can help your child develop this habit.

An easy way to do this is to have an open cup or cup with a straw available. While you are reading a book or playing with your child, have her take a sip approximately every 30 seconds. Have your own open cup or cup with a straw nearby, so you can act as a role model. This is also a good activity for hydration. Pam Marshalla has written a book for parents called *How to STOP Drooling*.[203] This and other resources for parents are listed in Appendix A.

5

Massage, "Jaws-ercise," Tooth-Grinding, Bubbles, and Horns

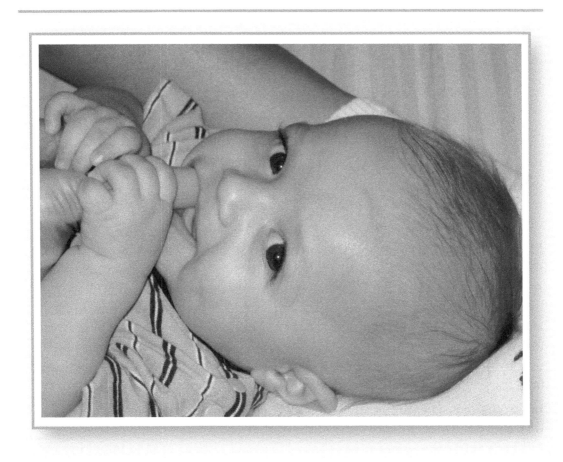

Y our baby learns about the world through touch and movement. Massage is becoming well known for its benefits and is one way that you can help your child learn about the world. Some of the benefits of massage include:[204–208]

- Helping you to bond with your baby

- Learning to communicate effectively with your baby

- Developing your baby's body awareness (which is important for movement development)

- Improving digestion, weight gain, and elimination (bowel movements)

- Improving sleep because of improved relaxation

For children who typically have difficulty feeding and gaining weight (such as preemies), full-body massage has been shown to help resolve these issues. Infant massage has also been used to help children with digestive concerns (such as reflux, colic, and excessive gas).

Massage can feel very natural for some parents but can feel unnatural for others. People are comfortable with differing levels of touch for a variety of reasons. As a parent, it is important for you to honor your comfort level, as well as your baby's comfort level when doing infant massage. Perhaps this is your first baby, and you haven't been around many babies. You may not be sure about how to touch and move your baby. This was my experience when I was a young mother over 30 years ago. It is important to be easy with yourself and know that there is help for you in this area.

In fact, there is an entire organization dedicated to infant massage, called the International Association of Infant Massage. If you are interested in learning full-body infant massage for your baby, you can locate a certified infant massage instructor. These are often people from other fields (such as nursing, massage therapy, occupational therapy, physical therapy, and speech-language pathology) who teach parents to massage their infants and young children.

Infant massage courses are usually offered in a small-group setting, where parents can learn massage and socialize with other parents. Parents bring their babies to the group and learn to massage their own babies. The book *Infant Massage: A Handbook for Loving Parents,* by Vimala Schneider McClure, is used as the text for these courses. Many community hospitals and other community organizations offer these courses. Contact the International Association of Infant Massage *(www.iaim.ws)* to locate instructors in your area.

Note: If your child has a medical condition that may contraindicate massage, please talk to your pediatrician before proceeding. Some medical conditions for which massage will need to be used with caution include skin problems such as rashes, infections involving fever, acquired immune deficiency syndrome, or AIDS, and stroke.[209]

Face, Jaw, and Mouth Massage with "Jaws-ercise"

As a certified speech-language pathologist, certified massage practitioner, and certified infant massage instructor, I found that I could easily teach parents face, jaw, and mouth massage in addition to full-body infant massage. The purpose of face, jaw, and mouth massage (called *oral massage*) is to bring awareness to these structures. "Jaws-ercise" can help balance the movements of the jaw. Remember that your baby uses his mouth to explore and learn, so oral massage and "jaws-ercise" can help your baby do this. They are systematic ways of providing the oral input your baby is seeking. However, oral massage and "jaws-ercise" *do not* replace the use of good feeding techniques or actual speech facilitation, covered in chapters 2, 6, and 7. Your baby needs to practice feeding and speech to learn these processes.

Face, jaw, and mouth massage can be used to prepare your baby's mouth for feeding and vocal interaction. Therefore, you should do the massage before a meal, during a break from feeding toward the beginning of the meal, or when you are playing with your baby. We want your baby to be calm and enjoy the massage. We don't want your baby to be hungry or frustrated during the massage. If you are doing the massage as part of feeding, you will want to make it part of your routine before feeding, if possible. However, if your baby is very hungry, you may want to do the oral massage when you and your baby take a break, near the beginning of feeding. You can also do the massage when you are interacting vocally with your baby (such as cooing and vocalizing together).

Some parents want to know when to use oral massage and/or exercise with their babies. You can use them during the first 2 years of life and beyond, as your child's mouth is developing. This would be particularly important for any child who drools or demonstrates some of the subtle concerns or differences discussed in chapter 2. You can eventually place oral massage work into your child's oral-hygiene routine. It can help to prepare him for eventual tooth-brushing. In fact, many adults include tongue brushing in their own tooth-brushing routine. Tongue stroking and brushing are part of the oral massage you will do with your child.

Face, jaw, and mouth massage and/or exercise can be a special time for dads to interact with their babies. This can help build communication between Dad and baby. If your baby is nursing, he may enjoy doing the massage and/or exercise with Dad before Mom feeds him. Some babies seem to be focused only on nursing when Mom picks them up. As you can see, having Dad perform the massage when he is available can have many benefits.

However, if Mom is having problems with nursing (because her baby has difficulty with oral awareness and jaw movement), it may be very important for her to complete a quick oral massage with her baby several times daily as part of feeding. Whether Dad or Mom does the massage, placing the baby on a towel or blanket for the massage will help him know the difference between massage time and feeding time. Babies are very smart and learn these differences with time and consistency.

Here is a simple face, jaw, and mouth massage that you can do with your baby (adapted from an unpublished protocol by Suzanne Wayson).[210–211] Remember that interacting with your baby in any way (such as feeding and massage) is like dancing. You are partners in this process. You may actually find ways that work best for you and your baby that are somewhat different from what is suggested in this book. This will help you learn to trust and follow your intuition as a parent.

While the description of the face, jaw, and mouth massage is detailed, it can be done very quickly (in 1 to 3 minutes) and easily with your baby. I will break the massage into several lessons for you, so that you will not feel overwhelmed. Give yourself several days on each lesson before trying to put it together.

Lesson 1: Positioning Your Baby for Face, Jaw, and Mouth Massage

Begin by finding a position in which you and your baby can interact comfortably face-to-face. I like to massage babies' faces, jaws, and mouths by positioning their heads on the heels and insteps of my feet. I learned this from a wonderful speech-language pathologist named Suzanne Evans Morris (coauthor of the book *Pre-Feeding Skills*[212]). Of course, I keep a supply of fresh socks on hand for this purpose!

You can sit on the floor or on a clean blanket or towel with your legs circled and the bottom of your toes touching each other. You will place your baby's head on the heels and insteps of your feet. The rest of your baby's body will be on the floor, inside the circle made by your legs. This allows you to make eye contact with your baby. It also places your baby's head into a slight chin-tuck or downward position, which keeps your baby from hyperextending the neck and body (ie, head, neck, and body arched backward).

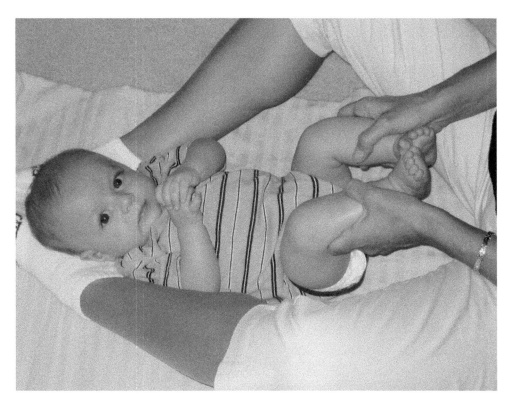

Photo 5.1: Anthony is positioned for face, jaw, and mouth massage.

If this position is not comfortable for you or your baby, find another position that is comfortable. If either you or your baby is uncomfortable, it will be communicated and will limit your experience. Once you find a comfortable face-to-face position with your baby, you can interact with one another through talking and touch.

Lesson 2: Helping You and Your Baby Become Accustomed to Massage

Begin talking to your baby, while giving some gentle on-off presses or gentle squeezes to your baby's arms. It is also a good idea to ask your baby's permission (eg, "Anthony, may I touch your arms?"). Tell your baby what you are doing (eg, "Anthony, I am touching your little arms. Doesn't that feel good?"). See Vimala McClure's book, *Infant Massage,* for more details about full-body infant massage. You can also create a song to go along with your massage. I like to use the melody of "The Farmer In the Dell." For example, "Massaging Anthony's arms, massaging Anthony's arms, hi-ho, the derry-o, massaging Anthony's arms."

You can increase the firmness of your touch as you become comfortable with massaging your baby. A firm but gentle touch (a term we will be using in this

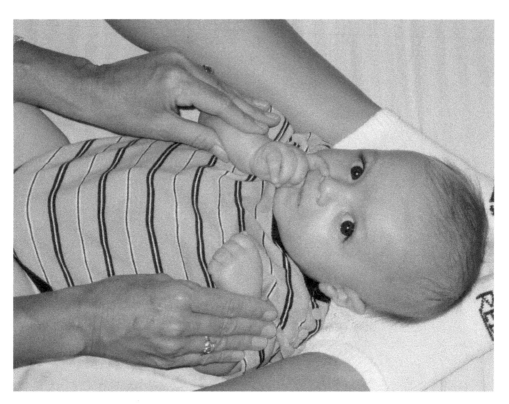

Photo 5.2: Diane massages Anthony's arms, helping him become accustomed to her touch.

section of the book) means that you want to press deeply enough for your baby to feel what you are doing, but you **never** want your touch to be uncomfortable for your baby.

Your baby will show you through body language and vocalization (such as cooing and fussing) how he or she feels about the touch. This is a wonderful way for you learn to communicate with your baby that can also empower you as a parent. You will learn to listen to your baby's signals and know what they mean.

Always listen to your baby's feedback as communication, and respect that communication. If your baby cries, squirms, or looks uncomfortable in any way, you can lighten or deepen your touch, as long as you are gentle. If your baby is uncomfortable with touch to the arms, begin by touching an area (such as the legs or back) where your baby likes touch. You will generally not begin with touch to the face or mouth, as your baby may feel more vulnerable in these areas.

If you are doing full-body massage as instructed by a certified infant massage instructor or by reading the book *Infant Massage* by Vimala McClure, you may choose to begin with a part of the massage you learned from your instructor or the book. Also, if you and/or your baby are uncomfortable with touch, it is a good idea for you and your baby to enroll in an infant massage class. You can also work with a certified infant massage instructor privately. Contact the

International Association of Infant Massage *(www.iaim.ws)* to locate instructors in your area.

Be creative about the sequence in which you do face, jaw, and mouth massage. There is no set sequence. It is most important that you read and respond to your baby's communication signals as you do this. Babies generally enjoy stimulation within the mouth. This activity should be fun for you and your baby.

If your baby seems sensitive to touch during a particular part of the massage, go back to massaging an area with which your child is comfortable. Do not stop massaging your child because he seems uncomfortable with one part of the massage. Slowly work toward massaging the area where your baby seems uncomfortable. You might have to change a part of the massage so your baby will enjoy it more.

For example, if your baby does not like little strokes, use little on-off presses. You can try the strokes later when you and your baby are more accustomed to the massage. You can try massaging an area up to three times per session. If your baby still does not seem to like that part of the massage, finish the massage by massaging an area that your baby enjoys.

Some babies are very sensitive in and around the mouth. Feeding therapists often see this in children who are experiencing some type of gastrointestinal concern (such as chronic reflux or belly pain). It is possible that these children demonstrate sensitivities in the mouth because they have learned to associate their discomfort with feeding. Some professionals believe that sensitivity in the mouth may be related to body memories of previous mouth experiences (such as deep suctioning at birth). Sensitivity in and around the mouth may also be inherited. You will work more slowly and carefully with your child if he is sensitive.

Some babies don't seem to feel things in the mouth in the same way as others. This is a common difference that is often seen in children with decreased muscle tone in the body. Many people have muscle tone that is on the low side of normal. This is often not a clinically significant concern, but may cause subtle difficulties with sensation and movement. Decreased muscle tone means that the muscles have less stiffness to stabilize or move the bones against gravity.[213–214] Children with decreased muscle tone may also need more sensory input or information to demonstrate their reflexes. If your child fits this description, you probably had to touch or press the areas around your child's mouth with greater intensity (a little firmer and longer but still gentle) to see the reflexes listed in chapters 1 and 4. Just like other traits, muscle tone seems to run in families.

Lessons 3–5: Massaging Your Baby's Face and Jaw

Here are some general guidelines that will help you with Lessons 3–5. When you and your baby feel comfortable, you can move the massage from your baby's arms or other parts of the body to your baby's face and jaw. This part of the massage will help your baby be more aware of structures that assist with feeding, as well as provide him with the oral information he naturally seeks. The face and jaw massage can help children who may seem overly sensitive to touch on the face and jaw. It can also help children who seem to have less sensitivity in these areas. Sometimes older babies demonstrate this decrease in sensitivity by not showing awareness of food or saliva (drool) on the face. You can always add other strokes that you learn in your infant massage class to the face and jaw massage.

I usually don't use creams, oils, or lotions when I massage babies' faces. However, you could carefully use a cream or lotion on your baby's face if needed. This would need to be a cream or lotion approved for use on babies' faces. Be aware that some children do not like the scents of some creams or lotions, so unscented products may be preferable.

When massaging near your baby's mouth, you will want clean hands and short fingernails. Likewise, if you have been giving your baby a full-body massage with oil or lotion prior to massaging your baby's face and jaw, you will want to wash your hands. If you only began with some on-off presses on your baby's arms, you will have washed your hands prior to beginning the massage. Your fingernails need to be short enough that you do not risk scratching your baby. I usually cut mine very short, because babies' faces and mouths are so small.

Some parents like to use gloves when their hands and fingers are in or near their baby's mouth. If your baby has a rash on her face or has chapped lips, gloves are recommended. Therapists, physicians, and nurses use gloves when touching broken skin, as well as lip and mouth areas, because they do not want to risk giving the baby a communicable disease. **If your baby has a rash, be sure to talk to your pediatrician about the use of massage.** One of the benefits of massage is to boost the immune system, so massage may help children who tend to have rashes. However, rashes can be a contraindication for massage.

If you have a communicable disease, wear gloves! I like the nonlatex, nonpowdered gloves we discussed in chapter 1. These can usually be purchased in pharmacies and medical supply stores. I don't feel comfortable using latex gloves, because so many people have latex allergies. See chapter 1 for more details.

As you massage your baby's face, you can continue singing your song if you like. I created a song to the tune of "The Farmer in the Dell," but you can create any song you like. ("Massaging Jacob's face, massaging Jacob's face, hi-ho, the derry-o, massaging Jacob's face").

Lesson 3: Massaging Your Baby's Face

To begin the face massage, anchor your thumbs lightly on your baby's chin, along the bony part of the jaw line, or on the chest area. You do not want your thumbs to poke your baby. Using your index and middle fingers, begin

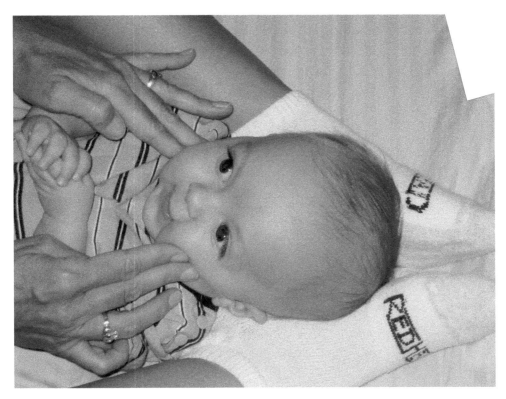

Photo 5.3: Anthony smiles at Diane during face massage.

the massage near your baby's earlobes, on both sides of the face. These are the masseter muscles, located between the jaw line and the cheekbones. The masseters are important for closing the mouth.

Massage your baby's face by making circles with your index and middle fingers. Instead of gliding over the skin, press firmly but gently into your baby's skin and the tissue underneath. It is easier if your circles are made toward the nose and lips, as this is the direction in which you are moving. Make two or three circles, then pick up your fingers and move them toward or onto your baby's cheeks. Make two or three circles, then pick up your fingers and move them toward the lips. Make as many stops as needed (possibly three to five) in the masseter and cheek areas as you progress toward your baby's lips. Your baby's cheeks consist of the buccinator muscles, which help to move your baby's lips.

Lesson 4: Massaging Your Baby's Lips

Continue to gently anchor your thumbs on your baby's chin, bony jaw line, or chest area. Using your index fingers, massage above the lips and below the lips from the corners to the center by making little circles with your index fingers. You will still be using both hands simultaneously. It seems easiest if your finger circles move toward the center of the lips. You will continue to press gently but firmly into the skin and tissue below it as you make the circles. You are now massaging the orbicularis oris muscle, which moves the lips.

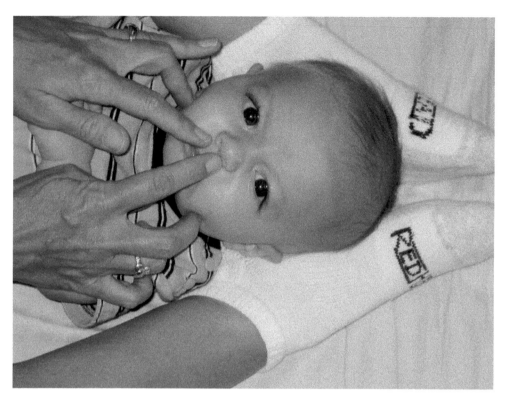

Photo 5.4: Anthony receives lip massage.

After you have massaged around the lips, massage the pink part of your baby's lips, called the *vermillion*. Again, use your index fingers and make little circles on your baby's top lip and little circles on your baby's bottom lip, moving from the corners to the center. You can use a glove for massaging the vermillion if you are concerned about getting dirt or bacteria from your finger into your child's mouth. This would be particularly important if you or your baby have an open cut or sore. Therapists, physicians, and nurses should always use gloves when touching your baby's lips. See information on gloves discussed previously and in chapter 1.

Lesson 5: Massaging under Your Baby's Chin

You can also massage under your baby's chin. This can be very relaxing for the muscles that work very hard while your baby is feeding. The muscles in the floor of the mouth (anterior belly of the digastric, geniohyoid, and mylohyoid) are responsible for opening the mouth and increased voice box elevation for swallowing as your child grows. The base of your baby's tongue is right above the floor of the mouth. Place the thumb of your dominant hand (eg, your right hand if you are right handed) on your baby's chin or jawbone. Then use the pad of your index finger to stroke gently under your baby's chin. Use small, back-to-front strokes, beginning near the chin and moving back toward the angle of the neck. Do not stroke beyond the angle of the neck, because your baby's very fragile larynx (voice box) is beyond this area in the throat.

Lessons 6–8: Massaging Your Baby's Mouth

You might want to use a glove for this part, because you will be placing your finger into your child's mouth. If you are having trouble with yeast infections in your breast or if your baby is susceptible to thrush, consider the use of a glove. (See previous information on gloves in this chapter and in chapter 1.)

Lesson 6: Massaging Your Baby's Tongue

Since babies are usually calm while suckling and sucking, you can begin by letting your baby suckle or suck on your finger. Some professionals will teach you to do this by orienting your index finger nail-side down and finger pad up. This is a fine method, as long as you are not inadvertently pressing the tip of your finger into the center of your baby's hard palate (the roof of the mouth).

Remember that your baby's hard palate is very flexible at birth. It will become more solid (like the roof of your mouth) over time. You don't want to apply pressure into the roof of your baby's mouth, because you don't want to press into an area that is flexible and still developing. We want the roof of your baby's mouth to remain fairly broad, with a slight arch. The roof of the mouth is the floor of the nasal and sinus areas. If the hard palate becomes high and narrow, the nasal and sinus areas can become misshapen. We want your baby's nasal areas and sinuses to remain open and clear.

Changing the orientation of your index finger by placing the finger pad down against the tongue can help you avoid this potential difficulty. It will also place your finger in a good position for tongue massage. While your baby is suckling on your finger, it is a good time to feel the natural rhythm of your baby's suckle or suck. It should be nice and rhythmic, occurring about once or twice per second.

While you have your finger on your baby's tongue, you can perform some tongue massage. Along with the rhythm of the suckle or suck, begin to stroke your baby's tongue with small back-to-front strokes. Begin near the tip of the tongue, and work your way back down the center. Some people call this "tongue walking." We want your baby's tongue to cup or groove around your finger. This cupping or grooving is important for both breast- and bottle-feeding. We do not want your baby's tongue to hump, as this does not support good feeding and swallowing skills. If this should occur, work with your baby's tongue to obtain the cupping or grooving motion during the suckle or suck.

As you work your way back on your baby's tongue, watch your baby's facial expressions carefully. Newborns have gag responses that are fairly forward on the tongue (occupying the back three-fourths of the tongue). This gag response is found further back on the tongue as your baby has an increasing number of mouth experiences.

Over time, as you massage your baby's tongue, you will notice that his gag reflex occurs further back toward the throat area. **You don't want to intentionally**

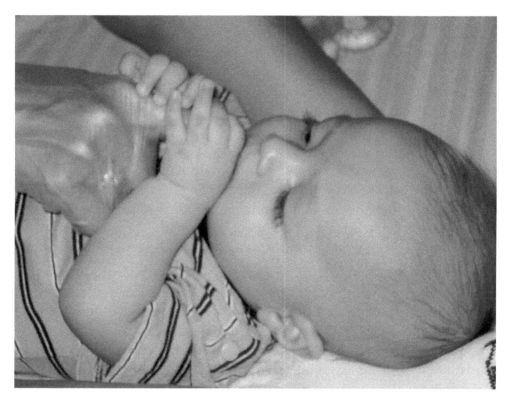

Photo 5.5: Anthony helps Diane with tongue massage.

gag your baby, so pay close attention to your baby's facial expressions. If your baby begins to look uncomfortable as you are walking your finger back on his tongue, move your finger forward and allow your baby to suckle. If your baby happens to gag, do not become overly concerned. Move your finger forward. You will massage your baby's tongue near the front if your baby is newborn. By 6 to 9 months of age, your child's gag reflex should occur on the back third of the tongue. You can then massage the front two-thirds of the tongue.

Initially, your baby will have the experience of the breast or bottle in the mouth. When your baby is drinking properly from the breast, it is drawn deeply into your child's mouth. As mentioned previously, this can help to maintain the shape of your child's hard palate (roof of the mouth). As your baby develops, he will hopefully participate in a wide variety of mouth experiences during feeding and mouth play. Appropriate oral experiences are very important for your baby's mouth development and have been discussed in great detail in chapter 4. The development of mature feeding patterns is discussed in chapter 6.

Lesson 7: Massaging Your Baby's Cheeks from Inside the Mouth

After your child has suckled or sucked on your finger and gotten accustomed to your finger being in his mouth, you can begin to stroke the inside of your baby's

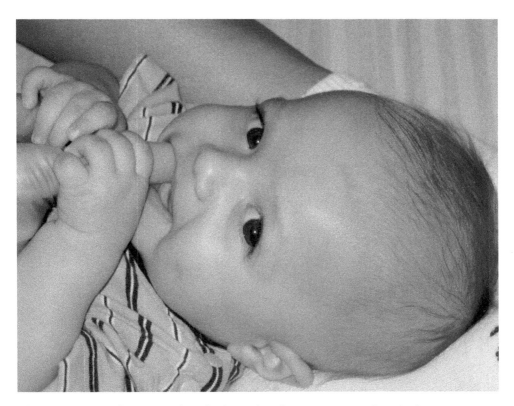

Photo 5.6: Anthony smiles during cheek massage with Infadent.

cheeks. Using small, firm but gentle, back-to-front strokes, stroke the inside of your baby's cheeks. This is similar to tongue walking. You might call it "cheek walking." You can begin near the inside lip corner and work your way back. To be sure you are covering the entire internal cheek surface, you may want to massage inside each cheek a couple of times.

You will be massaging the lateral pterygoids (for jaw opening), medial pterygoids (for jaw closing), and the inside of the buccinators (for good lip use and appropriate intraoral pressure). These muscles assist with the small, graded jaw and lip movements used during nursing, bottle-feeding, swallowing, and speech. The buccinators ultimately help keep the cheeks against the gum area, so that your baby can attain good intraoral pressure for swallowing and speech.

Remember that good intraoral pressure is important for the efficient flow of formula or breast milk through the mouth. If a baby is born without adequate sucking pads, the buccinators will need to quickly learn to do this work because sucking pads don't develop after birth. Your massage of the buccinators from the inside of the mouth can help your baby develop awareness of these muscles. As you massage inside the cheek areas, you may feel a little resistance (the cheeks pushing against your finger). These are the buccinator muscles working. We need good buccinator activity throughout life to effectively manage and swallow food and liquid. We also use these muscles to attain appropriate intraoral pressure for speech production.

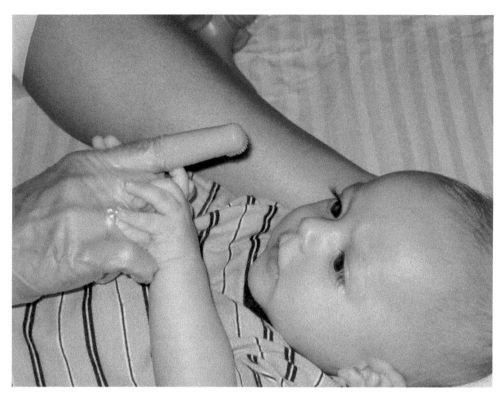

Photo 5.7: Anthony examines the Infadent Finger Toothbrush.

Note: Mouth massage may be used during the first 2 years of life and beyond. You can turn it into part of your child's oral hygiene routine, along with tooth brushing. Once your baby begins to get teeth, there are small brushes you can use for mouth massage (such as the Infadent Finger Toothbrush). My favorite brush is the Oral Probe, made by ARK. It has a very comfortable feel in the mouth. However, you can substitute other baby toothbrushes for this process. It is most important that your baby enjoys the feel of the brush in his mouth.

Lesson 8: Some Great Jaw Exercise ("Jaws-ercise") for Your Baby (Activities to Counteract Effects of Less-than-ideal Feeding Patterns)

Between massaging your baby's tongue and inner cheek, you can stop on your baby's back gum ridge (near where the back molars will eventually be), and allow your baby to chew on your finger. Babies are born with a phasic bite response that is believed to lead to the movements of chewing. If your baby has mild jaw weakness, unbalanced jaw movement, or underdeveloped sucking pads, your baby may have a tendency to stabilize the jaw by biting on the bottle or breast. This is one reason the breast shield was developed. However, the breast shield is not the best solution to this problem. We want your baby to stabilize the mouth without biting down.

Therefore, we do not want to teach your baby to bite or chew on your finger near the front of the mouth at this time. Instead, allowing your baby to chew on your finger in the back molar area is a preferred jaw activity with many benefits. This activity can assist the development of muscles that open and close the jaw. It can also encourage the tongue to pull back or retract (a movement needed for development of the mature swallowing pattern and speech).

When doing "jaws-ercise," it is important to note that our fingers are generally too big for our babies' small jaws. If you look at your index finger, you have small fleshy areas on either side of your fingernail. You can let your baby chew on these areas, but not the part with the fingernail. The part with the fingernail can hyperextend a baby's jaw (ie, cause the jaw to open too wide). This is very uncomfortable and may hurt your baby's jaw.

Place the side of your finger pad on your baby's back gum ridge. Press firmly but gently on your baby's gum with the fleshy part of your finger pad, and see how many times your baby can chew. Remember, your baby's phasic bite response can be stimulated on both the top and bottom gums.

By stimulating the back of the top gums with firm but gentle pressure, your baby's repetitive biting and chewing can possibly help to maintain the shape of the hard palate (roof of the mouth).[215] The gum ridge is firm, unlike the center of your baby's hard palate, which may remain flexible for some time. By pressing on the back of the top molar area, you may actually counteract the tendency of your child's palate to become high and narrow. This technique was originally developed by Sara Rosenfeld-Johnson and Lori Overland (two speech-language pathologists who work with babies).

You will initially notice how many times your baby will bite down or chew naturally without losing the rhythm. You can set a rhythm of about one per second, if that feels natural to you and your baby. If your baby can bite down on the fleshy part of your finger five times on each side, begin here. If your baby can bite down more times on one side than the other, move toward having your baby bite down the same number of times on both sides. As your baby can do this easily, move toward more repetitions.

Eventually, move toward having your baby bite down on the fleshy part of your finger 12 to 15 times in a row for three sets, alternating sides (eg, right back molar area, then left back molar area). This is an early form of exercise physiology. This up-down chewing exercise can be used in different forms as your baby's jaw grows to help him develop good jaw movement. Up-and-down jaw movement is needed for every process the jaw performs (such as speech, taking bites of food, and taking sips of liquid). See Activities 5.2 and 5.3 for information on the development of jaw movement through the use of appropriate mouth toys.

Mouth Toys and More "Jaws-ercise"

Your baby's jaw development is crucial to his development of sophisticated and mature eating, drinking, and speaking skills. The most pronounced jaw growth occurs in the first year of life, and jaw stability is established before 2 years of age. If the jaw is doing what it needs to be doing, then the lips and tongue can work properly.

Some babies have subtle or small difficulties with the jaw that affect eating, drinking, and ultimately speaking. In addition to the use of proper feeding techniques, the appropriate use of mouth toys (for biting and chewing) can help ensure that your baby's jaw develops properly.

By 5 to 6 months of age, your baby will be very interested in chewing. Chewing (or "jaws-ercise") is an excellent exercise for the jaw if done properly. Children will usually do this activity on their own if provided with the appropriate toys and foods. Remember that your baby is prewired neurologically for chewing via the phasic bite reflex.

The problem in today's world is that there are few commercially available items that will help your child learn to bite and chew properly. Safe, appropriate, chewable foods for infants are limited. Most commercially available mouth toys are too large for biting, chewing, and appropriate sensory exploration within the mouth.

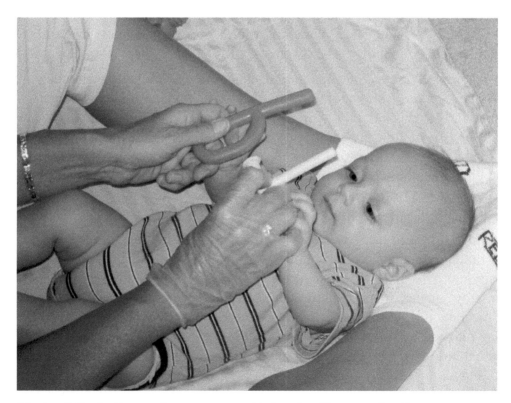

Photo 5.8: Anthony chooses a mouth toy for "jaws-ercise."

When choosing appropriate items for your child to chew, think of the following guidelines:

- Choose a safe toy that your child can hold and explore throughout the mouth without poking himself.
- Be sure that the toy fits your baby's jaw and does not cause him to open his jaw too wide. This means that the toy should fit comfortably and easily between your baby's gum surfaces in the back molar area. Jaw hyperextension places stress on the temporomandibular joint, or TMJ, and we do not want your baby to experience TMJ pain or discomfort. If you have ever experienced TMJ problems, you know what I mean.
- Be sure your child does not have to work too hard to bite and chew on a mouth toy. When children find things too difficult, they quickly stop doing the activity. However, some children really enjoy a harder surface for chewing. You will need to see what your child prefers, and his preferences may change over time as his mouth develops.
- Make sure that no part of the toy can break or be chewed off.
- Be sure that the toy is approved for mouth play. I recommend Chewy Tubes, Debra Beckman's Tri-Chews, and ARK's Grabbers. ARK products are manufactured in the United States with FDA-approved materials, scents, and colors. They are made without latex or phthalates. Chewy Tubes are nontoxic, latex free, and lead free, do not contain polyvinyl chloride, or PVC, or phthalates, and have FDA-approved colors. See the following chart for companies that carry these products.

COMPANIES THAT CARRY PRODUCTS FOR CHILDREN THAT CANNOT BE FOUND IN MOST STORES

Company	Phone Number	Web Site
ARK Therapeutic Services, Inc	(803) 438-9779	www.arktherapeutic.com
New Visions	(800) 606-7112	www.new-vis.com
The Speech Bin	(800) 850-8602	www.speechbin.com
SuperDuper Publications	(800) 277-8737	www.superduperinc.com

COMPANIES THAT CARRY PRODUCTS FOR CHILDREN THAT CANNOT BE FOUND IN MOST STORES (cont.)

Company	Phone Number	Web Site
TalkTools	(888) 529-2879	*www.talktools.net*
Therapro	(800) 257-5376	*www.theraproducts.com*

ACTIVITY 5.1: RECOMMENDED MOUTH TOYS

The mouth toys listed in Activity 5.1 are recommended as your baby grows. Most of these need to be ordered from the companies listed previously, because they are not available in stores. However, if you follow the guidelines listed previously and in chapter 4, you can find some appropriate mouth toys in stores. The guidelines are based on growth and individual mouth size, not on age or cognitive development. It is critical that you provide safe, appropriate mouth toys that fit your child's mouth. Toys that are too large or too difficult to chew will not give your child the desired result.

The toys listed in the Activity 5.1 are good for teething and exploration throughout the mouth (front, sides, and back). It is important that your baby bites and chews on appropriate toys by using the front, side, and back gum surfaces as part of teething. Mouth toy exploration and chewing activities do not need to be completed in isolation. They can be done as you look at books or view videos together. Remember, chewing can help increase attention, focus, and concentration in an individual of any age. See chapter 4 for a complete discussion of mouthing, teething, and calming.

Use the following chart to keep a record of the mouth toys you use with your child. Place a date by when you introduce mouth toys to your child. Make notes regarding your child's preferences.

Date	Age	Suggested Mouth Toys/Items
	Birth to 2 months (generalized mouthing)	Own hand, parent's finger Note:
	2–3 Months (generalized mouthing)	ARK's Baby Grabber and Debra Beckman's Tri-Chews by ARK (with a parent's help) Note:

	3–4 Months (generalized mouthing)	ARK's Baby Grabber and Debra Beckman's Tri-Chews by ARK (with a parent's help and supervision) Note:
	5–9 Months (discriminative mouthing)	ARK's Baby Grabber, Debra Beckman's Tri-Chews by ARK, yellow Chewy Tube, ARK's Soft Grabbers (eg, purple and soft), and other appropriately sized mouth toys approved for use with babies (with a parent's supervision) Note:
	9–12 Months (beginning true mouth play)	Yellow and red Chewy Tubes, P's and Q's; ARK's Grabbers, and other appropriately sized mouth toys approved for use with babies (with a parent's supervision); baby horns and bubbles (with a parent's activation and demonstration) Note:
	12–18 Months (true mouth play)	Yellow and red Chewy Tubes, P's and Q's, and ARK's Grabbers (with a parent's supervision); baby horns and bubbles (with a parent's activation, demonstration, and presentation to child) Note:
	18–24 Months (true mouth play)	Horns and bubbles (with parents and others); yellow and red Chewy Tubes, P's and Q's, and ARK's Grabbers (with a parent's supervision) Note:

Now, let's talk about a chewing activity (or "jaws-ercise") that can help to balance jaw structure and movement. Chewing and biting movements on appropriate mouth toys are typical jaw development processes that children can accomplish themselves when given the opportunity. This activity is particularly important if your child has subtle jaw problems that can also affect eating, drinking, or speech sound production. However, eating, drinking, and speaking are separate processes from chewing on mouth toys. See chapters 2, 6, and 7.

ACTIVITY 5.2: FUN WITH APPROPRIATE CHEWING AND BITING (MORE "JAWS-ERCISE")

Once you have found an appropriate item for your child's chewing and biting exercise, use the following steps:

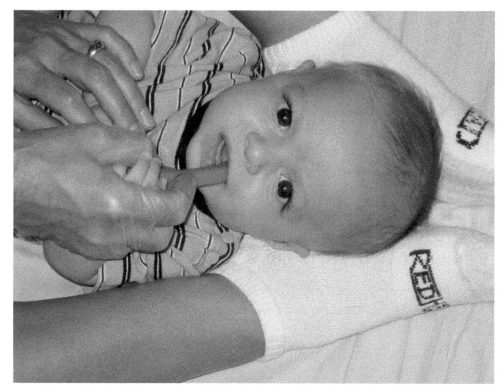

Photo 5.9: Anthony does hand-over-hand "jaws-ercise" with a Grabber.

- Begin by placing the toy or chewing item at the front of your child's mouth for exploration.

- Allow him to hold the toy with you. Don't forget about your child's hand-mouth connection.

- Allow your baby to bite on the toy or chewing item with the front gum surfaces.

- Then help him bite – bite – bite from the front gum surfaces toward the back molar area on each side.

- Play with this process, as your baby will naturally want to do this. We as humans are prewired to chew in the back molar area.

- Once your baby is chewing on the toy or chewing item, have him eventually chew on it 12–15 times on each side of the mouth in the back molar area. Then repeat two more times for three sets total. This is based on exercise physiology.

- If your baby cannot chew or does not seem interested in chewing as many times as I recommend, do what your baby likes to do. If your baby wants to chew only a couple of times on a side initially, this is quite natural. As your baby becomes more skilled, he will want to chew more. Your baby will eventually and naturally work his way toward chewing many more times on each side. It is important for you to be patient with this process, because you want these activities to be fun for you and your baby.

- If your child seems to have a weaker chew on one side than the other, you may want to give the weaker side more practice in chewing. However, the weaker side may fatigue more quickly, and we do not learn much when tired. We also want to have a good balance of function on both sides of the mouth, so we will want to move toward equal work and/or play on both sides of the mouth. It is during this process that you may notice your child prefers to chew on a particular side. This is quite natural.

- Vibration can also increase the interest some babies have in chewing. There are many vibrating mouth toys available, if you can find one that is an appropriate size and shape for this activity. Some parents hold a small battery-operated vibrating toy (such as a Garfield vibrator) at the handle of the Chewy Tube, which makes the Chewy Tube vibrate gently. ARK Therapeutic Services, Inc has also created some vibrating mouth toys and brushes.

  Note: Be very careful with the use of vibration. **Do not use vibration with babies who have a history of seizures or suspected seizures unless you have a doctor's permission.** Vibration in the mouth may go directly to the vestibular system and the brain. Also, we do not want our babies *hooked* on vibration when chewing or exploring items with the mouth. See if you can ultimately interest your baby in chewing and mouthing without vibration.

ACTIVITY 5.2: (cont.)

- When your baby is chewing or biting on a toy or chewing item, notice the alignment of his jaw. When your child is chewing on a toy, he will be doing what is called a *munch chew*. This means that his jaw will move straight up and down. You do not want to see your child's jaw sliding in any direction (front, back, right, or left). If you see this and it does not resolve with a little practice, it may be a good idea to visit a professional (such as an occupational therapist, speech-language pathologist, or other appropriate specialist) who can evaluate your child and advise you.

- Your child's chewing pattern on a toy or other appropriate chewing item will be different than the one he uses to chew food. At 5 to 7 months of age, your baby will begin to demonstrate lateral (side-to-side) and diagonal jaw movements on foods such as soft cookie pieces or food lumps. These patterns will eventually develop into the mature circular rotary chewing pattern that we use as adults when we chew foods. Chewing food is a different process than chewing on mouth toys during play.

- Remember, this is playtime for the mouth and should be enjoyable. The mouth is a very vulnerable area, and it is important that interactions in and around your baby's mouth be pleasant and fun.

- Listen to your baby's communication during this process, and follow his lead. Give your baby as much control as possible. Remember that all of the work and/or play we are discussing in this book is based upon the dance of communication and interaction. A dance is a partnership.

- Do this activity three to five times per week with your child. Again, this is based on the principles of exercise physiology.

Let's talk about what you are accomplishing when you are playing with your child in this manner. As your baby bites on the toy or chewing item along his gum surfaces, your baby's tongue is learning to move in the direction of the stimulation. This helps your baby's tongue learn to move independently of the jaw (called *dissociation* or *differentiation*). Side-to-side (lateral) tongue movement is a very important process for the placement and collection of food in the mouth.

As you and your child move the toy or chewing item further back in the mouth toward the back molar area, awareness develops in this area. The tongue will also learn to move in retraction (a backward motion) as your child chews at the back molar area. This motion is important for the development of the mature swallow. Graded tongue retraction is also very important for the development of connected, intelligible speech. Remember that graded means the structure moves just enough for the activity. While these activities will not guarantee good speech, they get the jaw and tongue moving in the right direction.

As your child chews on an appropriately sized toy or chewing item with the back molar area, he will learn to grade the up-and-down movements of the jaw. Graded up-and-down jaw movements are very important for the development of taking bites, taking sips, drinking from a cup, drinking from a straw, and speaking. During eating and drinking, the jaw should open only as far as needed for the cup, spoon, straw, other utensil, or food to enter. We don't want your child flinging his jaw open widely when utensils approach his mouth. We will discuss jaw grading for speech in chapter 7.

Appropriate biting and chewing work can help your child to appropriately strengthen the muscles of the jaw and tongue. I say appropriately, because the muscles need not be too strong, but strong enough. Strength is another form

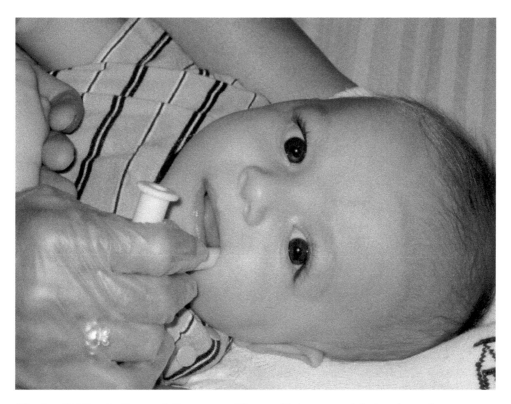

Photo 5.10: Anthony bites on a Chewy Tube near his back molar area with assistance.

of grading. Muscles need to be strong enough to learn the processes of eating, drinking, speaking, and maintaining a closed mouth at rest. Jaw work helps with mouth readiness for a variety of processes. Eating, drinking, and speaking are learned through the actual processes of eating, drinking, and speaking covered in chapters 2, 6, and 7.

We previously mentioned the idea that we do not want to place any stress on your child's temporomandibular joint, or TMJ, when we work or play with biting and chewing. Appropriate biting and chewing practice ("jaws-ercise") can help to bring your child's jaw into alignment and balance the movements of the jaw musculature. It can also help to realign the disk in the temporomandibular joint.[216] This is one reason that the jaw work and/or play is recommended for both sides of the mouth. If your child has had a subtle jaw weakness or difficulty on a particular side, these activities can help to resolve this issue. Remember that subtle jaw concerns often run in families.

Last, but not least, biting and chewing can help your baby's teeth come through on time. Today, we see many children who do not get their teeth on time. This may be related to the limited amount of biting and chewing experiences available to babies.

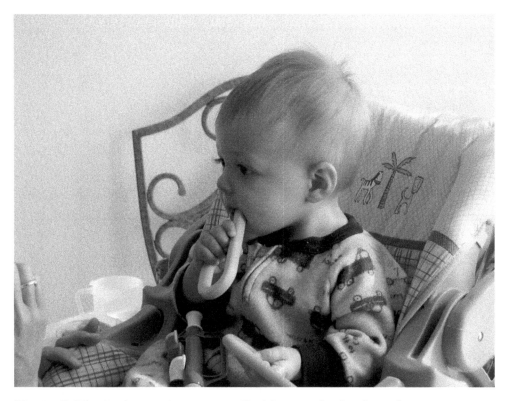

Photo 5.11: Anthony chews on a Grabber at the back molar area (age 12 months).

ACTIVITY 5.3: CHEWING EXERCISE SUMMARY

If your child has a subtle problem with the jaw, this activity and/or play routine can make a big difference. It summarizes the jaw exercise described in Activity 5.2. Mark the date you and your child begin working on this and the date you and your child accomplish the goal. Remember, this should be a fun activity. If your child gets tired or disinterested, come back to the activity at another time. Do "jaws-ercise" three to five times per week.

Dates	Age	Chewing Exercises
Begun: Accomplished:	Birth to 2 months	Chews on the fleshy part of a parent's index finger at the back molar area (working toward 12–15 times each side, three sets)
Begun: Accomplished:	2–3 Months	Chews on own fingers, fleshy part of a parent's finger, an appropriate toy with a parent's help at the back molar area (working toward 12–15 times each side, three sets)
Begun: Accomplished:	3–4 Months	Chews on own fingers, fleshy part of a parent's finger, appropriate toy with a parent's help and supervision at the back molar area (working toward 12–15 times each side, three sets)
Begun: Accomplished:	5–9 Months	Chews on own fingers, appropriate toy, or food in cheesecloth/safe feeder* with a parent's supervision at the back molar area (working toward 12–15 times each side, three sets)
Begun: Accomplished:	9+ Months	Chews on appropriate toy or food in cheesecloth/safe feeder* with a parent's supervision at the back molar area (working toward 12–15 times each side, three sets)

*Information about introducing foods in cheesecloth and safe feeders is found in chapter 6.

What to Do about Tooth-Grinding

We will talk about tooth-grinding in this chapter, because it is related to your child's jaw function. You will use mouth massage and jaw activities to help resolve this problem. Tooth-grinding can be an annoying habit. It is not only bad for your child's teeth, but it is bad for the jaw joint (known as the temporomandibular joint, or TMJ). When your child grinds his teeth, he moves his jaw back and forth, sideways. Your child may begin to grind or clench the teeth because of subtle jaw difficulties, which were discussed in chapter 2. Here are some suggestions to help your child move beyond the habit of tooth-grinding.

1. Once your child has teeth, you will use a brush instead of your finger for oral massage. See the note under Lesson 7, "Massaging Your Baby's Cheeks from Inside the Mouth."

2. Be sure you are using a brush that will not come apart. I like the ARK Oral Probe for this. It does not come apart like other brushes, and it is a good size. The Nuk Oral Massage brush is a two-piece brush that can come apart.

3. When you do oral massage in your child's mouth, let your child bite down and chew on the brush or gloved finger (if no teeth). You want to see up-and-down jaw movements during biting and chewing (no side jaw movement).

4. When your child is chewing on a jaw exerciser (eg, Chewy Tube or Grabber) with the back molar area, add some firm but gentle pressure up and down into the back gum and/or teeth to stimulate a munch chew.

5. Do "jaws-ercise" and/or chewing activities three to five times per week with your child (daily, if the grinding is bad).

6. Replace grinding with other more appropriate uses of the jaw. Use consistent parenting and behavioral techniques to help your child break the habit. See information in chapter 4 on breaking the habits of pacifier use and thumb-sucking for more detail.

Tooth-grinding moves your child's jaw in a manner that is detrimental to the jaw and teeth. By doing exercise that helps your child's jaw move up and down, you are working the muscles your child needs for most aspects of eating, drinking, and speaking. The only time your child needs to use the muscles that move the jaw side to side is while chewing food. Otherwise, your child needs up and down jaw movement. By doing oral massage, "jaws-ercise," and/or chewing activities, you can help your child break the habit of grinding.

Also, remember that habits are quickly established in 2 to 3 weeks. They can also be broken in 2 to 3 weeks. When your child grinds, offer him an appropriate mouth toy or a sip of water to interrupt or replace the pattern. Children tend to chew on mouth toys in the up-and-down manner we have described. This is very different than the side-to-side jaw movement seen in grinding.

When your child grinds his teeth, do not comment on it. Remember that ignoring a behavior is a good way to get rid of it. However, do comment when your child's mouth is still or when he is chewing on food or a mouth toy in an appropriate manner (eg, "Colin, you look so handsome right now").

If your child is grinding his teeth at night, massage and jaw exercise will hopefully help to break this habit. Have your child do some "jaws-ercise" just before bed as you read a book together.

You can also allow your child to go to bed with a safe mouth toy so he can chew on the toy in place of grinding. This approach is very similar to the one we used to help your child stop thumb-sucking and pacifier use in chapter 4. Take a look at the information in chapter 4 for more ideas about breaking unhealthy mouth habits. This is also a good approach to help children move past the habits of chewing on their own hair, clothing, and other items.

Now, let's talk about some activities that go beyond "jaws-ercise." Horn and bubble play can support the development of mature jaw, lip, cheek, and tongue movement. We will discuss how these activities also require dissociation, grading, and direction of movement (concepts discussed previously in Activity 5.2). However, the motor plans in your child's brain for horn-blowing and bubble play are different from those used (ie, sequencing of movements) in eating, drinking, and speaking.

Horn and Bubble Play

Children love horn- and bubble-blowing activities, and these are very good for their mouth and respiratory development. Blowing activities help your child learn to control breathing and other important mouth movements. You can understand this better by doing the activities yourself.

ACTIVITY 5.4: WHAT HAPPENS WHEN YOU BLOW INTO A HORN OR BLOW BUBBLES?

1. Place one hand on your abdomen, just below your belly button. Place your other hand on your diaphragm, just below your rib cage. Pretend you are blowing a horn or bubbles.

2. What are your abdomen and diaphragm doing? You will feel systematic contraction of the muscles in these areas. If you blow harder, you will feel greater contraction. Be careful, don't blow too hard.

ACTIVITY 5.4: (cont.)

3. Now, focus on your jaw when you blow. Is your jaw wide open or just open enough to blow? This is jaw grading.

4. Now, focus on your tongue when you blow. Is your tongue pulled back? This is tongue retraction, which is also a direction of tongue movement needed for eating, drinking, and speaking.

5. Focus on your lips when you blow. Are they round? This is graded lip movement.

6. Focus on your cheeks when you blow. Don't blow too hard. Are your cheeks lightly touching your teeth and gums? This is cheek grading to attain appropriate intraoral pressure.

We talked about your child beginning horn play between 9 and 12 months of age in chapter 4. I have found that many babies like to begin experimenting with baby horns around 10 months of age. Some baby horns work whether your child blows into them or sucks on them, like drinking from a straw. Whistle straws and baby harmonicas are examples of items that work this way and produce sound with little effort. If your child already knows how to drink from a straw (to be discussed in chapter 6), he may easily learn to activate this type of horn.

I recommend that you buy two of the same horns when you begin playing with horns with your child. You can help your child put the horn to his mouth, and you can blow on your horn at the same time. This shows your child what to expect. Most children enjoy playing with horns naturally. If your child has some of the subtle mouth movement problems discussed earlier in this chapter, this is a fun exercise that may help. Proper horn use can encourage more mature movements of the jaw, lips, cheeks, and tongue. In my practice, we often have horn races to see who can blow the longest. One of my graduate students came up with this idea.

Once your child learns to blow a horn, you can make sure he is getting the most from the activity with the following exercise, adapted from the work of Sara Rosenfeld-Johnson.[217] However, please do not make horn blowing a chore for your child—it should be fun for both of you. I am giving you this exercise because it systematically works many areas of the mouth and respiratory mechanism.

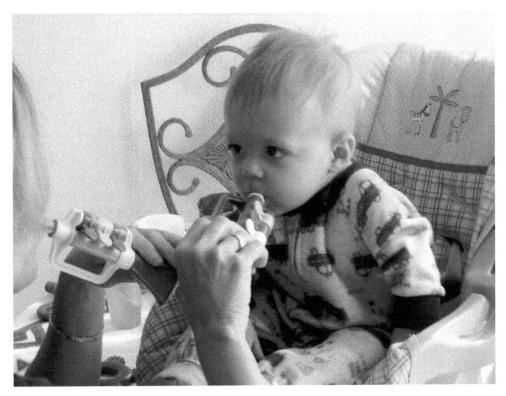

Photo 5.12: Anthony begins horn play with Diane at 12 months.

ACTIVITY 5.5: A HORN EXERCISE FOR YOUR CHILD[218]

(Adapted from the work of Sarah Rosenfeld-Johnson.)

You and your child can do this activity while sitting in appropriate chairs or on little benches. Be sure your child's feet are flat on the floor and he is sitting up straight. Do your best to be eye-to-eye with your child (ie, you don't want to be above him). You can stabilize your child's jaw if needed during this activity, but that makes it hard for you to blow your own horn. See chapter 6 for information on jaw support.

1. Once your child knows how to blow a horn, choose two easy horns for you and your child to use (such as a straight, recorder-like horn found in many party stores).

2. Show your child how to bring the horn to his mouth. Place your horn at your mouth at the same time. (**Note:** Between 18 and 24 months of age, you will hopefully notice that your child will stop biting down on the horn mouthpiece for stability. Prior to this time, your child might bite down for stability, and this is quite typical.)

ACTIVITY 5.5: (cont.)[218]

3. Blow into your horn at the same time your child does. See if your child can blow into the horn longer and longer as you blow into your horn longer and longer (ie, horn races).

4. See how many times in a row your child can blow into the horn before getting tired or bored. You can begin with very short toots in a row, and then make them longer. You can work toward 12–15 toots or blows in a row. You can even do three sets if your child really likes the activity. This makes horn blowing an exercise.

5. Take turns with your child. You blow your horn and then have your child blow his horn. As your child gets better at this, have your child imitate the number of times you blow (eg, one time, two times, three times). By age 2, your child will begin to understand the concept of numbers, because you use them in language (eg, "I am giving you just one cracker" or "One, two, three, jump").

6. See the TalkTools "Horn Hierarchy" by Sara Rosenfeld-Johnson for a more formalized program as your child gets older. This hierarchy will also show you which horns are easier to activate than others.

Note: When doing this activity, be sure your child is not blowing *too hard*. We want the air to come straight through the mouth without a lot of cheek puffing. **If your child has had a repaired cleft palate, DO NOT do this activity** unless you are working with a professional who knows something about changes in intraoral pressure.

ACTIVITY 5.5: A BUBBLE EXERCISE FOR YOU AND YOUR CHILD[219]

(Adapted from the work of Sara Rosenfeld-Johnson)

Many parents and therapists do not know how to teach a child to blow bubbles. This is a much more difficult task than it seems. Fortunately, Sara Rosenfeld-Johnson has figured this out for us through her use of task analysis. Here is an adapted form of her work. Be sure to use bubbles that are safe for children.

1. Begin by blowing the bubble through the wand. Then catch the bubble on the wand.

2. Pop the bubble on your child's lips. We want your child's lips to stay still for this. We don't want your child to "eat" the bubble.

3. Once your child becomes accustomed to the bubble coming toward his mouth, show your child how to move the bubble with air coming out of the mouth. I encourage the children with whom I work to open their mouths and make an "*h*" sound. This is a sound children make early in development, so your child should be able to make this sound (refer to chapter 7). However, there are some children who have trouble making the "*h*" sound. If that is the case, you can give some firm but gentle pressure to your child's diaphragm, just below the rib cage, to help your child make the "*h*" sound. Be sure your child's mouth is open, and be gentle.

4. Once your child knows how to move the bubble with air coming out of the mouth, begin to shape your child's lips. You will use the same strategy you used for getting a lip latch for better bottle drinking or pacifier use when your child was small. Take your thumb and index or middle finger and gently squeeze your child's cheeks inward and forward to round the lips.

5. Now, have your child blow the bubble off of the wand. Do this as many times in a row as your child can handle. Work toward 12 to 15 repetitions. If your child loves this activity, you can do three sets over time. Most children will blow bubbles over and over again. They just love it.

6. Once your child understands the idea of rounding the lips and keeping the cheeks against the gums and teeth, you can let your child blow bubbles toward targets that are further and further away from the mouth. Puppets make great targets.

7. Eventually, your child will learn to blow bubbles through a wand. This requires a lot of eye-hand coordination. However, I do know 2-year-olds who can do this.

8. See the TalkTools "Bubble Blowing Hierarchy" by Sara Rosenfeld-Johnson for a more formalized program as your child gets older.

Playing with horns and bubbles is a great part of growing up. You will have as much fun as your child when you do these activities. You can do them as an exercise if needed or just as part of play, keeping in mind some of the ideas mentioned previously. Blowing activities are very calming and can bring increased attention, focus, and concentration. What do you do when you are stressed? Do you ever find yourself blowing air from your mouth to relieve stress and get focused?

6

Secrets for Better Feeding Beginning around 5–6 Months of Age

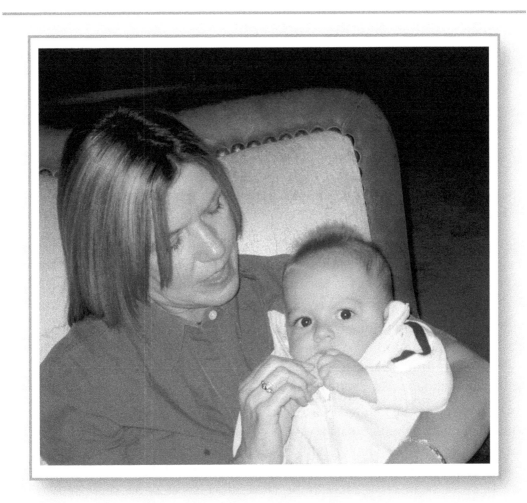

Key Topics in This Chapter

- Positioning Your Baby for Higher-Level Feeding Activities
- Jaw Support
- Spoon-Feeding
- Drinking from a Cup
- Drinking from a Straw
- Taking Bites and Chewing Safe, Appropriate Foods
- Introducing Foods and Liquids
- How Much Do I Feed My Child?
- Weaning from the Bottle and Breast
- Feeding Problems and Picky Eating
- Feeding Development from 5 to 24 Months of Age

When your baby is 5 to 6 months of age, you will begin to introduce new foods and liquids. You do not want to overwhelm yourself or your baby, so you have to make some choices. Ask yourself, "What do I feel most comfortable introducing to my baby first? Spoon-feeding, drinking from an open cup, drinking from a straw, or taking bites and chewing?"

Most parents choose spoon-feeding or drinking from an open cup. Your baby is ready for all of these processes around 5 to 6 months of age, but you do not want to begin too many at one time. However, you can introduce them within weeks of one another. Remember that it only takes 2 to 3 weeks of daily practice to develop a new habit.

Most parents successfully introduce spoon-feeding at 5 to 6 months of age. Two weeks later, they introduce drinking from a cup. After that, they may choose to teach drinking from a straw or taking bites of food. This way, all four skills can be taught in about a month and a half.

By using appropriate methods for spoon-feeding, drinking from a cup and straw, and chewing with your baby, you continue to encourage the best mouth development possible. Good mouth development supports adequate nutrition through effective food and liquid management and good digestion. Remember that digestion begins in the mouth, because saliva has enzymes that begin to break down food.

The methods discussed in this chapter, in conjunction with the ones you have learned in your baby's first 5 or 6 months of life, can also reduce the need for orthodontics (such as braces or a palatal expander) later on. If your child does require orthodontics at some point, you can minimize the work needed by helping your child develop the best mouth structures possible through good feeding experiences.

It may take a little time and practice for you and your baby to learn the skills discussed in this chapter. However, the techniques are easy to apply and can make feeding fun. In the long run, they save you time and aggravation. You are going to feed your baby anyway, so why not make it a pleasurable and successful experience? Remember, Dr Harvey Karp says that parents who succeed in feeding and calming their babies "feel proud, confident, and on top of the world!"[220]

As you and your baby learn the exciting new skills taught in this chapter, think about how you learn any new skill (such as a tennis serve, a golf swing, typing, or ballroom dancing). You need a certain amount of consistent practice and repetition to learn these skills. This is the same process you will use when you and your baby are learning the feeding dance. As feeding partners, you will both be learning new skills that will help you feel happy, satisfied, and successful.

Positioning Your Baby for Higher-Level Feeding Activities

If you begin spoon-feeding or drinking from a cup with your baby before 6 months of age, your baby will usually not be sitting up on her own. You can begin spoon-feeding or drinking from a cup with your baby placed securely in a baby seat. The baby seat can be placed on a secure table or countertop, and you can sit at eye level with your baby. It is important to position your baby so that you are sitting eye-to-eye. This allows you to make appropriate eye contact, keep your baby's head and neck in a good position, and communicate with your baby.

If your head is above your baby's head during feeding, your baby will look up at you to make eye contact. This will place your baby's neck into extension. Remember when you learned cardiopulmonary resuscitation, or CPR, how you extended the person's neck to open the airway? We don't want your baby's airway open too wide during feeding, because this may cause coughing or choking.

If you feed your baby by standing or sitting above her (called *bird feeding*), you are requiring your baby to open her airway. This makes swallowing more difficult to control and places your baby at risk for aspiration (choking). It also encourages extension patterns in the mouth, such as wide jaw movements and exaggerated tongue protrusion (sometimes called

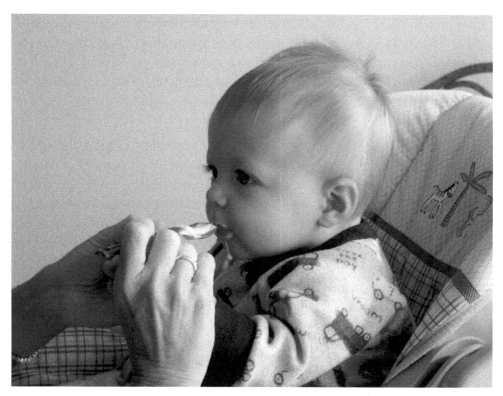

Photo 6.1: Anthony and feeder are sitting at eye level.

tongue thrusting). These movements can cause your child problems later in life.

By 6 months of age, most babies will sit on their own. However, many of the high chairs on the market are a little large for many babies. There are high chair inserts that you can purchase to make the high chair more comfortable and a better fit for your baby. I prefer the STOKKE Tripp Trapp chair *(www.stokke.com)* or other similar chairs (eg, Euro II Highchair from One Step Ahead, *www.onestepahead.com)* because they provide excellent postural support and can be adjusted as your child grows. If you are feeding your baby in a high chair, Tripp Trapp, or other chair, be sure that you are sitting at eye level with your baby.

In addition to a good feeding position, it is also a good practice to feed your baby with minimal external distractions. Try playing some soothing music in the background. Turn off the television. Talk to your baby.

ACTIVITY 6.1: HOW IS YOUR BABY POSITIONED DURING FEEDING?

Place a date in the column next to the description that matches what your baby is doing.

Date	What You Want My Baby:	Date	Things to Change My Baby:
	Sitting in a baby seat (before 6 months of age)		Not sitting in a stable seat, with her body at a 45°–90° angle to the earth
	Sitting in a high chair with an insert that fits my baby; sitting in an appropriately adjusted Tripp Trapp or other chair		Not sitting well supported in a high chair, Tripp Trapp, or other chair with her body at a 90° angle to the earth
	Looking straight into my eyes when we are feeding		Looking up at me when we are feeding

Jaw Support

In addition to getting your child into a supported position for feeding, you might find jaw support helpful during initial spoon-feeding and drinking from a cup or straw. Provide jaw stability with your nondominant hand (ie, your left hand if you are right handed and your right hand if you are left handed).

Never force or push on your baby's jaw in any direction, as this can hurt your baby. Instead, hold her jaw like you would hold a dance partner, and allow your baby's jaw to move naturally. Your baby is taking the lead in this dance, and you are following. Jaw support can help both of you feel more secure when learning new feeding skills.

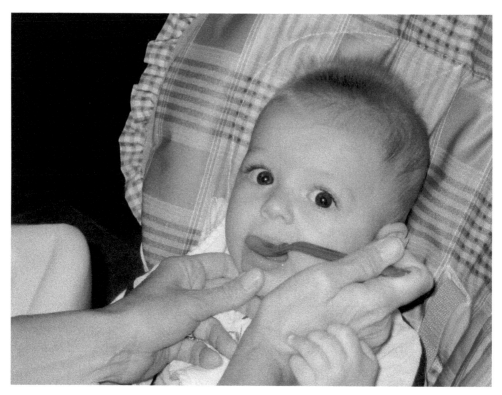

Photo 6.2: Anthony receives jaw support while learning to spoon-feed at 6 months.

As you face your baby at eye-to-eye level, you can stabilize your baby's jaw with your nondominant hand in a couple of ways. One way is to place your index finger under the bony part of your baby's chin and your thumb on her chin. Another way is to place your thumb and index finger along your baby's jawbone.

Then use your dominant hand (ie, your right hand if you are right handed and your left hand if you are left handed) to feed your baby by using the methods discussed in the next sections of this chapter. Jaw support can help both you and your baby feel more comfortable and controlled while learning these new feeding-skills. Your baby will also feel less vulnerable because you are providing some calming touch before moving toward your baby's mouth with a spoon, cup, or straw.

Spoon-Feeding

Before you feed your baby with a spoon, see how you use a spoon in your own mouth. Get some applesauce, yogurt, pudding, or another soft food you like to eat. Observe how you take the food off of the spoon and what you do with the food after you take it from the spoon. This exercise will give you more awareness regarding how the mouth works.

ACTIVITY 6.2: HOW DO YOU EAT FROM A SPOON?

Take some spoonfuls of applesauce or another soft food, and notice:

- Do you open your jaw really wide or just enough for the spoon?

- Do your lips move to take the food from the spoon?

- Is your tongue under the spoon or pulled back with just the tip touching the spoon?

- How far do you place the spoon into your mouth?

- Do you place the spoon straight into your mouth or at an angle?

If you tipped the spoon handle upward when you removed it from your mouth, you probably had a spoon with a bowl that was too deep. This is a very common problem with adult spoons that fortunately most baby spoons do not have.

Most people place the spoon partially into the mouth (half to three-quarters of the spoon, depending on the size of the spoon), allowing the tongue to move back, or retract. The spoon is often inserted at an angle (up to 45° from the left or right), depending on which hand you normally use to feed yourself. Most people place a reasonable amount of food on the spoon so the lips can work to remove the food from the spoon. The lips and the jaw provide the primary actions in removing food from the spoon. This is very different from suckling from a bottle or breast, where the tongue provides the primary action.

Up to this point, your baby has used a suckle swallow (a 50%-front and 50%-back wavelike tongue movement with the lips latched) or a three-dimensional suck to manage formula or breast milk. Taking food from a spoon is very different than taking liquid from the bottle or breast.

Many parents begin spoon-feeding with baby cereal (often rice). For successful early spoon-feeding, you can:

- Begin by mixing your rice cereal with water, formula, or breast milk so it has a pureed texture (not too thick or sticky).

- Help your baby become accustomed to the taste of the cereal by dipping your clean or gloved finger into the cereal and giving your baby tastes from your finger.

- Help your baby become accustomed to the spoon by letting your baby hold and mouth the spoon with your assistance.

- Begin spoon-feeding by dipping the spoon into the cereal mixture, and letting your baby taste the cereal from the tip of the spoon, rather than placing a typical amount of food on the spoon at first.

Don't forget to let your baby watch you eat food off a spoon. Babies are very tuned in to people's mouths. Eating is a social experience. Your baby will benefit by seeing you eat off the spoon. If you are eating something while your baby is eating, this will allow your baby some natural breaks between spoonfuls. You can alternate giving your baby a bite of her food with taking a spoonful yourself.

The pace of spoon-feeding your baby will depend on the personalities of you and your baby. However, it is important not to feed your baby too rapidly, as this sets up a pattern your baby may carry throughout life. Some babies appear to want to feed very rapidly. This is probably related to the habit of swallow after swallow during bottle- or breast-feeding. You don't want your baby to develop a rapid spoon-feeding pattern, so you will teach your baby about pacing the meal.

Pacing a spoon-fed meal is important for several reasons. First, it allows your child to fully experience the shape, size, and texture of food in the mouth. Second, the esophagus requires some time for the most efficient movement of food toward the stomach. Finally, the brain needs time to register the presence of food in the stomach so your child will know when she is full.

Avoid feeding your baby when you feel rushed. Try turning on some soft background music to relax you and your baby. Talk to your baby as you feed her.

Here are the characteristics of good spoon-feeding:

- The spoon is small enough to fit your baby's lip area comfortably.
- A small and/or reasonable amount of food is placed on the spoon.
- The spoon is placed into the mouth only far enough for the jaw and lips to close, so the food will be removed when the jaw and lips are closed.
- Food is removed by jaw and lip closure, so there is no need for the spoon to be tipped upward. Do not use your baby's upper lip or gum to scrape food off the spoon. If you find yourself doing this, slow down.

Be sure the spoon fits your baby's mouth. Regular, adult-sized spoons are too large. The bowls of those spoons are too deep for your baby's mouth. There are many small spoons available. My favorite spoon is the small Maroon Spoon. It has a small flat bowl that allows your baby to close the jaw and lips to remove the food.

The Maroon Spoon is fashioned after the Mothercare Spoon, which was originally developed for babies in Great Britain. It has become widely used all over the world with children who have special feeding concerns. However, don't let this deter you from using it. It is a wonderful, easy-to-use spoon. See the following list for further information on where to purchase Maroon Spoons and other feeding tools.

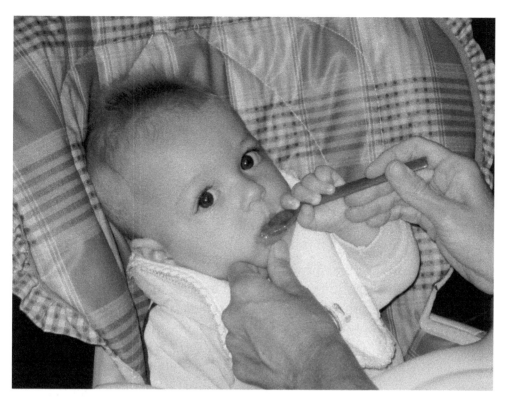

Photo 6.3: Anthony helps bring the Maroon Spoon to his mouth at 6 months.

COMPANIES THAT CARRY FEEDING PRODUCTS FOR CHILDREN THAT CANNOT BE FOUND IN MOST STORES

Company	Phone Number	Web Site
ARK Therapeutic Services, Inc	(803) 438-9779	www.arktherapeutic.com
New Visions	(800) 606-7112	www.new-vis.com
The Speech Bin	(800) 850-8602	www.speechbin.com
SuperDuper Publications	(800) 277-8737	www.superduperinc.com
TalkTools	(888) 529-2879	www.talktools.net
Therapro	(800) 257-5376	www.theraproducts.com

Your baby's upper lip will become more active over time, with development and the use of good feeding techniques. Some of your baby's more mature lip movements will begin to develop around 8 months of age. Therefore, you will need to work with your baby's less mature lip movement before that time.

At 5 to 6 months of age, your baby can close her lips on a spoon if you allow sufficient time. Over the next few months, your baby will begin to move her lips independently of her jaw. Independent lip and jaw movement is essential for the development of increasingly sophisticated eating, drinking, and speaking skills. Babies who do not learn this skill often have difficulty removing food from the spoon or extra food from the lips. The lip sound "*m*" is frequently heard when babies begin spoon-feeding. This may be one reason we say "mmm" when something tastes good.

When you spoon-feed your baby, place a small and/or reasonable amount of food on the spoon. Be careful not to overload it. A reasonable amount of food allows your baby to discriminate or feel the amount of food on the spoon and manage the food appropriately. Your baby can experience the texture, size, and shape of the food. The importance of oral discrimination was discussed in chapter 4. It is needed for manipulation of food and liquid within the mouth.

If you place too much food into your baby's mouth at one time, your baby may have difficulty learning to manage spoon-fed foods well. During spoon-feeding, we would like your baby to practice the sucking pattern, which involves increasingly active use of the lips, as well as up-down tongue movement. These are precursors of a mature swallowing pattern. Now let's learn a couple of effective spoon-feeding methods.

We will first learn *natural* spoon-feeding. This is how you feed yourself.

1. Place the front portion of the spoon straight into your baby's mouth. Allow the bottom of the spoon to touch your baby's lower lip. Do not place the spoon too far into your baby's mouth. Remember how far you typically place the spoon into your mouth.

2. When the spoon is placed on your baby's lower lip, wait for your baby's top lip to come down and close on the spoon. Once your baby's upper lip closes on the spoon, remove the spoon from your baby's mouth in a level manner. You will be pulling the spoon horizontally (ie, straight out) from your baby's mouth.

   Important Note: Do not tip the spoon upward to scrape the food off your baby's upper lip or gum. Babies who are fed in this way do not use the lips to manipulate the food and often have difficulty learning to use the lips properly at a later age. You can see some adults whose upper lips sit inactively at rest and do not close well when they eat. Your baby possesses the skill to close her jaw and lips on the spoon, so why not give her this practice?

The next method we will learn is *side-to-side* spoon-feeding. Sara Rosenfeld-Johnson and Lori Overland use this method.[221]

1. Place one side of the spoon onto your baby's lips, allowing your baby to take food off that side. The handle of the spoon may lightly contact your baby's lip corners if you are using a spoon like the Maroon Spoon.

2. Then turn your hand to allow your baby to take the food off the other side of the spoon. This may be similar to the way you eat from a soup or ice-cream spoon. It is still important that you use a small spoon with your baby. The small Maroon Spoon is ideal for this method of spoon-feeding.

ACTIVITY 6.3: HOW DOES YOUR BABY EAT FROM A SPOON?

Place a date in the column next to the description that matches what your baby is doing.

Date	What You Want — My Baby:	Date	Things to Change — My Baby:
	Eats from a spoon with a small, flat bowl that fits my baby's lips		Eats from a spoon that is too big or too deep (eg, a regular teaspoon)
	Watches me when I eat from a spoon		Does not have the opportunity to watch others eat from a spoon
	Has a good rhythm and rate when eating from a spoon		Eats too fast
	Eats a small and/or reasonable amount of food from the spoon		Eats large amounts from the spoon, and loses a lot of food from the mouth
	Closes the lips on the spoon, and waits for me to remove the spoon in a level manner		Lets me scrape food off of the upper lip or gum as I tip the spoon upward

ACTIVITY 6.3: (cont.)

Date	What You Want My Baby:	Date	Things to Change My Baby:
	Can take food from a spoon placed on the bottom lip, with the top lip coming down to meet the spoon		Lets me scrape food off of the upper lip or gum as I tip the spoon upward

Drinking from a Cup

Before you have your baby drink from an open cup, see how you drink from a cup. Try both thin liquid (like water) and a thicker liquid (such as tomato juice or a yogurt drink). Observe how you take liquid from a cup and what you do once the liquid is in your mouth.

ACTIVITY 6.4: HOW DO YOU DRINK FROM A CUP?

Take some sips and swallows of water from an open cup, and observe the following:

- Is the cup placed just on your lower lip, or is it pressed or jammed into the corners of your mouth?

- What happens if you press the cup rim into the corners of your mouth? Can you really drink this way?

- Are your lips helping you to keep from spilling the liquid when you drink?

- Is your tongue under the cup or pulled back a little in your mouth so the liquid can enter the mouth?

- What is the difference between taking one sip and drinking the liquid swallow after swallow?

- Does the tip of your tongue touch the bump behind your top front teeth when you swallow?

- Does the rest of your tongue hold the liquid and then "squeeze" the liquid to move it back for the swallow?

In a mature, sophisticated swallowing pattern, the tip of the tongue rises to the bump behind the top front teeth, the sides of the tongue rise, and the rest of the tongue "squeezes" the liquid back in a controlled manner. The tongue has a slight bowl shape. Some people either do not attain this mature pattern as children or they lose the ability to use this pattern (such as through stoke, brain injury, or aging). An immature or unsophisticated swallowing pattern can lead to significant orthodontic (eg, overbite, gaps between the teeth) and oral hygiene problems. This can also be associated with several speech problems (eg, lisps, "*r*" and/or "*l*" distortion). We will discuss this topic further in chapters 7 and 8.

Drinking from a cup is one of the easiest methods to use when feeding a baby. It has been used with babies born prematurely, as well as babies who are having difficulty learning to drink from a bottle. In my opinion, it is easier to teach than spoon-feeding.

Liquid is easily controlled in a small but wide-mouthed open cup, particularly if the liquid is slightly thickened. Medicine cups and clear plastic cocktail cups are frequently used as first cups because the parent can easily see and control the movement of the liquid.

Five to 6 months of age is a good time to begin drinking from an open cup. This is a time when your child's lip and tongue movements are becoming increasingly independent from her jaw movements. Your child is ready to begin taking single sips from an open cup.

Begin with a small but wide-mouthed open cup or a cutout cup (also called a *nosey cup*). Cutout or nosey cups have often been used with children who have feeding difficulties, but this means only that they are great cups for teaching the skill of drinking from a cup. The cutout portion of the cup is placed on top, so that you can see the liquid in the cup and your child can drink without moving her head and neck back into hyperextension. Cutout cups are available in a number of sizes. See the previous list of companies that carry feeding products for children that cannot be found in most stores.

Remember that when the head and neck are hyperextended, the airway is open (in a CPR position), and choking can occur more readily. When drinking from an open cup, your child's head needs to be in a neutral, aligned position, or your child's chin needs to be slightly tucked in (ie, the ears are just in front of the

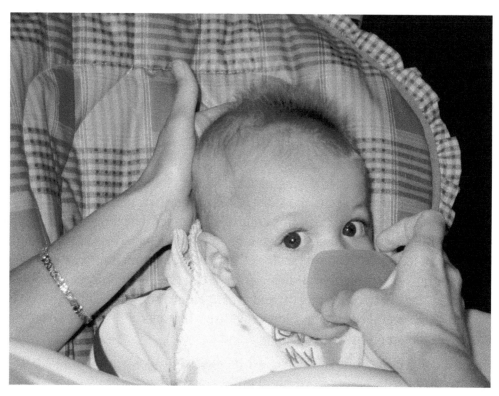

Photo 6.4: Anthony learns to drink from an open cup at 6 months.

shoulders). It is also important that you give your child a small and/or reasonable amount of liquid with each sip. You do not want to hear gulping or excessive coughing.

The rim of the open cup (the long side if using a cutout cup) is placed on your child's lower lip. Teach your child to drink from the cup by giving one sip at a time. Be sure that your child is not leaning into the cup and that the cup is not pressed or jammed into the corners of your child's lips. It is almost impossible to drink this way. Hold the cup during this process, but encourage your child over time to place her hands on the sides of the cup. This is a nice hand-mouth activity for your child.

I usually place a thickened liquid into the open cup when I teach the skill of drinking from a cup. This allows the parent to control the flow of the liquid. It also allows the child to receive greater sensory information from the liquid at first. First liquids could include formula or breast milk, thickened slightly with baby cereal (such as rice cereal). Also, stage-one baby-food fruits and sweet vegetables (such as carrots and squash) can be thinned with water and served from the open cup. When you and your child are comfortable with the single-sip drinking process, you can begin to use regular thin liquids (such as formula, breast milk, water, and juice).

When your child is taking single sips from an open cup, be sure that the cup rim is placed on the lower lip and that your child's tongue is not under the cup. Your child's tongue may occasionally slip under the cup because of the drinking pattern used previously with the bottle or breast (ie, suckle-swallow). However, I have found it is better to reposition the cup on the child's lower lip when giving her single sips so that poor drinking habits are not established.

After your child has become proficient at taking single sips from an open cup, she will begin taking longer drinks from the open cup by using more than one sip and swallow. This develops between 6 and 12 months of age, as your child's breathing and swallowing coordination is maturing. Your child will probably be drinking regular thin liquids (such as formula, breast milk, and water). However, if your child is having difficulty learning to swallow consecutively (ie, swallow after swallow), you may want to use a slightly thickened liquid until she becomes comfortable with this process.

Assist your child by holding the cup with her as she learns to consecutively swallow the liquid. She will begin by taking two or three consecutive swallows of liquid at one time. Your child's head should be in a neutral position (aligned with the body), and her chin may be slightly tucked in. Be sure she is not leaning into the cup. Again, you do not want to hear gulping or excessive coughing. Be sure you are giving her a reasonable amount of liquid during this process (not too much). See the "Feeding Development" checklist at the end of this chapter for further information.

You may have heard about the controversy surrounding the use of spouted (or "sippy") cups. The concern that many therapists have with these cups is they can promote the use of immature drinking and swallowing patterns. Children drink from sippy cups in a similar manner to a bottle. The pattern your child uses when drinking from a bottle is different from the pattern used in the more mature process of drinking from an open cup.

Drinking from a cup, like spoon-feeding, involves greater lip activity and more independent tongue jaw, lip, and tongue movement than the movements required for drinking from a bottle and breast-feeding. Sippy cups can impede your child's development of appropriate drinking and swallowing skills, because they can encourage the child to maintain old patterns used with drinking from a bottle.

This becomes a particular concern when the tip of the tongue should be learning to elevate or rise during the development of the mature swallowing pattern (around 12 months of age). The tip of the tongue cannot rise to the alveolar ridge behind the top front teeth for the mature swallow when the spout of the sippy cup is placed into the mouth. The spout is in the way. In some children, you can see the whole jaw moving front and back when they drink from a sippy cup. This is not the pattern we want to see when a child drinks from a cup. We want to see slight up-down jaw movement.

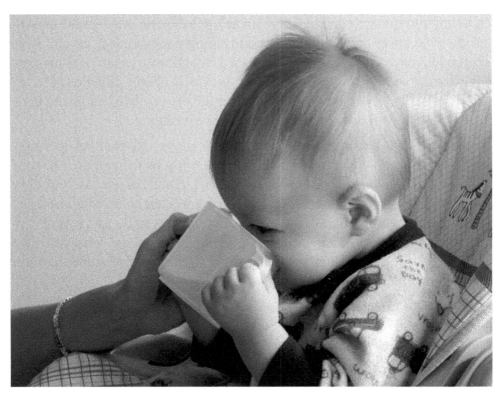

Photo 6.5: Anthony drinks from a cup with a recessed lid and handles at 12 months.

The potential problems caused by sippy cup use cannot be overstated. These include the interruption of the development of the mature swallowing pattern and liquid tending to sit in the mouth rather than being swallowed (which can lead to tooth decay). Dentists and therapists have long been concerned about the use of these cups for such reasons. Although they may be convenient, sippy cups should be avoided when possible.

There are actually a number of other spill-proof cup options (such as cups with recessed lids and straws from which your child can be taught to drink properly by 12 months of age). A cup with a recessed lid has a lip similar to an open cup and is used like one. However, the lid helps the child avoid spilling the liquid. These cups come with and without handles. See cups from ARK, TalkTools, and others in the previous list of companies that carry feeding products for children that cannot be found in most stores.

ACTIVITY 6.5: HOW DOES YOUR BABY DRINK FROM AN OPEN CUP?

Place a date in the column next to the description that matches what your baby is doing.

Date	What You Want My Baby:	Date	Things to Change My Baby:
	Drinks from an open cup that fits her mouth		Drinks from a cup that is too big or too small
	Allows the open cup to be placed just on her bottom lip		Leans into the cup with her lip corners pressed or jammed against the cup or has her tongue under the cup
	Takes one small sip of thickened liquid (such as stage-one baby food thinned with water) at a time		Gulps or chokes on liquid
	Takes one small sip of thin liquid		Gulps or chokes on liquid
	Drinks swallow after swallow in a coordinated manner		Has a lot of jaw movement and/or leans into the cup when trying to take swallow after swallow

Drinking from a Straw

Before you introduce your baby to drinking from a straw, observe how you drink liquid from a straw. What do you do once the liquid is in your mouth?

ACTIVITY 6.6: HOW DO YOU DRINK FROM A STRAW?

Take some sips and swallows from a straw, and observe:

- Is the straw placed far into your mouth onto your tongue, or just on your lips? If you place the straw far onto your tongue, then you are using an unsophisticated and/or immature swallowing pattern. See what it is like to just place the straw on your lips.

- Do you place the straw in the center of your lips or to the side? If you place the straw to the side you may have a stronger side, or this may be related to which side of your body is dominant. See what it is like to place the straw in the center of your lips.

- If you place the straw *just* onto your lips (not onto your tongue) to drink, do you pull your tongue back slightly? Can the tip of your tongue rise to the ridge behind your top front teeth to start the swallow?

- Can you drink swallow after swallow?

- Can you feel the muscles in your abdomen (just below your belly button) and diaphragm (at the bottom of your rib cage) working? Place your hands on these areas as you suck through the straw to feel your muscles working. These are the same muscles you use in breathing.

In addition to spoon-feeding and drinking from a cup, drinking from a straw can be taught around 6 months of age by using a bottle with a straw. These bottles are available from TalkTools, ARK, and others. See the previous list of companies that carry feeding products for children that cannot be found in most stores.

You can easily make a bottle with a straw. Here are the directions.

1. Use a bottle that is approved to contain food (such as a honey-bear bottle, sauce bottle, or cake-decorating bottle). While glue and hair color bottles look similar, they are not meant to hold food or consumable liquid!

2. Once you choose your bottle, make a straw from a piece of plumbing or refrigerator tubing (approximately a quarter of an inch in diameter and long enough to reach the bottom of the bottle). Plumbing and refrigerator tubing is designed to carry water, so it is considered safe to use as a straw. Place the plumbing tubing through the top of the bottle by cutting the bottle top to fit the tubing in a snug manner. You

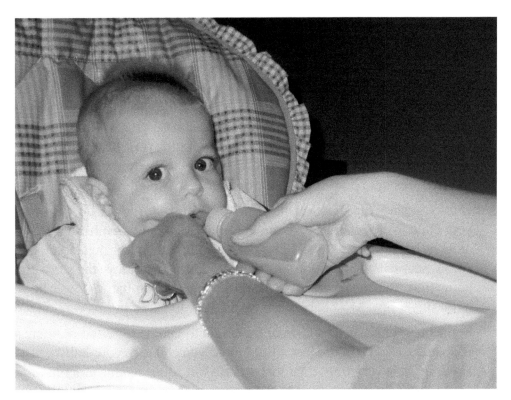

Photo 6.6: Anthony learns to drink from a bottle with a straw at 6 months.

can purchase plumbing or refrigerator tubing from a hardware store. **Please do not use aquarium tubing, as it may contain toxins.**

Here are the directions for teaching your child how to drink out of a bottle with a straw, beginning around 6 months of age:

1. Place a thickened liquid into the bottle. A thickened liquid will provide you with greater control and will give your child increased sensory information while learning this new skill. As mentioned previously with drinking from a cup, thickened liquids can include formula or breast milk thickened with rice baby cereal or appropriate stage-one baby foods thinned with water.

2. If you are teaching an older child how to drink from a straw, you can use a yogurt drink or fruit nectar. However, you must be careful about using these liquids with a 6-month-old child, who is just learning to digest a variety of new foods. Certain products (such as yogurt drinks) are not approved for young babies.

3. Once your thickened liquid is placed into your bottle, insert the straw and seal the bottle. Softly squeeze the thickened liquid so it reaches the top of the straw. Practice this several times before you present it to your baby. You do not want to accidentally squirt your baby in the face with

the liquid. There is a one-way straw mechanism available from ARK and others that can be attached to the bottom of the straw. This will keep the liquid from going back down the straw and into the bottle.

4. After you become skilled in squeezing the liquid to the top of the straw, place the end of the straw on the center of your child's lower lip. About one-quarter inch of the straw should be placed on your child's lip. The straw should not extend into your child's mouth. Your baby's tongue should not be under the straw, because this is the pattern that your child already uses on a bottle. We want to teach her something new.

5. Once you place the straw on the center of your baby's lower lip, wait for your child to close her lips around the straw. Many children learn this very quickly, because they already know how to close their lips on a bottle nipple. Allow your baby to take one sip from the straw, and remove the straw from her mouth. You can repeatedly place the straw on your baby's lower lip for more single sips. Most babies can easily learn to take sips this way.

6. Some babies may need a taste of the liquid to get them started or interested. If you squeeze the bottle just a little more you can give your baby a taste. However, it is very important that you **do not** squirt a large amount of liquid into your baby's mouth, as this can overwhelm your baby. We do not want to place more liquid into your child's mouth than she can handle.

7. After your child has learned to take single sips from the straw, she will learn to take consecutive sips and swallows on her own (ie, you will no longer need to squeeze the bottle). Many babies learn this very quickly, but some take more time. Consecutive swallowing (taking swallow after swallow) is a more complex task than taking single sips. However, your baby already does this with breast- or bottle-feeding. Your child will learn to take consecutive sips and swallows from a straw with a little consistent practice. Just be patient, and hold the straw at your child's lips during this process.

8. Again, try not to let the straw slip too far into your baby's mouth, or your baby will begin drinking from the straw the same way she drinks from a bottle. Always check to be sure that the straw is placed just on your child's lips, so the lips and cheeks can do the work instead of the tongue.

Once your child has learned to drink from a straw in the bottle, she can begin using a cup with a straw. This can be a cup with a flip-up straw or a cup with a hole for a regular straw (such as The First Years Take & Toss or TalkTools). I have worked with many children who were ready to drink from a cup with a regular straw between 9 and 12 months of age. You will place regular thin liquids into the cup when your child is ready (when she can drink thin liquids on her own from the straw in a bottle without excessive coughing or choking).

One problem with some cups with flip-up straws is that they are labeled for older children (eg, 2 years and up). However, I have taught many 12-month-old

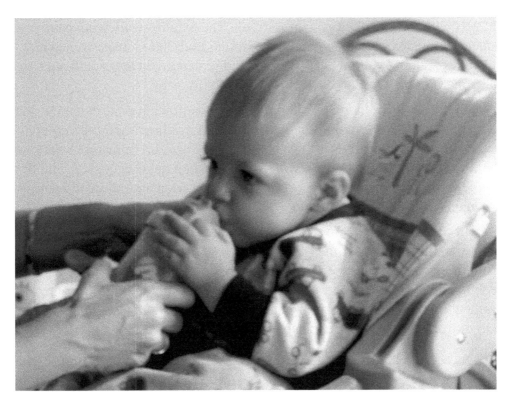

Photo 6.7: Anthony drinks from a flip-up straw cup at 12 months.

children to drink from these cups. Another problem with most flip-up straws is that they are too long and need to be shortened. You can cut the straw or place a bumper on the straw to help your child with this process, if you can do this safely (ie, we don't want loose parts that can become a choking hazard). Remember, appropriate straw use requires your child to place the straw only on the lips (not into the mouth and onto the tongue).

Lip bumpers can be made by drilling a straw-sized hole through a cork. The cork then fits snugly on the straw and only allows one-quarter inch of the straw to sit on your child's lips. You want a safe device that will keep the straw from going into your child's mouth onto her tongue. You do not want a device that will break into pieces and become a choking hazard. TalkTools carries ready-made lip bumpers for straws. They also carry a formalized straw program for older children.

Now let's summarize why you would want to begin teaching the skill of drinking from a straw to your baby around 6 months of age. First of all, it is a skill your baby can use throughout life. Also, drinking from cups with straws can replace spouted or sippy cup use. Remember, sippy cups encourage your child to use an immature swallowing pattern similar to the one used on the bottle.

The proper technique of drinking from a straw, like drinking from a cup, allows your child to lift the tip of her tongue to the bump or ridge behind the top front teeth to start the mature swallow. Sippy cups impede this process because the spout gets in the way of the tongue-tip lifting. The mature swallowing pattern is important for clearing the mouth of food and liquid. Individuals who do not develop this pattern tend to have food or liquid remaining in the mouth after swallowing. This can lead to difficulties with oral hygiene.

Also, individuals who do not develop a mature swallowing pattern tend to use other unsophisticated oral motor patterns (such as swallowing food whole, which can lead to poor digestion). When someone uses an immature swallowing pattern, the tongue tends to move with the jaw. When the tongue, jaw, and lips do not learn to work independently of one another, food and liquid are generally not managed well or efficiently.

The tip of the tongue rising to the bump behind the top front teeth is also an important movement for the speech sounds "*t*," "*d*," "*n*," and "*l*." Try making these sounds, and see where your tongue goes. While swallowing and speech require different motor patterns or sequences in your child's brain, the movements are similar in terms of placement and direction. We will discuss mouth movement for speech in chapter 7.

ACTIVITY 6.7: HOW DOES YOUR BABY DRINK FROM A STRAW?

Place a date in the column next to the description that matches what your baby is doing.

Date	What You Want My Baby:	Date	Things to Change My Baby:
	Drinks from a straw placed just on the lips		Drinks from a straw placed far into the mouth onto the tongue
	Drinks from a straw placed in the center of the lips		Drinks from a straw placed to one side of the lips
	Can take one sip at a time from a straw, with the straw placed just at the lips		Places the straw deeply into the mouth, like a baby bottle nipple
	Can drink swallow after swallow from a straw placed just on the lips		Places the straw far into the mouth to drink swallow after swallow

Taking Bites and Chewing Safe, Appropriate Foods

Before you give your baby food to bite and chew, see how you accomplish these processes. Get a soft cookie (such as an arrowroot, butter, or Lorna Doone cookie). Observe how you take bites of the cookie and what you do with the cookie after you take the bite.

ACTIVITY 6.8: HOW DO YOU TAKE BITES AND CHEW FOOD?

Take some bites of a soft cookie or cracker, and observe:

- Do you take bites of the cookie with your front teeth or those toward the side? If you take bites toward the side, this may have to do with the hand you are using to feed yourself or your dentition (how your teeth meet).

- How large of a bite do you take? Hopefully it's not too large.

- Notice how the tip of your tongue moves this bite of cookie to your back molars for chewing.

- After chewing, notice how the tip of your tongue collects the chewed cookie and brings it back to the center of your tongue for the swallow.

- Does the tip of your tongue then lift to the bump or ridge behind your top front teeth to start the swallow? If not, you may be using an unsophisticated swallowing pattern. A number of adults have never developed a fully mature swallowing pattern. This can ultimately lead to oral hygiene and dental concerns.

At 5 to 6 months of age, babies are ready to begin taking bites of soft cookies (such as arrowroot cookies) and learning to chew them. Your baby can also begin to have some lumps to chew in her baby food. This may happen automatically if you make your own baby food with a blender, grinder, or food processor.

When you are ready to give your baby safe foods for biting and chewing, consider the size of your baby's jaw. Soft cookies, such as arrowroot cookies, are a good place to start because they melt down easily in your baby's mouth. This decreases the risk of choking. Some baby cookies and toast (eg, teething biscuits and zwieback toast) are too large for the mouth of a 6-month-old child, and they are not considered soft cookies.

It is also important to give your baby cookies that are made for babies. You do not want to give your baby cookies or crackers that contain preservatives or foods that are not safe for babies. While many people think that Cheerios are safe first foods for babies, they have a rather crunchy, hard texture. I do not feel comfortable giving these to a child until she has developed some skill with chewing.

When you introduce a soft cookie to your baby, hold the cookie to his lips. Allow him to hold the cookie with you, if possible. He may use both hands. Don't forget the hand-mouth connection we discussed earlier. Remember, humans seem to be internally programmed to use hands and mouths together.

Let your baby explore the safe, soft cookie with his lips and gums. Your baby has an innate biting response that will help him to begin biting on the soft cookie when it touches and/or presses against his gums. He will bite, bite, bite on the cookie to soften it, and a piece will break off. The first time this occurs, your baby may appear surprised or make a funny face. It is important for you to monitor the size of the bite your baby takes. However, a soft baby cookie will usually soften and break down easily in the mouth.

Some parents are very concerned about giving their babies solid foods because they are afraid of choking. If soft, safe, solid foods are introduced appropriately, your baby will gain the skills he needs at the appropriate time. Some parents

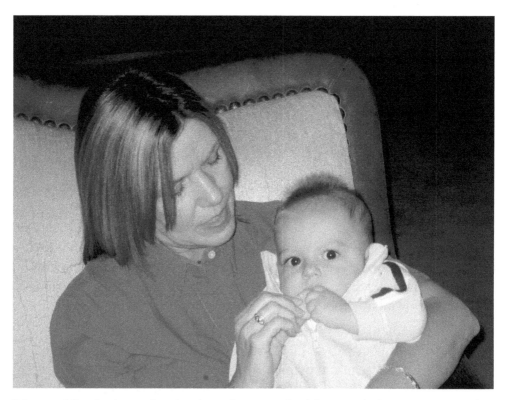

Photo 6.8: Anthony begins learning to take bites and chew at 6 months with a soft, baby cookie.

think that a baby cannot chew because he does not have teeth. However, teeth emerge as the gums are stimulated. Introducing safe and appropriate food textures for biting and chewing when your child is ready for them will help teeth develop.

Biting and chewing also help jaw development and independent tongue, lip, and jaw movement used in higher-level eating and drinking skills. Taking bites and chewing help your child to maintain adequate jaw strength as the jaw grows. The muscles of the jaw need to learn to readjust constantly as the jawbone grows. This is a relatively heavy bone, and muscle function of the jaw needs to keep up with the growth of the bone.

The lips need to move independently of the jaw to help get food and/or liquid into the mouth and to keep it in the mouth. The tongue will become increasingly skilled over time in placing and collecting food within the mouth. The tongue will also begin to move back or retract in a precise manner as part of the mature swallowing process. Controlled tongue retraction is very important for good speech production, as well. We will discuss this in chapter 7.

If you are afraid to introduce foods for your baby to bite or chew, use a safety net. A safe feeder allows you to place pieces of food into a mesh bag for chewing. Your baby can then chew on the foods in the mesh bag while holding onto a handle. As the food is broken down, it will come through the mesh in very small pieces for swallowing. There are several safe feeders on the market.

However, the mesh bags of some safe feeders are too large, allowing large pieces of food to be placed into the netting. This makes it difficult for your baby to bite and chew on food by using all gum surfaces (front, sides, and back). When you place food into one of these devices, be sure you only place a small, baby-bite-sized piece of food into the mesh. The bite-sized piece of food needs to fit your baby's mouth, so it will be much smaller than a bite you would take. A slightly longer mesh bag allows a child to bite on the food from the front gum surfaces to the back molar area, where actual chewing takes place.

Therapists have also used cheesecloth to create little pouches to hold food for chewing. Cheesecloth can often be purchased in grocery stores. Unwrap and cut a section of cheesecloth (which is packaged in a triple thickness). Place a baby-bite-sized piece of food into the center of the cheesecloth, and close the cheesecloth around it. Twist the cheesecloth into a sack or pouch, so you can hold onto it without losing the food while your baby chews on the food in the cheesecloth. Unlike the safe feeder, you will need to hold the cheesecloth as your baby chews. If your baby places his hands on your hands, this again represents the hand-mouth connection.

Now, here is an activity you can do with baby-bite-sized pieces of food wrapped in cheesecloth or placed into a safe feeder.

1. Place the baby-bite-sized piece of food onto your baby's gums in the cheesecloth or safe feeder.

2. Let your baby hold the cheesecloth or safe feeder with you.

3. Press gently but firmly into the bottom or top gum with the food in the cheesecloth or feeder to remind your baby to begin biting or chewing.

4. Work the bite-sized piece of food in the cheesecloth or mesh bag from the front of your baby's mouth to the back, where the molars will eventually emerge. Your baby will be taking little bites all along the way, as the food in the cheesecloth or mesh feeder is worked toward the molar area.

5. You can let your baby chew naturally on one back molar area and then the other.

6. You can encourage your baby to chew food placed in the cheesecloth or mesh feeder 12 to 15 times in each back molar area, alternating sides. However, if your baby only wants to chew six times on a side, that is fine. Maybe he will want to chew seven times the next time. Follow his lead.

7. You can alternate chewing sides two more times (for three sets total) if your baby is interested and having fun. However, be sensitive to your baby's interest level, abilities, and communication. If your baby becomes fatigued (if his chewing begins to feel weak) or disorganized (if he loses the chewing rhythm), stop and move to the other side, or take a break.

8. While your child may demonstrate a preferred side of the mouth for chewing, try to have him chew the same number of times on each side. This will help to balance the movements of the jaw. Does this sound like the "jaws-ercise" we did in chapter 5?

As food moves through the mesh, replace it with another baby-bite-sized piece of food. If you are using a mesh bag or placing food in cheesecloth, you can introduce foods other than the soft baby cookies we discussed earlier. You can place baby bite-sized pieces of cooled, soft, steamed vegetables (such as carrots or squash) or cooled, parboiled fruit without skin (such as apples, peaches, and pears) into the mesh or cheesecloth. As your child's abilities to take bites and chew foods become more sophisticated, you can begin to give your child these and other foods without the cheesecloth or mesh bag. See guidelines on when to introduce foods in the next section.

This activity is excellent exercise for your baby's jaw muscles. It helps your baby to develop graded jaw movement (the ability to move the jaw as needed for the particular activity) and separation of lip and tongue movement from the jaw. These skills are important in the development of mature eating and drinking.

As your baby begins to chew on foods and appropriate toys at 5 to 6 months of age, chewing can begin to replace sucking and suckling for calming. This is the time when you can begin to wean your baby from the pacifier if he is using one. We talked about pacifier use and weaning in chapter 4.

ACTIVITY 6.9: HOW DOES YOUR BABY TAKE BITES AND CHEW FOODS?

Place a date in the column next to the description that matches what your baby is doing.

Date	What You Want My 5- to 7-month-old baby:	Date	Things to Change My 5- to 7-month-old baby:
	Takes little phasic bites (a rhythmic bite, bite, bite) of a soft cookie held by baby and me at the front of his mouth		Only sucks or suckles on the soft cookie
	Chews on lumps of food in the mouth, even without teeth		Only sucks or suckles lumps of food
	Moves his tongue toward food in the side of the mouth		Tongue does not move independently from the jaw

Introducing Foods and Liquids

Now you know the mechanics of feeding. Here are some guidelines for introducing foods and liquids from a variety of resources:[222–225]

ACTIVITY 6.10: SOME GUIDELINES FOR WHEN TO INTRODUCE FOODS AND LIQUIDS

Suggested Foods and Liquids	Date
Birth to 4–6 Months	
Breast milk or infant formula	

ACTIVITY 6.10: (cont.)

Suggested Foods and Liquids	Date
No extra water normally needed (breast milk usually has plenty of water; bottle-fed babies may need extra water if you live in a hot, dry climate). Boil water for 3 minutes and cool for children under 6 months. Talk to your pediatrician about this; too much water can harm small babies.[226]	
4–6 Months	
Fortified baby cereal mixed with the breast milk or formula to start	
Nonwheat cereals (eg, rice, oat, millet, barley, rye, soy)	
Pureed fruits and vegetables	
Sips of water (boiled for 3 minutes and cooled), formula, or breast milk from an open cup held by you	
Soft baby cookie (eg, nonwheat, arrowroot) held by you and baby at 5–6 months	
Breast milk from the breast or formula from a bottle (let baby self-limit)	
6–8 Months	
Milled, blended, or well-mashed vegetables and fruits (well cooked with small, soft lumps)	
Wheat-free soft cookies and crackers, teething biscuits	
Cooked rice (sticky)	

Suggested Foods and Liquids	Date
Sips of water, very diluted fruit juices, formula, or breast milk from an open cup and a cup with a straw	
Breast milk from the breast or formula from a bottle (let baby self-limit)	
7–10 Months	
Chopped cooked fruits and vegetables (includes canned fruits, no citrus)	
Soft cheese	
Mashed cooked beans or tofu	
Wheat and corn products (eg, bread, toast, soft tortilla strips, crackers, dry cereals without sugar, well-cooked pasta)	
Sips of water, very diluted fruit or vegetable juices, formula, or breast milk from an open cup and a cup with a straw	
Breast milk from the breast or formula from a bottle (let baby self-limit)	
9–12 Months	
Soft, cut-up cooked and raw foods (eg, bananas, skinned peaches); introduce citrus slowly	
Cooked fruits or vegetable strips	
Soft, chopped meats (eg, stewed chicken, no bone; ground meat; no fish)	

ACTIVITY 6.10: (cont.)

Suggested Foods and Liquids	Date
Casseroles with noodles, pasta, or rice	
Bread, toast, crackers, dry cereal without sugar (no chocolate)	
Eggs (yolks at 9 months, whites at 12 months) and cheese (soft cheese strips, cottage cheese, yogurt formulated for babies)	
Sips of water, very diluted fruit or vegetable juices, formula, or breast milk from an open cup and a cup with a straw	
Breast milk from the breast or formula from a bottle (let baby self-limit)	
12–18 Months	
Chopped table food (avoid round foods, such as whole grapes and hotdog pieces)	
Soft meats, including fish (no bones)	
Cookies and crackers (can bite through)	
Drinks of milk, water, very diluted fruit or vegetable juices from an open cup, a recessed-lid cup, and a straw	
Weaning from the bottle; breast-feeding may continue	
18–21 Months	
Chopped table food, including many meats and raw vegetables	

Suggested Foods and Liquids	Date
Can bite through a hard cookie or cracker but may struggle a little	
Drinks of milk, water, very diluted fruit or vegetable juices from an open cup, a recessed-lid cup, and a straw	
Weaned from bottle; breast-feeding may continue	
24 Months	
Can bite through a hard cookie with ease	
Can chew with lips closed and uses mature chewing patterns; can manage most foods in bite-sized pieces cut by a parent or created by taking bites	
Uses lips actively when drinking from an open cup, can hold an open cup with one hand, and does not spill liquid from an open cup	

As you introduce foods to your baby, introduce one food at a time. Wait 3 to 4 days before introducing another food. Look for any sensitivity to the food, such as wheezing and/or dry cough, apparent stomach pain, excessive burping and/or reflux, diarrhea, or any type of rash.

The first time many parents and pediatricians see food sensitivities in some babies is right after birth. The sensitivity is often indicated by excessive spit-up and apparent gastrointestinal discomfort. This is one reason why pediatricians have parents try different formulas. Breast-fed babies tend to have fewer food allergies and sensitivities. However, some breast-fed babies are sensitive to certain foods or liquids that Mom eats or drinks. Pediatricians and lactation consultants will often recommend that Mom eliminate certain foods from her diet. See chapter 3 for more information.

When introducing a new food, do not expect your child to like the taste and texture immediately. Think of when you first try a food, particularly a food from another culture. Do you always like foods when you first taste them? Your baby's food culture has been different than yours from birth if you are bottle-feeding. Your baby has been eating basically the same thing every day if she is drinking formula. If you are breast-feeding, your baby is more likely to be getting some different tastes, based on what Mom is eating and drinking.

It may take 10 to 15 opportunities or exposures to a new food or liquid for your child to begin to enjoy it. This is an important idea for you to understand, because this is where many of our picky eaters seem to start. See the section toward the end of this chapter on feeding problems and picky eating for more information. If you see your baby make a face or spit out food or liquid when she first tastes it, it may just mean that she is not used to the taste or texture. Your baby may actually like this food if given more opportunities.

Also, be careful with what you say about food and liquid. Babies understand more language than many people think. They also understand body language and tone of voice. If you don't like a food or liquid, or you comment about your baby disliking a food or liquid, this can become a self-fulfilling prophecy (ie, your baby may not like the food or liquid because of messages she is receiving from you or others who feed her). You can be a good role model by eating, drinking, and talking about different foods and liquids with your child. Meals are a social experience.

How Much Do I Feed My Child?

Once your baby begins eating solid food between 4 and 6 months of age, all of his nutritional requirements change. First, you must remember that your child's stomach is about as big as his fist. Therefore, your child's portion sizes will be nowhere near your portion sizes.

Some portion guidelines are listed in the following chart.[227–228] According to Morris and Klein,[229] a serving size is approximately one tablespoon per year of the child's life (eg, a 2-year-old would have a serving size of 2 tablespoons). According to the following portion guidelines from Satter[230] and Morris and Klein,[231] your child should be eating six servings of rice, cereal, or pasta per day. He should be eating five servings from the fruit and vegetable group; two servings from the meat, poultry, fish, eggs, and cooked beans group; and two to three servings from the milk, yogurt, and cheese group.

Please check the following chart with your pediatrician to determine when to introduce certain foods. Some foods like wheat, citrus fruits, eggs, cow's milk, and fish will be introduced later than other foods in the same food group. **Do not give your baby raw honey or foods containing raw honey during the first 12 months because of the risk of botulism.**

SERVING SIZES AND NUMBER OF SERVINGS PER DAY[232-233]

Food	6–12 Months of Age	1–2 Years of Age	Total Servings Per Day
Bread Group			**Six**
Rice	½–1 Tablespoon	1–2 Tablespoons	
Cereal	½–1 Tablespoon	1–2 Tablespoons	
Pasta	½–1 Tablespoon	1–2 Tablespoons	
Bread	⅛–¼ Slice	¼ Slice	
Fruit and Vegetable Group			**Five**
Fruit	½–1 Tablespoon or ⅛–¼ piece	1–2 Tablespoons or ¼ piece	Two to three
Vegetables	½–1 Tablespoon	1–2 Tablespoons	Two to three
Meat Group			**Two**
Meat, poultry, fish	½–1 Tablespoon	1–2 Tablespoons	
Eggs	Yolks at 9 months, whites at 12 months	¼ Egg	
Cooked beans	½–1 Tablespoon	1–2 Tablespoons	

SERVING SIZES AND NUMBER OF SERVINGS PER DAY[232-233] (cont.)

Food	6–12 Months of Age	1–2 Years of Age	Total Servings Per Day
Cooked beans	½–1 Tablespoon	1–2 Tablespoons	
Dairy Group			**Two to Three**
Milk	No cow's milk	¼–⅓ cup	
Yogurt	½–1 Tablespoon (baby yogurt product, according to product labeling)	1–2 Tablespoons (baby yogurt product)	
Cheese	½–1 Tablespoon	¼–⅓ ounce	

Note: Don't forget about hydration. Water regulates all functions of the body.[234] It helps keep body chemistry in balance by carrying hormones, nutrients, and other important substances to the cells of the body. Water also removes waste from these cells. Your child should drink two-thirds of his body weight in ounces (eg, a 36-lb child needs 24 oz of water per day).[235-236] There is water in breast milk, formula, other liquids, and stage-one baby foods. There is also some water in fruits, vegetables, and other foods. See Activity 6.10 for some guidelines for when to introduce foods and liquids, including water.

Weaning from the Bottle and Breast

This part of the chapter will help you wean your child from the bottle and/or breast. The process starts when your baby begins to drink from open cups, cups with recessed lids, and straws, around 6 months of age.

You will initially place breast milk and/or formula into these cups as your child learns to use them, until your pediatrician tells you to offer other liquids (such as water and diluted juice). You will use these cups more frequently as your child becomes skilled in their use. By 12 to 15 months of age, your child will primarily be taking the breast or bottle in the evening before bed. Most of your child's liquid will be given by cup.

As your child learns to drink from a cup and straw, praise him. Be sure to provide your baby with appropriate mouth activities to replace the stimulation he received from the bottle and/or breast. Spoon-feeding and taking bites of a soft baby cookie will help to fulfill this need, in addition to drinking activities. Also, see chapters 4 and 5 for information on the appropriate use of mouth toys.

Every child is unique, so the weaning process is different for each child. Do not stress yourself or your child during this process. Go slowly. Replace bottle- and breast-feedings throughout the day, as you and your child are ready. You have 6 to 9 months to wean your child from the bottle (ie, 6 months of age until 12 to 15 months). You may choose to breast-feed longer.

If your pediatrician is in agreement, you can add water to formula in the bottle during the weaning process and present the undiluted formula or breast milk in a cup. This way, your child is rewarded with the full taste of the formula or breast milk while drinking from the cup.[237]

Note: It is very important that you work closely with your pediatrician on this process to ensure that your child is getting proper nutrition and hydration.

By 12 to 15 months of age, your child will take the bottle or breast primarily around bedtime. All other liquid will be taken from an open cup, a cup with a recessed lid, or a straw. During the weaning process, we want your baby to breast- or bottle-feed before bed, not in bed. Remember, you have not allowed your baby to take a bottle while lying down because of the related risk of ear infections. See chapter 2 for more information.

If your baby has reflux or a history of reflux, you might want to give your child the bottle or breast before a bath and reading time. This will allow him to be upright for a while before sleep. If you have experienced reflux, you know that it is worse at night when you eat or drink just before lying down in bed.

If your child is still seeking comfort to fall asleep at night, you can provide him with safe mouth toys. He can appropriately mouth or chew on these prior to sleep. You have already weaned your child from the pacifier between 6 and 10 months of age. See chapter 4 for further information on this topic.

When weaning your child from the bottle or breast, you can start to skip some evening feedings by replacing them with a snack before bedtime. This can include a drink from an open cup, a cup with a recessed lid, or a straw, and some food. Do this when your child is in a good mood and not too tired. Remember, children often derive comfort from suckling at the breast or on a bottle.

While you read a story with your child and look at books after a snack and bath time, allow him to chew on and mouth appropriate mouth toys. This will help to satisfy your child's need for oral stimulation and can

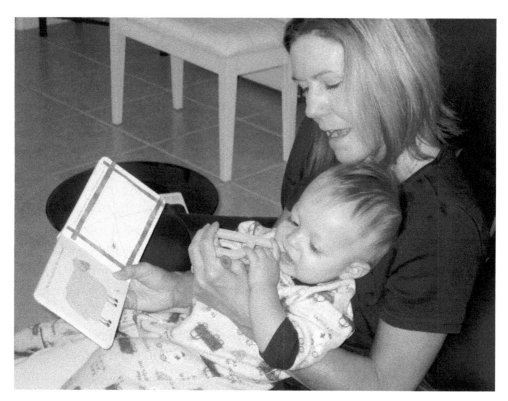

Photo 6.9: Chewing on a mouth toy can improve attention, focus, and concentration as well as satisfy the need for oral stimulation.

improve attention, focus, and concentration. See chapters 4 and 5 for more detail.

If your child asks for the breast or bottle on an evening where you have replaced the feeding with a snack and drink, explain to him that he is getting to be a big boy. Reassure and praise him by saying how proud and happy you are. As you go through this process, be patient and supportive of yourself and your child. Offer your child choices of snacks, drinks, and mouth toys (eg, "Jonathan, do you want a cookie or cracker?" "Do you want milk or juice?"). You can offer one preferred item and one that is less preferred to increase your child's incentive to choose. This helps him become part of the process and makes life easier for you.

Twelve to 15 months of age is a good time to finish weaning your child from the bottle to ensure good mouth development. You may choose to breast-feed longer. You have been giving your child experiences with the open cup, a cup with a recessed lid, and a straw since 6 months of age. These are important skills your child will use throughout life.

Your child never needs to use a sippy cup. The problem with sippy cup use at 12 to 15 months of age and beyond is that it is used like a bottle. If a straw is used improperly (placed too far into the mouth), it is also used like a bottle. However, you have learned about proper cup and straw use previously in this chapter.

Congratulations! You are ready to wean your child from the breast and/or bottle. You are also helping your child develop the mature swallowing pattern he will use throughout life.

<table>
<tr><td colspan="2">ACTIVITY 6.11: WEANING FROM THE BREAST OR BOTTLE</td></tr>
<tr><td colspan="2">Place a date in the column next to the description that matches what you and your child are doing during the weaning process. Work with your baby's pediatrician on the weaning process.</td></tr>
<tr><td>Weaning Guidelines</td><td>Date</td></tr>
<tr><td>4–6 Months</td><td></td></tr>
<tr><td>Begin having your baby drink from an open cup by using formula or breast milk (can thicken with rice or other baby cereal when given the OK from your baby's pediatrician)</td><td></td></tr>
<tr><td>Begin having your baby drink from an open cup by using stage-one baby food thinned with water (boiled for 3 minutes and cooled) when given the OK from your baby's pediatrician</td><td></td></tr>
<tr><td>Provide other appropriate mouth activities for your baby</td><td></td></tr>
<tr><td>6–9 Months</td><td></td></tr>
<tr><td>Continue having your baby drink from an open cup by using thickened or regular liquid (eg, formula, breast milk, very diluted fruit juices)</td><td></td></tr>
<tr><td>Begin teaching your baby to drink from a straw by using a specially made bottle with thickened liquids (eg, formula or breast milk thickened with baby cereal, or stage-one baby food thinned with water)</td><td></td></tr>
<tr><td>Provide other appropriate mouth activities for your baby</td><td></td></tr>
</table>

ACTIVITY 6.11: (cont.)

Weaning Guidelines	Date
9–12 Months	
Provide drinks (formula, breast milk, very diluted fruit or vegetable juice) throughout the day with an open cup, straw, and/or cup with a recessed lid	
Provide other appropriate mouth activities for your baby	
12–15 Months	
Only give your baby the bottle at nighttime before bed, with the child sitting upright (can dilute the milk in a bottle with water if pediatrician says it's OK)	
Give remaining liquid (milk, water, very diluted fruit or vegetable juice) throughout the day from an open cup, cup with a recessed lid, or straw (your child should be able to drink from a cup with a straw on her own)	
You may also want to give your child a cup with handles	
Provide other appropriate mouth activities for your child	
15–18 Months	
Your child is weaned from the bottle and is drinking from an open cup, a cup with a recessed lid, or a straw; may continue some breast-feeding	
Provide other appropriate mouth activities for your baby	

For more ideas on weaning, go to "The Weaning Room" at *www.theweaningroom.com*. The information on the "Baby-Led" feeding approach by Gill Rapley can be very useful for parents.

Feeding Problems and Picky Eating

Feeding problems, including picky eating, are usually very stressful for parents and their children. If your child has any of the following feeding problems, talk to your child's pediatrician:

- My child does not eat enough.
- My child wants to eat all the time.
- My child will eat only certain foods.

You may also need to work with a nutritionist and/or feeding therapist (eg, an occupational therapist or speech-language pathologist who specializes in feeding).

Some children do not eat what is considered to be "enough" because they have small stomachs. Remember, the size of your child's stomach is about the size of your child's fist. For these children, your child's pediatrician may recommend that you feed your child smaller meals throughout the day. We already know that this is a good practice for most of us.

Some children may not seem to eat enough because they get distracted by other things in the environment. These children may begin to feel full because they don't stay focused on the meal. Look at the environment in which your child eats. Are other people being appropriate role models while eating? What is the conversation at the table? Are topics neutral and calm? Is calming music playing as a background, or are there other distractions, such as TV? Some young children zone out or are overstimulated by TV.

Some children may not eat enough because they begin to feel sick when they eat. These may be children who have some type of food sensitivity or allergy. They may also have reflux. Chapter 3 has information on these topics. Infant massage can be helpful for children with digestive problems and has been shown to improve weight gain.[238]

Some children may want to eat all the time. It is important to evaluate these children for reflux. I have worked with many children who have chronic reflux. When a person swallows, the esophagus is set into motion toward the stomach. This makes it impossible for the child to reflux. Therefore, a child may want to eat all the time because it stops reflux.

There are children who "graze" throughout the day. Some of these children have difficulty gaining weight. Grazing is not the same as eating small meals every 2–3 hours.

ACTIVITY 6.12: WHAT TO DO IF MY CHILD HAS FEEDING PROBLEMS

Identify and date the problem you are seeing, and place a date in the column next to what you want to try.

Problem My child:	Date	Things to Try My child:	Date
Does not eat enough		Provide smaller meals throughout the day; eliminate distractions from the environment; work toward a neutral, soothing environment with good role models; notice how your child is acting (eg, does she burp a lot or seem to have belly problems?); work with your child's pediatrician, nutritionist, and/or feeding specialist	
Wants to eat all the time		Have your child evaluated for possible food allergies, sensitivities, and/or reflux; work with your child's pediatrician, nutritionist, and/or feeding specialist	

If your child is a picky eater, look for:

- Problems with mouth movements
- Problems with sensation in or around the mouth
- Any medical issues (such as reflux or sinus concerns) that may be related to the problem
- Whether food textures were introduced on schedule
- Behavioral problems that have become related to picky eating

ACTIVITY 6.13: WHAT TO DO IF MY CHILD IS A PICKY EATER

Identify and date the problem you are seeing, and place a date in the column next to what you want to try.

Problem	Date	Things to Try	Date
Inadequate mouth movements for eating and drinking		See a feeding specialist who knows about mouth movement (eg, a speech-language pathologist or occupational therapist)	
Inadequate sensation in or around the mouth (taste, texture, temperature, smell, etc)		See a feeding specialist who knows about sensation (eg, a speech-language pathologist or occupational therapist); systematically change your child's food and liquid textures, tastes, and smells over time	
Reflux, sinus, or other medical conditions that may be related to the problem		See your child's pediatrician and an appropriate specialist (see "Health Problems and Possible Treatments" in chapter 3)	
Behavior that has become related to picky eating		See a feeding specialist who knows about behavior in addition to sensory and motor problems (eg, a speech-language pathologist or occupational therapist)	

Note: If your child is a picky eater, talk with your child's pediatrician. If this is a serious concern (if your child is not getting adequate hydration and nutrition), your child's pediatrician will usually refer you to a feeding specialist and nutritionist. The feeding specialist should be someone who can evaluate the problems listed in Activity 6.13. Therefore, you will probably see a speech-language pathologist or occupational therapist specifically trained in feeding. The nutritionist or dietician will guide you, the feeding therapist, and your child's pediatrician in food, liquid, and supplement selection for your child.

From reading this book, you already know a lot about how your child's mouth is supposed to move. If your child does not seem to have the ability to move her mouth appropriately for the feeding activity, you will need someone to evaluate this for you. A feeding specialist can evaluate your child and provide you and your child with activities to do at home. This way, your child can develop the movement needed for good feeding, eating, and drinking.

You also know something about the importance of sensation within and around your child's mouth. We talked a lot about this in chapters 4 and 5. A feeding specialist can evaluate this area and give you specific activities to do with your child, if needed.

In addition, you can systematically change your child's food and liquid textures to see if your child improves. For example, thickened liquids provide more information to the mouth than regular thin liquids. Your child may improve with drinking if you thicken the liquid. You can also change the texture of a food by using your blender or food processor. See if your child does better if you change the texture (either thinner or thicker).

Some children also prefer to have more taste. Baby foods tend to be very bland. Babies typically prefer sweet and salty tastes, but you don't want to add too much sugar or salt to the food. As your child gets older, you can add some

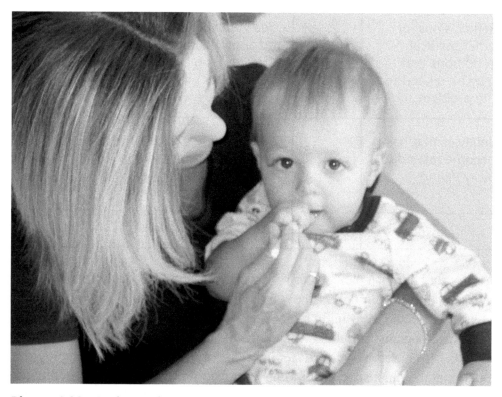

Photo 6.10: Anthony demonstrates oral massage, used to improve oral sensation in some children.

tastes that you have in your diet (such as garlic, onion, cinnamon, and other appropriate spices). If you are breast-feeding, your baby is probably getting many different tastes already. You can add breast milk to the cereal to see if your baby prefers that combination to cereal made with water only.

It is also important that you look to see if your child has any medical problems that may be causing her to be picky. A child who has reflux may realize at some level that certain foods make her feel sick. However, she may not know which foods are causing the problem. This can also change from day to day. Reflux and other digestive problems may provide at least part of the explanation for picky eating in some children with autism.

If your child has sinus problems, this can change the taste of foods. (If you've ever noticed that food tastes different when you have a sinus infection or cold, then you know what I mean.) Therefore, it is very important to take care of any nasal and sinus problems your child may be having. The smell of food is an important aspect of being able to experience taste. We taste sweet, salty, sour, and bitter with the tongue. It is the smell of food that allows us to taste the difference between flavors, such as cherry and strawberry. When children are picky eaters, it can often be the smell of the food that does not appeal to them.

If your child is having difficulties accepting particular food or liquid tastes or textures, a food record is an important starting point. You need to keep a record of at least 3 full days of everything your child eats and drinks. Once you have this, you can begin to systematically make some changes to your child's diet.

ACTIVITY 6.14: FOOD AND LIQUID RECORD

Record the approximate amounts of food and fluid consumed by your child below. Enter the date next to the appropriate day.

	Breakfast	Lunch	Dinner	Snacks
Day 1 Date:				
Day 2 Date:				
Day 3 Date:				

ACTIVITY 6.15: MY CHILD'S EATING AND DRINKING PATTERNS

Look at your child's food record, and take note of any patterns. Use the following chart to help you discover your child's individual patterns. You may also discover through this process that your child is doing better than you thought when you compare your child's intake to the information found in the previous section, "How Much Do I Feed My Child?"

Food and Liquid Characteristics	What Is Similar about My Child's Foods and Liquids?	What Could We Try?
Taste		
Smell		
Texture		
Temperature		
Color		
Shape		
Other		

Example: Emily, Aged 12 Months

Emily is a healthy child, who is developing well. Emily's mom and dad kept a 3-day food and liquid record. She basically had adequate nutrition, according to the guidelines in the section entitled, "How Much Do I Feed My Child?" However, Emily was eating many foods with sweet tastes (such as applesauce and squash baby food). When green vegetables were offered to her to smell, she made a face. She was also only eating foods with a relatively fine texture (such as ground and pureed foods). She preferred her foods and liquids warmed.

Emily's information is presented in the following chart. You can see how the use of the chart helped Emily's parents pinpoint a solution.

PROBLEM SOLVING FOR EMILY AND HER FAMILY		
Food and Liquid Characteristics	What Is Similar about My Child's Foods and Liquids?	What Could We Try?
Taste	Sweet tastes	Puree or grind appropriate mashes or casseroles made of foods preferred by Emily (eg, mashed potatoes and squash, rice and carrots)
Smell	Does not like the smell of green vegetables	Give Emily experiences with vegetables outside of feeding (eg, let her handle some green vegetables when you are not trying to get her to eat them)
Texture	Soft textures	Begin slowly thickening the textures of the foods (adding more lumps over time)
Temperature	Warmed	Present new foods warmed if appropriate
Color	N/A	
Shape	N/A	
Other	N/A	

Note: If Emily had serious feeding problems, I would want her to work with a feeding specialist and/or dietician on a regular basis. Because she is a healthy child who is developing well, these are my four recommendations for Emily's parents:

1. Begin to thicken food textures by grinding and pureeing her food less over time. I would recommend that the family stop using baby food as Emily becomes more accustomed to eating food prepared by Mom and Dad.

2. Give Emily experience with vegetables outside of feeding. I would suggest a time when Mom, Dad, and Emily can look at and talk about green vegetables when there is no pressure on Emily to eat them. Since Emily is 12 months of age, Mom and Dad can let Emily look at, touch, and smell the vegetables before cooking as an experience activity. Many 12-month-old children love to go to the grocery store. Emily's parents can talk to her about these vegetables as they are placed into the shopping cart.

3. Many people like vegetable mashes and casseroles. Make some appropriate mashes or casseroles for Emily (such as mashed potatoes and squash, or rice and carrots). Since Emily likes soft textures, the mashes and casseroles may need to be pureed or ground at first. Other appropriate foods can be mixed with the foods she likes in the mashes and casseroles. Don't mix foods you would not eat (such as applesauce and eggs). Don't try to fool Emily. Show her the foods before and as you cook them. Talk about them.

4. Present new foods warmed if appropriate. Many foods are appropriately served warm (eg, steamed or mashed fruits and vegetables, casseroles, etc).

In addition to mouth movement problems, sensation problems, and medical problems, **behavioral problems quickly become associated with feeding problems**. This occurs because **behavior is a way of communicating**. If your child cannot let you know something in words, she will let you know through behavior and body language.

I am often concerned when parents and professionals assume that picky eating is purely a behavioral problem. It is important to look at what your child's behavior is communicating. This way, you can find ways to change the situation and let your child know you understand her communication. Also, involve your child in the food preparation process. This may seem a bit odd for you to do with a very young child, but she is learning a lot from what is happening in the environment around her. It helps the child become part of the process.

It can be as simple as having your child sit in the highchair as you prepare some of the meal. Your child does not need to sit there the entire time. You can show your child the foods you are about to prepare, or talk about the food. Let your child see, smell, and touch the food. Praise your child for doing this. Give your child a choice of which food you will prepare. Even very small babies (6-month-old children) make choices with their eyes and body language. For example, you can say, "Katie, pick one for Mommy to cook." as you show her broccoli and asparagus. You let her look at, smell, and touch the one she picks. Praise her for helping you.

As mentioned previously, many children like going to the grocery store with Mom and Dad. This is a great time to talk about the foods you are picking out for your family meals. Your child can help you make some choices. Of course, you will be offering healthy food choices that support your family's nutritional needs. ("Emily, should we get apples or oranges?").

Some parents also give their children too many choices of foods. When giving choices, limit your choices to two items at first. Too many choices can overwhelm your child. I once worked with a mom who had 15 jars of baby food on the table as choices for her baby. This was very overwhelming for the child and for the mom.

Having your child make food choices and become involved in food preparation is a way to gain cooperation and participation. This can help your child develop a wonderful relationship with food for life. As you feed your child, remember that meals are social experiences. Take your time. Talk to your child. Have some food to eat or liquid to drink with your child. This will help you and your child pace the meal, another important life skill.

Parents also need to remember that their child may not like a food the first time he tastes it. Do you like every food you taste the first time you taste it? How many times does it take? You may need to provide your child with 10 to 15 exposures of a food to help him accommodate to the taste or texture of a food. Be patient with this process, and **do not force-feed** your child. We talked about this briefly in the section entitled "Introducing Foods and Liquids."

If your child initially spits out a food, don't assume he will never like it. This may only be his reaction to something new. Also, don't react by getting upset with your child, as this can inadvertently reinforce the spitting. Remember to ignore behaviors you don't want (when possible), and praise behaviors you do want.

When children are being exposed to new food tastes, smells, and textures, it is important to give them as much structured control over the situation as possible. This is a good time to let your child dip a finger into a food or pick up the food to try. There are spoons that allow your child to dip the spoon into the food to taste it. This allows him to experiment with new foods at his own pace, using his own ideas. Again, choices of foods (beginning with two) are important. These techniques do not spoil your child. They show him you respect his communication and his choices.

There are many good books on nutrition, and this book is not meant to replace them. In fact, I recommend that you buy one. Ellyn Satter has written two books on nutrition that I often recommend to parents:

1. *Child of Mine: Feeding with Love and Good Sense*[239]
2. *How to Get Your Kid to Eat...But Not Too Much*[240]

There is also a book written specifically to address picky eating entitled, *Just Take a Bite: Easy, Effective, Answers to Food Aversion and Eating Challenges,* by Lori Ernsperger and Tania Stegen-Hanson.[241]

Feeding Development from 5 to 24 Months of Age[242-252]

Here is a summary of the feeding skills we have discussed. Place a date next to the skills your baby is accomplishing. Circle the items your baby needs to accomplish. Know that these checklists are approximate, and not absolute. Every baby has his own unique developmental sequence. These checklists are a guide to let you know if your baby is basically on track or not. The detail presented in these lists is available to therapists, but most parents and pediatricians do not have the benefit of this level of detail. I think it is important information for you to have. If you have questions or concerns regarding your child's feeding development, please discuss these with your child's pediatrician and appropriate others as needed.

Date	Feeding Checklist: 5–9 Months
	Involuntary suckling reflex is seen less and less; seems to be disappearing (6–12 months)
	Suckles or sucks liquid from the breast and/or bottle; long suck, swallow, breathe sequences from the breast and/or bottle (6–12 months)
	Drinking from an open cup: wide jaw movements on the cup are common at first (5–7 months); better control of the jaw develops (6–8 months); baby develops continuous, consecutive sucks (three or more) (6–12 months)
	Learns to drink from an open cup and straw (6–12 months)
	Gag reflex is located on the back third of the tongue (6–9 months)[253]

Date	Feeding Checklist: 5–9 Months
	Soft baby cookie, thicker puree or cereal, and foods with very small, soft lumps are introduced (5–7 months)
	Baby learns to manage many different food and liquid textures; relies less on breast- and bottle-feeding (6–12 months)
	By 6–7 months, baby looks at the spoon and holds mouth still prior to taking food from spoon; lips move inward slightly when food remains on them
	Around 8 months, the upper lip finally becomes active enough to remove food from the spoon
	Baby can pick up food pieces with a fist and hold a soft baby cookie to eat it (6–8 months)
	Can pass a piece of food from one hand to the other (8–9 months)
	Bottom two front teeth (central incisors) come in (5–9 months)
	Top two front teeth (central incisors) come in (6–10 months)
	Bottom lateral incisors erupt (7–20 months)
	Top lateral incisors erupt (8–10 months)
	Control of the bite reflex develops; more diagonal rotary jaw movement is seen
	Jaw movements during biting and chewing begin to match the shape and size of food (beginning around 6 months)
	The lip and cheek begin to tighten to keep food in place during chewing on the side where food is placed (around 6 months)

Date	Feeding Checklist: 5–9 Months
	The tongue moves up and down with the jaw but begins to move toward small pieces of food on the side gums (around 6 months)
	The tongue moves toward food placed on the side of the gum area with a rolling or shifting motion (around 7 months)
	Control develops over the transverse (side) tongue reflex (6–8 months)

Many changes will occur in your child's feeding skills during the 5- to 9-month period. The involuntary suckling reflex that your baby had at birth seems to be disappearing between 6 and 12 months. While your baby will continue to suckle and suck liquid from the breast and bottle, an increase in true sucking will occur over time. The suck has more up-and-down jaw and tongue movement than suckling. Your child now manages long periods of sucking, swallowing, and breathing while breast- or bottle-feeding.

You will introduce the open cup to your baby between 5 and 7 months of age by giving her single sips of liquid. Between 6 and 12 months of age, your child develops the ability to sequence three or more consecutive sucks from the open cup. Between 6 and 12 months, your child can also learn to drink from a straw. See information on drinking from an open cup and straw in previous sections of this chapter.

Between 6 and 9 months, your baby's gag reflex will be located on the back third of the tongue. This occurs through the mouthing of appropriate toys and objects, as well as through exposure to different feeding experiences. Between 6 and 12 months of age, your baby learns to manage many different food and liquid textures. She relies less on breast- or bottle-feeding.

Between 5 and 7 months of age, your baby will be eating soft baby cookies, thicker purees and cereals, and foods with very small, soft lumps. By 6 to 7 months, your baby will look at the spoon and make her mouth quiet or still before taking food from the spoon. If food is left on your baby's lips, her lips will move inward slightly to remove the food. Around 8 months of age, your baby's upper lip will finally become active enough to remove food from the spoon. Up to this point, your baby has closed her lips to do this.

Your baby will pick up food pieces in her fist and feed herself a soft baby cookie between 6 and 8 months. By 8 to 9 months, she can pass food pieces from one hand to the other.

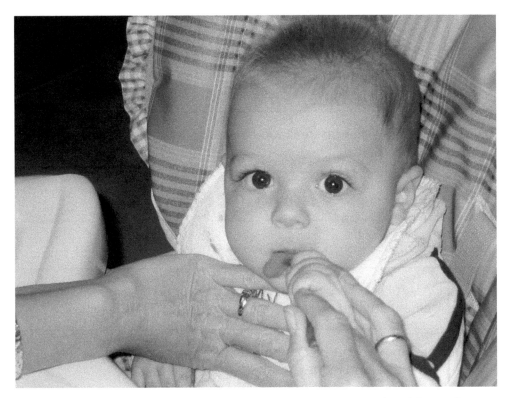

Photo 6.11: Anthony's mouth was quiet before taking food from the spoon.

Your baby will begin to get teeth during the 5- to 9-month period. The bottom two front teeth (central incisors) will usually come in between 5 and 9 months, the top two front teeth (central incisors) will usually come in between 6 and 10 months, the bottom lateral incisors will usually come in between 7 and 20 months, and the top lateral incisors will usually come in between 8 and 10 months.

The development of teeth is directly related to the control that is developing in your baby's jaw. As your baby develops control of the bite reflex, more diagonal rotary movement is seen in the jaw during the chewing process. Your baby's jaw movements while taking bites of food and chewing foods will begin to match the shape and size of the food within the mouth beginning around 6 months. You will also begin to see your baby's lips and cheeks tighten to keep food in place within the mouth around 6 months of age.

Between 6 and 8 months, your baby develops control over the transverse (side) tongue reflex. At 6 months of age, the tongue moves up and down with the jaw but also begins to move toward small pieces of food on the side of the gums with some control. Around 7 months of age, your baby's tongue moves with a rolling and shifting motion toward food placed on the side of the gum area. The development of lateral (side) tongue movement is critical for the manipulation and management of solid foods.

Date	Feeding Checklist: 9–12 Months
	Holds and/or bangs spoon (9 months); imitates stirring with spoon (9½ months)
	Begins to pick up small food pieces with thumb and fingers instead of fist
	Bottom first molars come in (10–12 months)
	Bite reflex is seen less and less; seems to be disappearing
	A soft cookie is initially held with the gums and/or teeth while the parent or child breaks off the rest of the cookie
	Jaw movements increasingly mature and match the size and shape of food in the mouth
	Diagonal rotary jaw movement is seen increasingly during chewing
	From 9–24 months, the transverse (side) tongue reflex is seen less and less; seems to be disappearing
	Side-to-side tongue movements become increasingly sophisticated and mature
	Food is moved from the center of the tongue to the side of the mouth for chewing
	Lip movements continue to mature (upper lip moves forward and down, lower lip moves inward) to remove food from a spoon
	Continuous, consecutive sucks (three or more) occur while drinking from an open cup, a cup with a recessed lid, and a straw

At 9 months of age, your baby will hold and bang the spoon. By 9½ months, she will begin to imitate stirring with the spoon. This is also when your baby will begin to pick up small pieces of food with the thumb and fingers instead of the fist.

Your baby's jaw is continuing to develop, and the bottom first molars usually come in between 10 and 12 months of age. The bite reflex is seen less often as diagonal rotary chewing develops. Your baby will hold a soft cookie with the gums while you or she breaks off the rest of the cookie. Your baby's jaw movements match the size and shape of the food when taking bites and chewing.

Between 9 and 24 months, the transverse (side) tongue reflex is seen less often, while increasingly mature, side-to-side tongue movements are seen more often. Between 9 and 12 months, your child can move food from the center of the mouth to each side for chewing. Lip movements continue to develop (the upper lip moves forward and down; the lower lip moves inward) to remove food from the spoon. Continuous and consecutive sucks (three or more) are seen while drinking from an open cup, a cup with a recessed lid, and a straw.

Date	Feeding Checklist: 12–15 Months
	Can pick up small food pieces with thumb and index finger
	Puts food pieces into a bowl
	Begins to feed self with a spoon, but may turn it over on the way to the mouth (12–14 months)
	Jaw, lips, and tongue continue to learn to move independently of one another
	The different parts of each structure continue to learn to move separately (eg, the tip of the tongue begins to move independently of the rest of the tongue; each lip corner contracts independently of the rest of the lips)
	The tongue (front-back) reflex is seen less and less, seems to be disappearing (12–18 months); the transverse (side) tongue reflex is seen less and less, seems to be disappearing (9–24 months)
	The tip of the tongue begins to move independently of the rest of the tongue as part of the mature swallowing pattern (ie, the tip of the tongue intermittently rises to the ridge behind the top front teeth to initiate the swallow)

Date	Feeding Checklist: 12–15 Months
	Lips may close during the swallow
	Lip movements become increasingly mature and/or sophisticated (eg, lip corners and cheeks move to control food manipulation within the mouth by 15 months)
	Top front teeth can remove food from bottom lip
	Can easily bite through a soft cookie with the front teeth
	Eats chopped-up table food and very soft meats (eg, stewed chicken, ground meat)
	Top first molars come in (14–16 months)
	Continuous, consecutive sucks (three or more) occur while drinking from an open cup, a cup with a recessed lid, and a straw
	Child is ready for weaning from the bottle (only given before bed); mostly drinks from an open cup, a cup with a recessed lid, and a straw; some breast-feeding may continue
	Holds an open cup and drinks with some spillage (12 months)
	If cup has handle(s), holds handle(s) when drinking (12 months)

Between 12 and 15 months, your child will pick up small food pieces with the tips of the thumb and index finger. You will also see your child put food pieces into a bowl. Self-feeding with a spoon will usually begin between 12 and 14 months; however, you may see your child turn the spoon over on the way to the mouth.

Your child's jaw, lips, and tongue are continuing to learn to move independently of one another. The tongue (front-back) and the transverse (side) tongue reflexes are seen less. The tip of the tongue is also continuing to learn to move independently of the rest of the tongue. This is important for the development of the mature swallowing pattern and for effective food manipulation within the

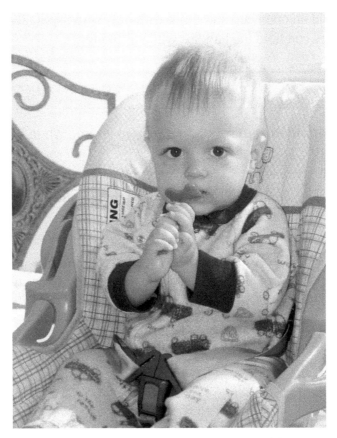

Photo 6.12: Anthony is learning to self-feed with a spoon at 12 months.

mouth. At this time, the tip of your child's tongue will intermittently rise to the ridge behind the top front teeth to begin the swallow.

Lip movements continue to develop. The lips may close during the swallow. In addition to increased lip movement necessary to clear the spoon, each lip corner is learning to move independently of the rest of the lips. By around 15 months, the lip corners and cheeks help control where food goes within the mouth.

During the 12- to 15-month period, the top front teeth can now remove food from the bottom lip, and your child can easily bite through a soft cookie with the front teeth. Your child will be eating chopped-up table food and very soft meats (such as stewed chicken and ground meat). The top first molars usually come in between 14 and 16 months of age.

Your child's breathing patterns continue to mature, allowing her to drink from an open cup or straw with three or more sucks in a row. The 12- to 15-month period is when most parents wean their children from the bottle. The bottle or breast is provided primarily as a snack before bedtime, and drinks throughout the day are given with an open cup, a cup with a recessed lid, or a straw. By around 12 months, your baby can hold an open cup and drink with only some spillage. If the cup has handles, your baby can hold the handles while drinking.

Date	Feeding Checklist: 15–18 Months
	Scoops food with spoon, but may spill some when bringing to the mouth
	Jaw, lips, and tongue continue to learn to move independently of one another
	The tongue (front-back) reflex is seen less and less, seems to be disappearing (12–18 months); the transverse (side) tongue reflex is seen less and less, seems to be disappearing (9–24 months)
	Different parts of each structure continue to learn to move separately (eg, the tip of the tongue moves independently of the rest of the tongue; each lip corner contracts independently of the rest of the lips)
	The top front teeth remove food from the bottom lip as the lip moves inward
	Continuous, consecutive sucks (three or more) occur while drinking from an open cup, a cup with a recessed lid, and a straw; may bite on the rim of an open cup for jaw stability
	Bottom cuspids come in (16–18 months)
	Coordinates diagonal rotary jaw movement for chewing
	Lips are quite active during chewing; lip corners and cheeks work independently of the rest of the lips and jaw to help to place and collect food

Between 15 and 18 months, your child will scoop food with a spoon but may spill some food while bringing the spoon to the mouth. The jaw, lips, and tongue continue to learn to move independently of one another. The different parts of each structure also continue to learn to move independently of one another. The top front teeth remove food from the bottom lip as this lip moves inward. The tongue (front-back) and transverse (side) tongue reflexes are seen less.

Maturing breathing patterns help your child drink from an open cup, a cup with a recessed lid, and a straw with continuous sucks and swallows. However, your child may still bite on the cup rim to stabilize the jaw. The bottom cuspids emerge between 16 and 18 months. Your child will use coordinated diagonal rotary chewing with food. Your child's lips become even more active during chewing. The lip corners and cheeks now work independently of the rest of the lips and jaw to help place and collect food within the mouth.

Date	Feeding Checklist: 18–21 Months
	Good control of swallowing develops by 18 months
	The tongue (front-back) reflex is seen less and less, seems to be disappearing (12–18 months); the transverse (side) tongue reflex is seen less and less, seems to be disappearing (9–24 months)
	Jaw, lips, and tongue continue learning to move independently of one another
	Different parts of each structure continue learning to move separately (eg, the tip of the tongue moves independently of the rest of the tongue; each lip corner contracts independently of the rest of the lips)
	Eats chopped foods, including many meats and raw vegetables
	May still bite down on cup rim to stabilize jaw
	Top cuspids come in (18–20 months)
	Jaw stability increases substantially (16–24 months)
	Can bite through a hard cookie but may struggle a little with this
	Can chew with closed lips

Date	Feeding Checklist: 18–21 Months
	Development of the mature swallowing pattern continues (mature, adultlike tip of the tongue elevation during swallowing that began at 12 months is becoming well established); coughing and/or choking is seldom seen
	Can take all liquids from an open cup, a cup with a recessed lid, or a straw (is weaned from the bottle; may continue some breast-feeding)
	Tries to feed Mom, Dad, or care provider
	Tries to wash and dry hands

Maturing respiration supports good control of swallowing by 18 months. By 18 months, the tongue (front-back) reflex is usually not seen, and the transverse (side) tongue reflex is seen less. Your child's jaw, lips, and tongue continue learning to work independently of one another. Different parts of each structure also continue learning to work separately.

Now your child can eat chopped table foods, including many meats and raw vegetables. Your child may continue to bite down on the open cup rim to stabilize the jaw. The top cuspids emerge between 18 and 20 months. Your child can now chew with closed lips. The tip of the tongue frequently rises to the area behind the top front teeth during the swallow. The mature, adultlike swallow is becoming well established. Coughing and choking are seldom seen.

Your child can now drink all liquids from an open cup, a cup with a recessed lid, or a straw. You have weaned your child from the bottle, but some moms may choose to continue some breast-feeding. Your child may try to feed you, and she will try to wash and dry her hands as part of the meal process.

Date	Feeding Checklist: 24 Months
	Jaw, lips, and tongue continue learning to move independently of one another
	Different parts of each structure continue learning to move separately (eg, the tip of the tongue moves independently of the rest of the tongue; each lip corner contracts independently of the rest of the lips)

Date	Feeding Checklist: 24 Months
	Bottom second molars come in (20–24 months)
	Top second molars come in (24–30 months)
	Jaw stability increases substantially (16–24 months)
	All first (primary) teeth come in by 24–30 months
	Can bite through a hard cookie with ease
	Uses lips on cup rim (no longer needs to bite on cup rim for stability)
	Does not spill liquid from an open cup when drinking
	Can drink from a small open cup held in one hand (20–22 months)
	Has palm up when bringing a spoon or fork to the mouth (parent still stabs food for the child with a fork)
	The transverse (side) tongue reflex is seen less and less, seems to have disappeared by 24 months
	Can easily move the tongue tip to place and collect food for chewing and swallowing
	Can chew with closed lips by using both diagonal rotary and circular rotary jaw movements
	Mature swallowing pattern is established (ie, the tip of the tongue touches the area behind the top front teeth to initiate the swallow)

By 24 months of age, your child's jaw, lips, and tongue are working independently of one another. The different parts of each structure are also skilled at moving separately. The bottom second molars come in between 20 and 24 months. The top second molars come in between 24 and 30 months. All first or primary teeth come in by 24 to 30 months. This helps to complete the development of jaw stability, which has increased substantially between 16 and 24 months. This jaw stability allows your child to bite though a hard cookie with ease.

The development of jaw stability and lip growth allows your child to drink from an open cup by using her lips only. Your child will no longer need to bite down on the cup rim to stabilize her jaw. Also, your child can now drink from an open cup without spilling the contents. By 20 to 22 months, your child can drink from a small open cup held in one hand.

Your child can now bring a spoon or fork to the mouth with the palm of the hand up. You will still have to help your child stab food with the fork, and you will need to closely monitor your child's use of the fork. We don't want your child to poke herself.

Your child's transverse (side) tongue reflex will seem to disappear by 24 months. She can easily move the tongue tip to place and collect food for chewing and swallowing. Your child can now chew with closed lips by using both diagonal rotary and circular rotary jaw movement. Diagonal rotary jaw movement means that your child moves the jaw to each side diagonally and then back to the center. Circular rotary jaw movement means that your child moves her jaw in a circle. This is the most sophisticated pattern of chewing and the one you (hopefully) use as an adult.

Your child now has a mature swallowing pattern and seldom loses control of the swallow. The mature swallowing pattern involves touching the tip of the tongue to the ridge behind the top front teeth to begin the swallow, with the tongue slightly cupped, the sides of the tongue sealing against the sides of the palate, and the tongue systematically moving the food or liquid back to the throat.

Now you have an appreciation for all that your child accomplishes in feeding development by the age of 2 years. Let's move on to speech development in chapter 7. This is another truly amazing process.

The Secrets to Good Speech Development

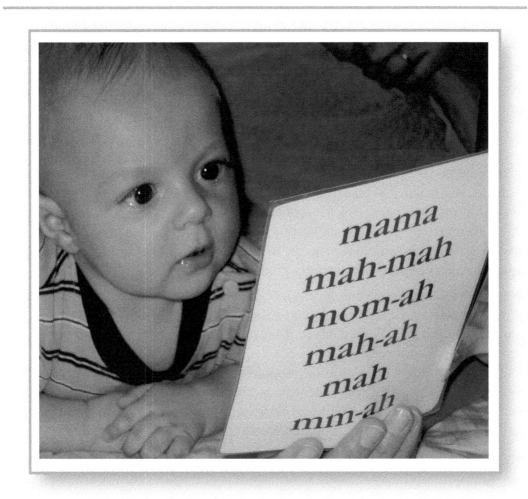

Key Topics in This Chapter

■ Tips to Encourage Good Vocal Development from Birth

■ Speech Sound Development from 1 Month of Age to 8 Years

■ Essentials for Intelligible Speech Production and Communication

■ Speech and Communication Development Up to 3 Years of Age

■ What to Do If Your Child Is Not on Track with Speech and Communication Development

■ Combination of Specific Treatment Ideas for Young Children with Speech and Communication Problems

Speech is one of the most refined fine motor functions in the body, and we are often judged by our speaking abilities. When a baby is born, the mouth moves basically as a unit (the jaw, lips, and tongue move together). However, babies do communicate from birth through vocalization and body language.

During the first 3 years of life, your child learns to move the mouth in a very sophisticated manner to produce speech. Your baby will produce many speech sounds during the first year. First words appear around 1 year of age. Two-word phrases and/or sentences appear around 2 years of age. Your 3-year-old child is usually speaking in simple sentences. Between the ages of 3 and 8 years, your child's speech becomes increasingly precise.

However, if the parts of your child's mouth do not learn to move independently of one another with appropriate awareness, skill, and direction of movement, your child's speech may be delayed. Many children have delayed speech development for this reason. In this chapter, we will talk about how to keep your child on track with speech development. We begin with tips to encourage good vocal and speech development from birth. If your child happens to have a problem with speech, you will find information in this chapter that can guide you in getting the help your child may need.

Tips to Encourage Good Vocal and Speech Development from Birth

I have included checklists in this chapter to help you know what to expect as your child develops speech and communication skills. However, here are some general ideas to encourage your child's vocal and speech development from birth:

1. From birth, give your child plenty of opportunities to interact and vocalize with you. These will naturally occur throughout the day when your baby is awake. Be sure to set aside some time each day to interact and communicate with your baby. This is the fun part of having a baby.

2. If using a pacifier, use it only for calming. Take the pacifier out of your baby's mouth when your baby has calmed. This allows your baby to play with vocalization. The suckle and sucking movements used with the pacifier and thumb-sucking are different from movements used for speech.

3. Start taking turns with vocalization from the beginning. When your baby vocalizes, listen. Then talk to your baby. Wait for your baby to vocalize. You can have early "pretend" conversations with your baby. For example, the baby vocalizes. The parent says, "Is that right?" The baby vocalizes. The parent says, "And what happened next?" The baby vocalizes. The parent says, "Really? And then what?" You are following your baby's lead in this "pretend" conversation. This is very empowering for you and your baby.

4. You can also imitate what your baby says. For example, if baby says, "ba ba ba," you say, "ba ba ba." This is another way to follow your baby's lead.

5. You can make positive statements to your child during your "pretend" conversation, such as, "You really are a happy boy!" Then wait for your baby to respond.

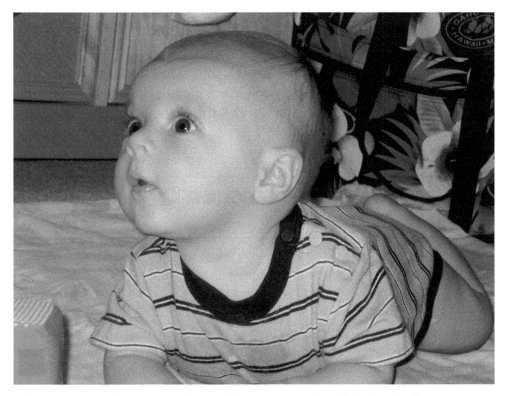

Photo 7.1: Anthony vocalizes with Mom and Dad during belly time.

6. By responding positively in a conversational manner to your baby, you encourage more vocalization. Your baby gets the idea that vocalization is communication.

7. Around 6 months of age, you can introduce pictures to your child. You can look at simple picture books (such as *Moo, Baa, La La La!* by Sandra Boynton[254]) or picture cards with your child, while naming and talking about the pictures. After you have done this for a while, you can start to ask your child to locate a picture with his eyes (eg, "Where is the cow?"). You will be surprised at how much language your child will learn this way. Reading to your child is one of the most important language development activities you can do. **I recommend that you read to your child daily.**

See information in the speech and communication development section of this chapter for more ideas on what to expect from your interactions with your baby at different ages. Other resources for parents on this topic include:

- *Beyond Baby Talk: From Sounds to Sentences—A Parent's Complete Guide to Language Development* by Kenn Apel, PhD, CCC-SLP, and Julie J. Masterson, PhD, CCC-SLP

- *Look Who's Talking! How to Enhance Your Child's Language Development Starting at Birth* by Laura Dyer, MCD, CCC-SLP

Speech Sound Development from 1 Month of Age to 8 Years[255-267]

The following chart will help you track your child's speech sound development from 1 month to 8 years of age, when speech sound development is complete. This is a unique compilation of information and materials. Parents, pediatricians, and therapists do not usually see all of this information on speech development in one place.

ACTIVITY 7.1: TRACK YOUR CHILD'S SPEECH SOUND PROGRESS

Place a date next to the skills your child is accomplishing. Circle the skills your child needs to accomplish. Know that the checklists in this book are approximate, and not absolute. Every child has his own unique developmental process.

This checklist is a guide to let you know if your child is basically on track or not. If you are concerned about your child's development, speak with your pediatrician and other appropriate professionals (such as a speech-language pathologist).

Date	Age	Speech Sound Skills
	1 Month	Makes vowel-like sounds similar to short "*a*" and long "*e,*" with sound coming mostly through the nose instead of the mouth
	2–3 Months	Vocalizes mostly vowel-like sounds (up to five different vowel-like sounds, with sound often coming through the nose); vowel-like sounds include short "*e,*" "*i,*" "*u,*" "*a,*" and "oo" as in the word "book"[268–269]
	2–3 Months	Makes consonant-like sounds "*h,*" "*k,*" and "*g,*" heard from the back of the mouth/throat
	2–3 Months	May begin to vocalize simple sound combinations (eg, "ba ba," "da da")[270] during crying or cooing
	3–4 Months	Makes long vowel-like sounds with cooing (eg, long "*e*" and "*a*")
	3–4 Months	May hear consonant-like sounds "*p,*" "*b,*" and "*m,*" made with the lips
	3–4 Months	Babbling may include "ba ba ba," "da da da," or "ma ma ma,"[271] particularly when a parent or care provider is not interacting
	4–6 Months	Changes in consonantlike and vowel vocalizations are heard with consonant-vowel and vowel-consonant syllables developing; typical-sounding vowels heard
	4–6 Months	"Raspberry," "*k,*" "*g,*" "*p,*" and "*b*" sounds heard
	4–6 Months	May hear long "*o*" and "oo" and other vowels

ACTIVITY 7.1: (cont.)

Date	Age	Speech Sound Skills
	5–6 Months	Produces vowels made in the back of the mouth, such as long "*u*" and "*o*," short "*u*" and "*o*," and "*ough*," as in "bought"[272]
	5–6 Months	Babbles four syllables or more (eg, "ba ba ba ba"); may use different intonations and/or inflections with the same sounds
	5–6 Months	Plays with and/or practices putting different speech sounds together (eg, "bee," "daa," "moh," and "paa")[273]
	6–7 Months	Occasionally may combine two or more unique syllables when babbling (eg, "ba da"); says four unique syllables (eg, "ma ma ma," "pa pa pa," "ba ba ba," "da da da")
	6–7 Months	Begins to imitate two-syllable babbling; coos and/or babbles in 2–3–second segments[274]
	6–7 Months	Lip sounds "*p*," "*b*," and "*w*," tongue-tip sounds "*t*" and "*d*," "*m*" and "*n*" nasal sounds, "*k*" and "*g*" back-of-mouth sounds, and the gliding sound "*y*" are heard[275–276]
	7–9 Months	Begins to string vowels together in conversational, sentencelike vocalizations
	7–9 Months	Begins to imitate a parent's or care provider's speech sounds (eg, "ba ba ba") and other sounds (eg, cough)
	7–9 Months	More consonant sounds are heard; vowels and consonants are more distinguishable; often says the same syllable over and over (eg, ba ba ba ba)

Date	Age	Speech Sound Skills
	9–12 Months	First words with meaning are heard (eg, "dada," "mama," "bye bye," "no," "go," "me"); three or more words are heard by 10–11 months; descriptive words begin at 11–12 months (eg, "all gone")
	9–12 Months	Puts together four or more syllables in his or her own language (ie, jargon); "*d*" and "*b*" sounds are heard frequently in babbling (10–12 months); syllables may be the same ("ba ba") or may vary ("ba da"); sounds like adult sentences without real words (11–14 months)
	9–12 Months	Peak of typical echolalia period occurs (ie, child parrots others' speech and intonation patterns)
	9–12 Months	Imitates simple sound combinations (eg, "mah," "bah," "dah," "doh"), as well some animal and other sounds
	9–12 Months	Occasionally attempts to imitate new and/or simple words (eg, names of toys or objects)
	12–15 Months	May use the same sound combinations for different words (eg, "ba" for "bottle" or "ball")
	12–15 Months	Uses five or more meaningful words; at 14–15 months will use at least seven meaningful words
	12–15 Months	Jargon consists of three to four syllables with a variety of sounds (eg, "ba da bo")
	12–15 Months	Says real words within conversational jargon
	12–15 Months	Spontaneously imitates words he or she has not said before

ACTIVITY 7.1: (cont.)

Date	Age	Speech Sound Skills
	12–15 Months	Produces many consonant speech sounds by 14–15 months, including lip sounds "p," "b," "m," and "w;" tongue-tip sounds "t," "d," and "n;" back-of-the-mouth sounds "k," "g," and "h," as well as the gliding sound "y"
	15–18 Months	Can imitate or repeat unfamiliar words with new sounds and/or sound combinations heard in conversation
	15–18 Months	Learns many new words slowly but constantly over time (about 10 new words per month)
	15–18 Months	Can say at least 15–20 words with meaning by 18 months, name five to seven items when asked, and use words to identify objects or events
	15–18 Months	Words consist primarily of consonant-vowel (eg, "me") and consonant-vowel-consonant-vowel (eg, "puppy") sounds[277–278]
	15–18 Months	Uses many consonant sounds in words by 18 months, including lip sounds "p," "b," "m," and "w;" lip and teeth sounds "f" and "v;" tongue-tip sounds "t," "d," "l," and "n;" as well as back-of-the-mouth sounds "g," "k," and "h"
	18–21 Months	Two-word stage begins; child imitates two- to three-word sentences with appropriate intonation but primarily speaks in single words; participates in conversation with adults
	18–21 Months	Can clearly and appropriately use 10–20 words

Date	Age	Speech Sound Skills
	18–21 Months	Begins using consonant-vowel-consonant words (eg, "cat") around 18 months
	18–21 Months	Uses many consonant sounds in words by 18 months, including lip sounds "*p*," "*b*," "*m*," and "*w*;" teeth-to-lip sounds "*f*" and "*v*;" tongue-tip sounds "*t*," "*d*," "*l*," and "*n*;" as well as back-of-the-mouth sounds "*g*," "*k*," and "*h*"
	18–21 Months	Vowel sounds developed early and are generally accurate; greatest difficulties occur with short "*e*" and "*i*"[279]
	21–24 Months	Says two or more words in simple sentences (eg, "Go bye bye," "No cookie")
	21–24 Months	Echolalia and parroting decrease
	21–24 Months	Clearly and appropriately uses 20+ words
	21–24 Months	Tries to talk about experiences or events by using words and jargon
	21–24 Months	Is more likely to imitate speech when a variety of interesting toys and materials are present[280]
	21–24 Months	Can say between 50 and 270 words (mostly nouns with some verbs, adjectives, adverbs, and pronouns)
	21–24 Months	Primarily uses speech to express self and is understood by an unfamiliar person 50% of the time (22 months)[281]

ACTIVITY 7.1: (cont.)

Date	Age	Speech Sound Skills
	21–24 Months	Uses a full range of vowel, diphthong, and consonant sounds in speech[282]
	21–24 Months	By 24 months, the following sounds are heard in the beginning of words: lip sounds "*b*," "*p*," "*m*," and "*w*;" tongue-tip sounds "*t*," "*d*," and "*n*;" back-of-the-mouth sounds "*k*," "*g*," and "*h*;" teeth-to-lip sounds "*f*" and "*v*;" and the noisy sound "*s*"[283–285]
	21–24 Months	By 24 months, the following sounds are heard at the end of words: lip sound "*p*," tongue-tip sounds "*t*" and "*n*," back-of-the-mouth sounds "*k*" and "*r*," and the noisy sound "*s*"[286–288]
	21–24 Months	May leave final sounds out of words (eg, "ca" instead of "cat"), may simplify words (eg, "cown" instead of "clown"), may say "*t*" or "*d*" in place of "*k*" or "*g*" (eg, "tat" instead of "cat"), may say "*w*" for "*r*" ("wed" instead of "red")
	2–3 Years[289–290]	Says words clearly; speech is understandable
	2–3 Years	Speaks in simple two- and three-word sentences
	2–3 Years	Can say at least "*p*," "*b*," "*m*," "*h*," "*n*," "*w*," "*t*," "*d*," "*k*," "*g*," and "*ng*" sounds
	2–3 Years	Says vowels, including diphthongs
	2–3 Years	Varies loudness of voice

Date	Age	Speech Sound Skills
	2–3 Years	May leave out unstressed syllable (eg, "nana" for "banana") or last sound in a word (eg, "ca" for "cat")
	2–3 Years	May say "w" for "r" (eg, "wed" for "red")
	2–3 Years	May simplify words (eg, "side" instead of "slide")
	3–4 Years	Speech becomes more precise
	3–4 Years	Speaks in simple sentences
	3–4 Years	Vocabulary increases to 900-1000 words, using about 12,000 words per day[291–292]
	3–4 Years	Most vowel sounds are accurate[293–295]
	3–4 Years	Can say at least "p," "b," "m," "h," "n," "w," "k," "g," and "d" sounds accurately
	3–4 Years	At least 50% of children can say "t," "ng," "f," "y," "r," "l," and "s" sounds accurately[296]
	3–4 Years	Consonant blends (eg, "bl," "br," "dr") appear and are established[297]
	4 Years	Begins to form increasingly complex sentences
	4 Years	Vocabulary increases to 1500-1600 words, using about 15,000 per day[298–299]
	4 Years	Can say "p," "b," "m," "h," "n," "w," "k," "g," "d," "t," "ng," "f," and "y" sounds accurately

ACTIVITY 7.1: (cont.)

Date	Age	Speech Sound Skills
	4 Years	At least 50% of children can say "r," "l," "s," "ch," "sh," and "z" sounds accurately[300]
	5 Years	Uses adultlike language
	5 Years	Vocabulary increases to around 2200 words
	5 Years	Can say "p," "m," "h," "n," "w," "b," "k," "g," "d," "t," "ng," "f," "y," "r," "l," "s," "ch," "sh," "z," and "v" sounds accurately
	5 Years	At least 50% of children can say "th," as in the word "this," accurately[301]
	6 Years	Vocabulary increases to around 2600 words
	6 Years	Can say most speech sounds, including "th," as in "think," and the "zh" sound that is in the middle of words like "measure" and the end of words like "garage" accurately[302]
	7 Years	Speech sound production continues to mature
	7 Years	Some children continue to work on saying consonant blends; the speech sounds "s," "z," "v," and "th," as in the word "this;" as well as the "zh" sound that is in the middle of words like "measure" and the end of words like "garage"[303–304]
	8 Years	Can say complicated consonant blends (eg, "str," "sl," "sk," "st," and "dr") accurately
	8 Years	Speech sound production is mature

Essentials for Intelligible Speech Production and Communication

Speech is a "light-touch act,"[305] requiring that appropriate sensory information be sent through the tactile (touch) and proprioceptive (inner awareness in muscles and joints) systems. The functioning of the tactile and proprioceptive systems affects many of the processes used in good speech production. Speech does not require a great deal of strength. It requires only enough strength.

The following are all very important for intelligible speech communication: accurate consonant and vowel sound production; good speech breathing; appropriate intraoral pressure; adequate dissociation, grading, and direction of mouth movement; tongue retraction; hand-mouth connection; and other nonverbal forms of communication. These areas must be treated systematically when a child has a speech problem. Many speech-language pathologists have been trained to work with consonant sounds and nonverbal communication. However, fewer have been adequately trained to treat problems with vowel sounds; speech breathing; intraoral pressure; and dissociation, grading, and direction of mouth movement.

While appropriate consonant sound production is important for intelligible speech, vowel sound production is at least equally important for speech intelligibility. Vowels require significant jaw grading and breath control. Children who don't develop good vowel sounds are often very difficult to understand. Let's see how this works.

ACTIVITY 7.2: WHAT DO YOU DO WHEN YOU MAKE VOWEL SOUNDS?

- Place your hand under your chin.

- Now say the following vowels, and see what your jaw does: long "*e*" as in "eat," short "*i*" as in "it," long "*a*" as in "ate," short "*e*" as in "Ed," and short "*a*" as in "at."

- Do you feel your jaw gradually dropping (ie, grading)? Your tongue is pulled back in your mouth, and these vowels are made by the front of the tongue. Your lips are spread, similar to a smile.

- Place your hand under your chin again.

ACTIVITY 7.2: (cont.)

- Now say the following vowels, and see what your jaw does: long "*u*" as in "due," short "*u*" as in "put," long "*o*" as in "bow," "ough" as in "ought," and short "*o*" as in "odd."

- Do you feel your jaw gradually dropping (ie, grading) again? Your tongue is pulled back in your mouth, and these vowels are made by the back of the tongue. Your lips are round.

- Now speak a short sentence in just vowel sounds, with appropriate rhythm and intonation (eg, "Hello, how are you?"). In vowels, this would be "*-e-o, -ow a- u?*" Now try the same thing with just consonant sounds (ie, "*H-ll-, h-, -r, y-?*"). Which sentence can you understand? In this case, you understand the sentence with the vowel sounds, because the vowels carry much of the content of this message. Appropriate production of consonant sounds is equally important for intelligible speech. It is difficult to have intelligible speech without both.

You can now see why children who cannot produce vowels properly have significant speech problems. If your child has a problem saying vowel sounds, find a speech-language pathologist who knows how to treat these.

ACTIVITY 7.3: SPEECH BREATHING

- Place one hand on your abdomen, and one hand on your diaphragm (just below your ribs).

- Take a large breath in through your nose.

- Now, say the "ah" sound for 3 seconds. You can count in your mind ("one one-thousand, two one-thousand, three one-thousand").

- What do you feel in your abdomen and diaphragm? Do you feel the slow contraction of each area as you let the air out?

This type of breath control is similar to what you use when you speak. Speech requires a large inhalation (breath in) and a slow, controlled exhalation (breath out). According to Dr Raymond D. Kent, "speech breathing is relatively more work for young children than for adults."[306] Here, we will talk about your child's respiratory development.

Your child will experience significant respiratory development between birth and approximately 18 years of age. Your newborn baby breathes shallow and fast (between 30 and 80 breaths per minute at rest)[307] and appears to breathe with his belly. This is because the structures of the chest, head, and neck are small and close together. They have not yet developed.

When your baby was born, he had few "terminal air sacs" in the lungs.[308] Development of these sacs (ie, alveoli) begins around 2 months of age and is complete around 8 years of age. These air sacs are responsible for getting oxygen to your baby's bloodstream. Oxygen is important for every life process.

Between 3 and 5 months, your infant develops head control. While your infant is learning to control his head, neck, and upper spine relative to gravity, he is also strengthening the muscles throughout the body needed for more mature breathing. You will see your baby leaning on his forearms when he is on his belly. As your baby rocks the body from side to side, the lower chest, abdominal musculature, and pelvis are working. These activities help to move the shoulders and ribcage downward. Now your baby has a neck, his upper chest area is more open, his breathing will slow down, and he will produce more vocal sounds.[309]

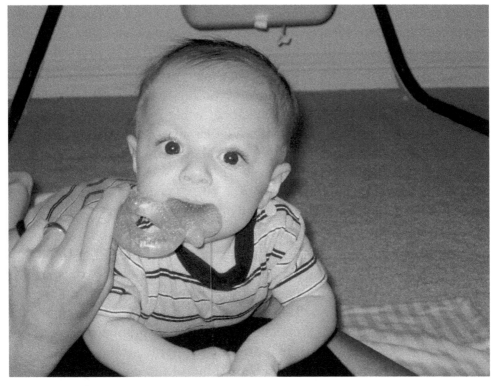

Photo 7.2: Belly time is important for the development of speech breathing.

Your baby's ability to "grade air flow"[310] begins with coordinated sucking, swallowing, and breathing during feeding. It develops or matures significantly during the first year of life, as your child simultaneously develops postural control. Postural control develops as your baby experiences different body positions and movement patterns. Having belly time while your baby is awake is critical for this development. See chapter 3 to read more about the importance of belly time.

As your baby experiences different positions and movements in the body (such as having belly time and lying on his side while awake, learning to roll, and learning to crawl), your baby is also developing breath control. During this period of time, you will hear a constant increase in your baby's amount and type of "vocal play."[311]

Between 6 and 12 months, your baby will experiment with much vocal sound play, including changes in pitch, intonation, and loudness. Your baby can now hold his spine up against gravity (ie, sit up), reach across the center of his body, get on his hands and knees, and crawl. These activities are very important for the development of good breath control, because they work the back, chest, rib, abdominal, and diaphragm muscles. This leads to three-dimensional breathing movements by 12 months.[312]

Your 1-year-old child has a breathing rate of 15 to 40 breaths per minute (the adult rate is 10 to 22 breaths per minute). By the time your child is 3 years old, breathing is well coordinated with speech. Between 3 and 10 years of age, your child's respiratory system will continue to mature. According to Dr Raymond D. Kent, the general breathing pattern for speech is fairly close to that of adults by age 7.[313] Your child's respiratory system will continue to develop until 15 to 18 years of age.

When your child's respiratory system reaches maturity, 40% of quiet breathing time is inhalation, and 60% is exhalation, according to Oetter, Richter, and Frick. Ten percent of speech time is inhalation, while 90% is exhalation.[314] Breathing for speech production requires a larger air volume than breathing at rest (ie, conversational speech uses 25% of vital capacity, loud speech uses 40% of vital capacity, and quiet breathing uses 10% to 15% of vital capacity).[315] Vital capacity is the largest quantity of air that can be exhaled from the lungs and airways after a person breathes in as much air as possible.[316]

Good speech breathing is not only important for speech sound development, it is important for the other vocal features that express meaning. Intonation, inflection, rate, rhythm, and stress are called *prosodic features* by speech-language pathologists. If someone speaks with appropriate rhythm, intonation, and inflection (eg, "Hel↑ lo↓. How are you?↑"), you can understand him better than if someone speaks in a monotone voice with poor rhythm. If someone speaks with inappropriate syllable stress, this will also affect your ability to understand him. Just think of the word "syllable," for example. Which is easier to understand? When someone says "syl´able," or when someone says "syl a´ ble?"

Similarly, it is difficult to understand someone who speaks too quickly and/or with poor rhythm. It is much easier to understand someone who speaks slowly. Many children with speech problems do not have appropriate breath control and try to speak more rapidly than their motor ability will allow. They also tend to speak without appropriate rhythm.

Air for speech needs to come straight through the mouth (no cheek puffing) with appropriate intraoral pressure. The tongue, lips, and cheeks stop, restrict, or shape the sounds of speech. If your child does not have the ability to maintain appropriate intraoral pressure, his speech will not be precise. We need appropriate intraoral pressure for adequate breast-feeding; drinking from a bottle, cup, and straw; swallowing; bubble blowing; horn blowing; and speech.

Good intraoral pressure for speech production is created primarily by the cheeks maintaining dynamic stability against the gums and teeth (ie, keeping the cheeks against the teeth and gums while maintaining the ability to make needed adjustments). It is also related to the precision of jaw, lip, and tongue movements. The lips, jaw, and tongue need to have appropriate dissociation (ie, one structure moving separately from another), grading (ie, structure moving just enough for the task or activity), and direction of movement. These processes are all important for good speech production.

You can experience differences in intraoral pressure during speech by completing Activity 7.4.

ACTIVITY 7.4: INTRAORAL PRESSURE DURING SPEECH

1. Say the words "Penelope" and "bugaboo." Notice that you seal the inner borders of your lips for the "*p*" and "*b*" sounds so that air pressure can build in your mouth.

2. Feel how your cheeks stay against your gums and teeth. They are not stuck there. They are dynamically stable.

3. Now, say the same words and let your cheeks and lips puff out as you say them.

4. How do you sound now?

Children who have not developed the ability to dynamically stabilize the cheeks during speech have a problem maintaining appropriate intraoral pressure for speech. This significantly affects intelligibility.

ACTIVITY 7.5: TONGUE RETRACTION DURING SPEECH

(Adapted from an exercise by Sara Rosenfeld-Johnson)[317]

1. Say a long "*e*," as in the word "eat." Keep saying this sound until you can feel where your tongue moves and touches.

2. Do you feel your tongue pulled back in your mouth? Do you feel your tongue touching your teeth and gums in the back?

3. Now, I want you to say the alphabet quickly and naturally. This is something you don't need to think about because you know this automatically. As you say the alphabet, where is your tongue most of the time?

4. Do you feel your tongue "holding on" at or near the same location in the back of the mouth where you said the long "*e*" sound?

5. Is your tongue stuck back there, or is it dynamically stable (ie, holding relatively still while maintaining the ability to make needed adjustments)? Your tongue is dynamically stable and is not stuck. Your tongue stabilizes for speech production in retraction (ie, pulled back).

Children who have difficulty dynamically stabilizing their tongues in retraction during speech have significant speech intelligibility problems. Children with Down syndrome often have this difficulty. However, I have seen this problem in many other children. For example, children with enlarged tonsils often do not retract their tongues, as this may block their airways.

ACTIVITY 7.6: DISSOCIATION, GRADING, AND DIRECTION OF MOVEMENT FOR SPEECH

1. Hold your tongue in the bottom of your mouth as you say the words, "Hello. How are you?"

2. How does this sound? It sounds very imprecise.

3. When you do this, you are not separating your tongue movement from your jaw. That means that your tongue and jaw are not dissociated. Your jaw movements may be graded appropriately (ie, moving just enough for the speech sounds), but your tongue movements are not graded, dissociated, or properly directed.

4. What about direction of tongue movement? Your tongue is not retracted (pulled back) to the place where your tongue typically stabilizes in a dynamic way for connected speech. The tip of your tongue does not move up for the "l" sound, which is another problem with direction of movement.

5. This greatly affects your speech intelligibility when you try to speak this way.

You can see why children who do not learn the skills of dissociation, grading, and direction of movement in the mouth have difficulty being understood. As a therapist, I have treated many children with speech problems who had these underlying problems.

ACTIVITY 7.7: THE HAND-MOUTH CONNECTION FOR SPEECH

1. Restrict the use of your hands while you try to explain to your spouse or significant other a story you heard today on the news.

2. Now tell your spouse or significant other about another story you heard on the news while your hands are free.

3. Which story was easier to tell? Don't forget that we, as humans, have a hand-mouth connection neurologically, from birth. The use of our hands is a natural part of our expression.

According to Oetter, Richter, and Frick, it has been suggested that between 87% and 95% of communication is nonverbal.[318] Nonverbal communication includes facial expression and body language. Your infant will show you a full range of facial expressions within the first few months of life. Before your infant can talk, your infant will communicate with you primarily through facial expression and body language. As your child develops, he will add speech to facial expression and body language for clear and effective communication. Speech is the most efficient and effective means of communication, particularly when appropriate facial expression and body language are used.

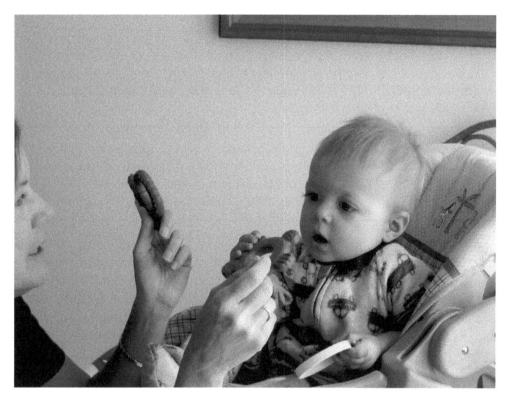

Photo 7.3: Communication often begins with making choices.

Therapists and other early intervention specialists often teach children sign language and other forms of self-cueing when children have difficulty expressing themselves verbally. When the child uses a hand signal or another hand movement for self-cueing, the child often produces a word or word approximation at the same time. The use of sign language and other hand movements in self-cueing are examples of the hand-mouth connection to facilitate communication. See the section of this chapter entitled, "A Combination of Specific Ideas for Young Children with Speech and Communication Problems" for more detail.

Speech and Communication Development Up to 3 Years of Age

In this section, you will find checklists for speech and communication development from 1 month to 3 years of age. It includes some of the information from the previous speech sound development checklist. You can see how this information fits into your child's entire communication-development picture.

Again, these checklists are not absolute. All children have their own unique developmental patterns. However, you can use these checklists to see if your child is basically on track. You can also get ideas for interacting with your child. If you have any concern about your child's development, speak with your child's pediatrician and other appropriate professionals (such as a speech-language pathologist or other early intervention specialist). Place dates next to the skills your child accomplishes.

DEVELOPMENTAL CHECKLISTS: COMMUNICATION DEVELOPMENT[319-338]	
Date	**Age: 1 Month**
	Prefers to look at human faces
	Begins to smile socially
	Can imitate some mouth movements (open mouth, tongue out)
	Significant jaw growth occurs (birth to 1 year)[339-341]
	Jaw stability is developing; lip and tongue stability follows (birth to 1 year)[342-343]
	Significant lip and tongue growth occurs (birth to 2 years)
	Baby cries during inhalation and exhalation, with exhalation getting longer over time[344]
	Cries vary (may begin to hear a short "hunger cry" of approximately 1.3 seconds, a longer "pain cry" of approximately 2.6 seconds, or an "angry cry")[345-346]
	Baby gets quiet when he hears human voices and vocalizes when he hears Mom's voice
	Baby can match the voice pitch and duration of that of a care provider[347]
	Baby makes vowel-like sounds similar to a short "*a*" and a long "*e*," with sound coming mostly through the nose instead of the mouth

Your 1-month-old baby prefers to look at human faces rather than objects. You will see your baby start to smile socially. You may even see him imitate some mouth movements, such as an open mouth or the tongue out. No, this is not your imagination.

Your baby's most significant jaw growth will occur during his first year of life. Jaw stability is developing during this time, with lip and tongue stability following. Your baby will have significant lip and tongue growth between birth and 2 years of age. See chapter 8 for further details on mouth development.

Your baby will cry when breathing in and breathing out. The cry when breathing out gets longer over time. This is important for speech development, as discussed previously, because vocalization for speech requires a large inhalation and a slow, controlled exhalation. You can also begin to tell the difference between your baby's short cry for hunger, his longer cry for pain, and his angry cry.

Your baby will get quiet when he hears human voices but may vocalize when hearing Mom's voice. He may match the pitch (high or low sound) and length of Mom's voice or that of another care provider. He makes vowel-like sounds (short "*a*" as in "at" and long "*e*" as in "eat") that mostly come through his nose. The sound may come through your baby's nose instead of his mouth because the space within the mouth is still very small.

Date	Age: 2–3 Months
	Baby begins to show anticipation of feeding and being held through body language, including sustained eye contact and looking at items of interest (eg, a bottle)
	Baby follows a parent's or care provider's movements with his eyes
	Baby's mouth begins to change shape, and his tongue begins to move more within the mouth
	Baby learns to send air through the mouth when cooing
	Baby learns to control the flow of air across the vocal cords in the voice box

Date	Age: 2–3 Months
	Baby vocalizes in response to speech, environmental sounds, or a smile
	Baby has an increased range of vocal sounds and a strong-sounding cry
	Baby has cries for hunger, discomfort, sleepiness, and attention
	Baby makes soft sounds for pleasure and a loud "*a*" sound for distress
	Baby may laugh, chuckle, or coo
	Baby vocalizes with mostly vowel-like sounds (up to five different vowel-like sounds, with sound often coming through the nose); vowel-like sounds include short "*e*," "*i*," "*u*," "*a*," and "*oo*" sounds[348-349]
	Baby makes consonant-like sounds "*h*," "*k*," and "*g*," heard from the back of the mouth or throat
	Baby may begin to vocalize simple sound combinations (eg, "ba ba," "da da")[350] during crying or cooing

At 2 to 3 months, your baby will begin to show you he is anticipating or looking forward to being held or fed. You will see this in his body language (eg, his body is alert and moving) and eye contact. He will begin to maintain eye contact with you and will look at items of interest, such as the bottle. He will also begin to watch you as you move.

Around 2 to 3 months of age, you will hear your baby make more vocal sounds in response to your speech, your smile, and sounds in the environment. He now has a wider range of vocal sounds and a strong-sounding cry. He is learning to manipulate the increasing space within his mouth; to control some movements of his jaw, tongue, lips, and cheeks; and to send air across the vocal cords in the voice box in an increasingly controlled way. You will hear a difference between your baby's cries for hunger, discomfort, sleepiness, and attention. He will make soft vocal sounds to express pleasure and a loud "*a*" sound to indicate distress.

Your baby will begin to laugh, chuckle, and coo. He is learning to direct air through his mouth instead of his nose during cooing (due to having more space in his mouth and increasing control of his oral structures). You will hear your baby produce up to five different vowel-like sounds, including a short "*e*" as in "Ed," short "*i*" as in "it," short "*u*" as in "put," short "*a*" as in "at," and "oo" as in book. You may also hear back-of-the-mouth and/or throat sounds, such as "*h*," "*k*," and "*g*," as well as some simple sound combinations, such as "ba ba" or "da da" during crying or cooing.

Date	Age: 3–4 Months
	Baby vocalizes when he sees objects move (eg, a mobile)
	Vocal turn-taking begins
	Baby listens to speech addressed to him
	Games of facial expression and body language begin
	Baby can manage more space developing between the structures in the mouth (jaw, lips, cheeks, and tongue) and in the throat (soft palate, epiglottis, and larynx)
	Baby laughs during play with body or objects
	Baby makes long vowel-like sounds with cooing (eg, long "*e*" and "*a*")
	May hear consonant-like sounds "*p*," "*b*," and "*m*" made with lips
	Babbling may include "ba ba ba," "da da da," or "ma ma ma,"[351] particularly when a parent or care provider is not interacting

At 3 to 4 months of age, your baby will often vocalize when he sees objects (such as a mobile) move. When you talk to your baby, you will notice the beginning of vocal turn-taking (you vocalize, then your baby vocalizes) and that your baby listens to your speech when you talk to him. You will also begin to play games with your baby by using different facial expressions and body movements (eg, the game "sooo big").

You will hear your baby laugh during play with his own body or toys. Now your baby has more control over the space developing between the structures in the mouth (jaw, lips, cheeks, and tongue) and in the throat (soft palate, epiglottis, and larynx). He is also learning to control his breathing and his voice. You will hear long, vowel-like sounds, such as "*e*" in "eat" and "*a*" in "ate," more frequently. You may also hear him produce the lip sounds "*p*," "*b*," and "*m*," or other consonant-like sounds. His babbling may include the sound combinations "ba ba ba," "da da da," or "ma ma ma," particularly if he is playing with a toy or his own body.

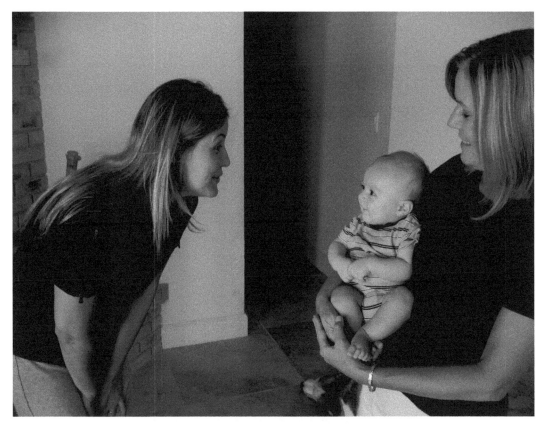

Photo 7.4: Anthony listens and makes eye contact as his mom Cris talks to him.

Date	Age: 4–6 Months
	Space between the mouth and nasal area increases (4–6 months)
	Open space in the mouth continues to increase through jaw growth and the reduction of sucking pads (4–6 months)
	The tongue moves up and down down and front-to-back with a little less cupping (4–6 months)
	Increased lip control develops (4–6 months)
	The gag reflex moves from the back ¾ of the tongue toward the back ¼ of the tongue (4–6 months)
	Teeth begin to come in with increased chewing and biting experiences (5–6 months)
	Appropriate intraoral air pressure is developing; changes are noted in voice, pitch, and babbling (4–6 months)
	The voice becomes louder as coordination improves between breathing and movements of the voice box (4–6 months)
	The voice is used to express a range of emotions (happy, mad, irritated, protesting, eager, satisfied); pitch and loudness changes are heard at 4–5 months
	Baby vocalizes when another person is singing and when others make new or unique vocalizations (3–6 months)
	Baby vocalizes when looking in the mirror or playing with a toy, when a person approaches without talking, or when he plays on his own (5–6 months)

Date	Age: 4–6 Months
	Baby can look where a caregiver is looking and look at an object with another person (4–6 months)
	Baby looks at the faces of his parents and care providers and imitates expressions (3–6 months)
	Baby begins taking conversation-like turns while vocalizing with a parent or care provider (ie, initiates vocalization, stops to hear vocalization, interrupts other person's vocalization) at 3–6 months
	Changes in consonant-like and vowel vocalizations are heard, with consonant-vowel and vowel-consonant syllables developing (4–6 months)
	"Raspberry" sounds and "*k*," "*g*," "*p*," and "*b*" sounds are heard (4–6 months)
	Typical-sounding vowels are heard; may hear long "*o*," "*oo*," and other vowels (4–6 months)
	Baby produces vowels made by the back of the tongue, such as long "*u*" and "*o*," short "*u*" and "*o*," and "*ough*" as in "bought" (5–6 months)[352]
	Baby babbles four syllables or more (eg, "ba ba ba ba"); may use different intonations or inflections with the same sounds (5–6 months)
	Baby plays with and/or practices putting different speech sounds together (eg, "bee," "daa," "moh," and "paa")[353] at 5–6 months

Your baby's mouth and vocal structures are undergoing significant changes between 4 and 6 months. The space in your baby's mouth and nasal area is increasing. This allows your child's resonance (quality of vocal sound) to begin to mature. Your child's jaw is growing, and the sucking pads are getting smaller.

Your baby has increasing control of the jaw, lips, and cheeks. The gag reflex is moving toward the back of the tongue. Now, your baby can begin to move different parts of the tongue without gagging.

Your baby is learning to build appropriate pressure within the mouth, which is needed to produce many speech sounds and eventually connected speech. You will hear changes in your baby's voice as the voice box is now lower in the neck and your baby starts to develop increasing control over breathing and the small muscles of the voice box. Your baby will change pitch and loudness, which is important for the development of vocal inflection, intonation, and stress. These are characteristics that speech-language pathologists call *prosodic features*. In addition to the production of consonant sounds, vowel sounds, and body language, these features carry a significant amount of the speech message.

Between 5 and 6 months of age, your child's teeth begin to come in with increased chewing and biting experiences. Your child's teeth are important structures for jaw development and stabilization. Jaw stabilization will be complete when the majority of your child's primary teeth are in, around 24 months of age.

Your baby participates in conversation-like turn-taking while he is vocalizing with you (he begins vocalizing so you will vocalize, he stops to hear your vocalizing, and he may interrupt your vocalizing). Your baby will also start to vocalize when you sing or make different and/or interesting sounds. It is fun to see how your baby imitates your facial expressions. Looking at faces and imitating facial expressions are very important skills that lead to a child's ability to interpret facial expression during communication interactions.

By 4 to 6 months, your baby will look where you are looking and look at an object with you. These are indicators that your baby is learning to interact appropriately with others. With all of the children currently being identified with autism, these early communication abilities are being scrutinized by professionals. Often, children with autism do not show these abilities.

At 4 to 5 months, your baby can use his voice to express a range of emotions, such as happiness, anger, irritation, eagerness, and satisfaction. You will notice your baby's voice getting louder. He also uses a variety of pitches (high, middle, and low) when babbling. The voice box is lower in the neck, and the muscles of the voice box are developing, allowing these pitch changes. At 5 to 6 months, your baby will vocalize while looking into a mirror, when playing with a toy, and when a person approaches your baby without talking.

Between 4 and 6 months, you will hear changes in your baby's consonant-like and vowel-like vocalizations. Your child is developing appropriate control of intraoral pressure within the mouth. You will remember from our previous

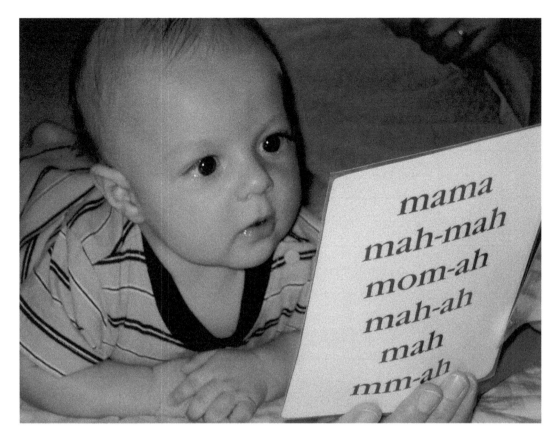

Photo 7.5: Anthony looks at a picture with his mom.

discussions of intraoral pressure that air for speech needs to come straight through the mouth (no cheek puffing). The tongue, lips, and cheeks stop, restrict, and shape the sounds of speech. The jaw also shapes the sounds of speech by being in the right position. You will hear both consonant-vowel (eg, "ba") and vowel-consonant (eg, "ab") syllables. Your baby will produce "raspberry" sounds and "*k*," "*g*," "*p*," and "*b*" sounds more consistently. You may also hear longer vowel sounds, such as "*o*" as in "bow" and "oo" as in "boo."

At 5 to 6 months of age, you may hear your child produce the full range of back vowel sounds (ie, long "*u*" as in "due," long "*o*" as in "bow," short "*u*" as in "put," short "*o*" as in "odd," and "ough" as in "ought"). When your child produces these vowels, his tongue is pulled back, and these sounds are produced by the back of his tongue. His length of babbling will move from three to four syllables (eg, "ba ba ba ba") using different intonations and inflections. This occurs because your baby's vocal (ie, voice box) and respiratory systems (ie, lungs and muscles that control breathing) are developing. You will also hear your baby play with or practice different sound combinations (eg, "bee," "daa," "moh," and "paa").[354]

Date	Mouth Development from 6–9 Months
	Most pronounced period of mouthing occurs (5–7 months)
	Bottom two front teeth (central incisors) come in (5–9 months)
	Top two front teeth (central incisors) come in (6–10 months)
	Bottom lateral incisors come in (7–20 months)
	Top lateral incisors come in (8–10 months)
	Gag reflex is located on the back third of the tongue (6–9 months)[355]
	Increased control of air through the throat, mouth, and nose develops

Date	Communication Development from 6–7 Months
	Baby may occasionally combine two or more unique syllables when babbling (eg, "ba da"); says four unique syllables (eg, "ma ma ma," "pa pa pa," "ba ba ba," "da da da")
	Baby begins to imitate two-syllable babbling; coos and babbles in 2–3–second segments[356]
	May hear lip sounds "p," "b," and "w;" tongue-tip sounds "t" and "d;" "m" and "n" sounds coming through the nose; back-of-the-tongue sounds "k" and "g;" and the gliding sound "y"[357–358]
	Baby vocalizes 50% of the time when he hears his name
	Baby appears to be naming things with his own sounds by using the same sounds for certain objects

Date	Communication Development from 6–7 Months
	Baby may begin to be less interactive around strangers (5½–8 months) and "checks in" with care provider when exploring independently[359–360]
	Between 6 and 8 months, interest in objects increases significantly (looking at, pointing to, reaching for, and using gestures to show use, such as picking up a telephone and putting it to the ear)

Date	Communication Development from 7–9 Months
	Baby plays speech and gesture games (eg, pat-a-cake, peek-a-boo)
	Baby sings with a parent or care provider with an occasional "real" word heard
	Baby vocalizes or raises voice to get attention or protest
	Baby begins using some standard gestures and body language (eg, head shaking for "no," waving hand for "bye-bye")
	Baby begins to string vowels together in conversational, sentence-like vocalizations
	Baby begins to imitate a parent's or care provider's speech sounds (eg, "ba ba ba") and other sounds (eg, a cough)
	More consonant sounds are heard; vowels and consonants are more distinguishable; baby often says same syllable over and over (eg, ba ba ba ba)
	Baby responds to parents' or care providers' vocalizations at least 80% of the time

The 6- to 9-month period is another significant period of mouth development for your baby. As you know, the most pronounced period of mouthing occurs between 5 and 7 months of age, when your baby is learning to discriminate shape, size, taste, and texture throughout the mouth. This helps your baby integrate his gag reflex so it is found toward the back of the tongue. Then the gag does not inhibit tongue movements for eating, drinking, or speech sound production. Good discrimination within the mouth is needed for placement of the mouth structures for good speech sound production.

During the 6- to 9-month period, your baby is developing increased control of the air flow through the voice box, mouth, and nose. This is important for the development of good resonance, intraoral pressure, loudness, inflection, intonation, stress, and rate, which are all key elements for intelligible speech production. If your child is missing any of these components, his speech intelligibility can be significantly affected. You will also notice the nice rhythm your child is developing during babbling. A good speech rhythm is important for adequate speech intelligibility.

Your child is getting his front teeth during this period of time. This will not only help your child begin to take bites of food, but tooth development is crucial for jaw development. Dynamic (active) jaw stability is very important for speech production. Vowels require graded jaw positions based on dynamic jaw stability. Remember the number of jaw positions you experienced when you produced the different vowel sounds in Activity 7.2? Vowels are found in just about every word in English and most other languages. Vowels, consonants, body language, vocal intonation and inflection, rate, rhythm, and stress carry the content of the message in speech.

The 6- to-12 month period is a time for increased vocal play, when your baby will experiment with many speech and nonspeech sounds, changes in tone of voice, and differing volume levels. You will hear longer sequences of speech sounds because your baby is developing increasing breath control.

Between 6 and 7 months, you may hear your baby combine two or more unique syllables (eg, "ba da"). You will hear four unique syllables in what therapists call "reduplicative babbling" (eg, "ma ma ma," "pa pa pa," "ba ba ba," and "da da da."). Your baby will also begin to imitate two-syllable combinations. His cooing and babbling now occurs in 2- to 3-second segments. In addition to vowel sounds, you will hear the lip sounds "*p*," "*b*," and "*w*;" the tongue-tip sounds "*t*" and "*d*;" the nasal sounds "*m*" and "*n*;" the back-of-the-tongue sounds "*k*" and "*g*;" and the gliding sound "*y*."

If you call your baby's name, he will vocalize about 50% of the time. Your baby will also seem to name things with his own sounds by using the same sounds over and over for certain objects or toys. However, your baby may become less interactive with strangers between 5½ and 8 months of age.

Between 6 and 8 months of age, you will notice your baby's interest in objects increase significantly. This is when your baby will look at, point to, reach for, and show the use of objects (eg, trying to push the buttons on the remote, putting a telephone receiver to his ear).

Between 7 and 9 months of age, your baby will begin to string vowel sounds together in conversational, sentence-like vocalizations. This is the beginning of what we call "jargon." This is also a really fun time with your baby because he will begin to play speech games involving gesturing and body language, such as "pat-a-cake" and "peek-a-boo." He will attempt to sing along with you, and you may hear an occasional "real" word in his singing.

Your baby will vocalize or raise his voice to get your attention or to protest during the 7- to 9-month period. He will begin using standard gestures and body language, such as shaking his head for "no" and waving his hand for "bye-bye." You may hear your baby begin to imitate more of your sounds (eg, "ba ba ba" or a cough). You will also hear your baby say more consonant sounds. Now, your baby will respond to your vocalizations most of the time. These, again, are important characteristics to observe if you have any concern regarding your child's development of interaction skills, which is a big concern for parents of children with autism.

Date	Age: 9–12 Months
	Bottom first molars come in (10–12 months)
	Baby says first words with meaning (eg, "dada," "mama," "bye-bye," "no," "go," or "me"), three or more words by 10–11 months, descriptive words at 11–12 months (eg, "all gone")
	Baby vocalizes to express surprise (eg, "ut oh") or frustration, to greet someone, or make a request
	Baby will call to parents or care providers with a word or answer a call from them
	Baby puts together at least four syllables in his own language (ie, jargon); "d" and "b" sounds are heard frequently in babbling (10–12 months); syllables may be the same ("ba ba") or may vary ("ba da"); adultlike sentences without real words are heard (11–14 months)

Date	Age: 9–12 Months
	Baby practices changes in speech volume, intonation, timing, patterns, and rate when playing on his own; begins to use these when vocalizing with others; peak of typical echolalia or parroting period occurs
	Baby imitates simple sound combinations (eg, "mah," "bah," "dah," "doh"), as well some animal and other sounds
	Baby occasionally attempts to imitate new or simple words (eg, names of toys or objects)
	Baby answers simple questions (eg, "Where's Mommy?") with gestures, body language, and/or vocalization
	Baby participates vocally in songs and rhymes
	Baby attempts communication as much as one time each minute (11–12 months)[361]
	Baby uses appropriate gestures for wants, needs, and desires (eg, pointing, reaching, and pantomime)
	Baby uses gestures and vocal sounds to get attention or help; makes vocal sounds while reaching for objects[362]
	Baby begins to point or reach to show or identify toys and objects when named
	Baby initiates gesture games with others (eg, peek-a-boo)
	Baby looks at toys and books with others; plays early games, such a knocking over blocks[363]

The 9- to 12-month period is a time when your child's mouth and vocal structures continue to grow and develop. Your child's bottom first molars come in between 10 and 12 months of age. You already know the importance of tooth development for jaw development. Molars not only allow your child to chew foods of increased texture, they seem critical for the development of jaw stability. Jaw stability is complete around the time that your child has most of his primary teeth, including the molars.

Between 9 and 12 months of age, you will hear your baby's first meaningful words (eg, "dada," "mama," bye-bye," "no," "go," or "me"). By 10 to 11 months, you will hear three or more words. By 11 to 12 months, you will hear descriptive words, such as "all gone." Your baby may say "ut oh" to express surprise. He will vocalize to express frustration, to greet someone, or to make a request. Your baby may also call to you with a word or answer you when you call to him.

Your baby's jargon increases with better breath control and support. You will hear him string four or more syllables together, producing long vocalizations that sound like conversation. You will frequently hear the sounds "*b*" and "*d*" in his babbling at 10 to 12 months. The syllables may contain the same or different consonant sounds (eg, "ba ba" or "ba da"). By 11 to 14 months, your baby's jargon sounds like adult sentences without real words.

Nine to 12 months is the peak of the typical echolalia period, when your baby immediately repeats many speech patterns he hears. You may be reminded of a talking parrot when you hear your baby do this. He will imitate simple sound combinations (eg, "mah," "bah," "dah," "doh"), occasional simple new words,

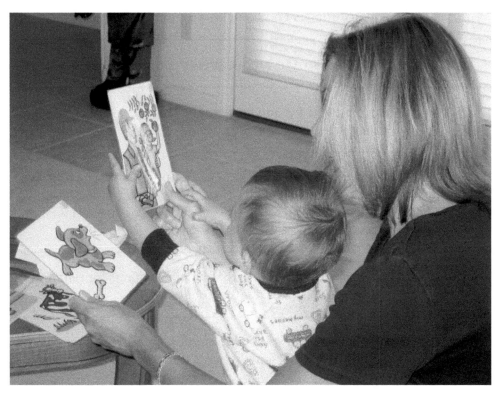

Photo 7.6: Anthony reaches for the picture of "dada" being named.

as well as some animal and other nonspeech sounds. The development of vocal imitation is another important milestone for your baby. Children with autism often have great difficulty with vocal imitation.

In addition to speech, your baby will use a number of appropriate gestures to indicate his wants, needs, and desires. These include pointing, reaching, and pantomime. When you name toys or objects, your baby may also point to or reach for them. He will begin to answer simple questions, such as "Where's Mommy?" by using gestures, body language, and/or vocalization. When he is playing on his own, you will hear changes in his speech volume, intonation, pattern, and rate. Your baby will also begin to use these when interacting with others, particularly if he is participating in singing and rhymes.

Your baby may attempt to communicate as often as one time per minute by 11 to 12 months of age. He will look at toys and books with you and other familiar people. You can play games together, such as knocking over blocks. Your child will also start a game like "peek-a-boo" with you.

Date	Age: 12–15 Months
	Respiration is maturing
	Top first molars come in (14–16 months)
	Significant lip and tongue growth occurs (12–24 months)
	Jaw, lips, and tongue continue to learn to move independently of one another
	Different parts of each structure continue to learn to move separately (eg, the tip of the tongue moves independently of the rest of the tongue, each lip corner contracts independently of the rest of the lips)
	Baby may use the same sound combinations for different words (eg, "ba" for "bottle" or "ball")
	Baby uses five or more meaningful words; by 14–15 months will use at least seven meaningful words

Date	Age: 12–15 Months
	Baby gestures and points with sounds and words to make requests; can name at least one object consistently
	Baby has a variety of gestures (eg, waving, blowing kisses, pointing)
	Jargon consists of three to four syllables with a variety of sounds (eg, "ba da bo")
	Baby says "real" words within conversational jargon
	Baby spontaneously imitates words not said before
	Baby produces many consonant speech sounds, including lip sounds "p," "b," "m," and "w;" tongue-tip sounds "t," "d," and "n;" back-of-mouth sounds "k," "g," and "h," as well as the gliding sound "y" by 14–15 months
	Baby can imitate at least three animal or other environmental, nonspeech sounds
	Baby tries to sing along with music or when playing by himself
	Baby changes pitch, loudness, rate, stress, and intonation when vocalizing (eg, pitch goes up for request, attention, and curiosity, and goes down for greetings, surprise, persistence, and attempts to be recognized)[364]
	Baby communicates frequently with real words and gestures (eg, shaking head "no")
	Baby interacts vocally with other children
	Conversational and gestural turn-taking becomes more routine

Date	Age: 12–15 Months
	Baby gives hugs and kisses to familiar people; is shy with strangers[365]
	Baby begins to go to adults for help or assistance, takes pride in accomplishments, and role plays or pretends[366]

Between 12 and 15 months of age, your child's mouth and vocal structures continue to mature. His lips and tongue grow rapidly between 12 and 24 months of age. His lips continue to learn to move independently of the jaw. Your child's tongue will not only move independently of the jaw, but the tip of the tongue and sides learn to move independently of the rest of the tongue. Independent movement of the tip of the tongue is used in speech sounds such as "*t*," "*d*," and "*n*," as well as the later-developing "*l*." The sides of your child's tongue also lift to stabilize the tongue for sounds such as "*t*," "*d*," and "*n*," as well as the later-developing sounds "*s*," "*z*," "*sh*," "*ch*," and soft "*g*." The tongue movements used in speech-sound production have been tracked via a process called *palatometry*.[367–368] Between 14 and 16 months, your child's top first molars will emerge, contributing to his jaw stability.

Your baby's overall communication skills also increase during the 12- to 15-month period. He will use five or more meaningful words (increasing to seven or more by 14 to 15 months) and will communicate frequently with "real" words and gestures (eg, shaking his head "no"). He may use the same sound combinations for different words (such as "ba" for "bottle" or "ball"). In addition to vowel sounds, your child will produce many consonant sounds, including lip sounds "*p*," "*b*," "*m*," and "*w*;" tongue-tip sounds "*t*," "*d*," and "*n*;" back-of-the-mouth sounds "*k*," "*g*," and "*h*;" and the gliding sound "*y*" by 14 to 15 months of age.

Your child will point and gesture along with sounds and words to request something he wants. Conversational and gestural turn-taking becomes increasingly routine for your child. Some of his gestures may include waving, blowing kisses, and pointing. You will also hear him name at least one toy or object consistently. You will hear "real" words within your child's conversational jargon. His jargon will consist of three to four syllables with a variety of speech sounds (eg, "ba da bo"). He can now imitate words he has not said before, as well as three or more animal or environmental sounds (such as the sound of a car).

Your child will interact with other children vocally when given the opportunity and give hugs and kisses to familiar people. However, he may be shy with strangers. You will notice him coming to you for help or assistance (eg, to open a box he cannot open). His vocalizations and body language will demonstrate pride in his accomplishments, and you will begin to see pretend play.

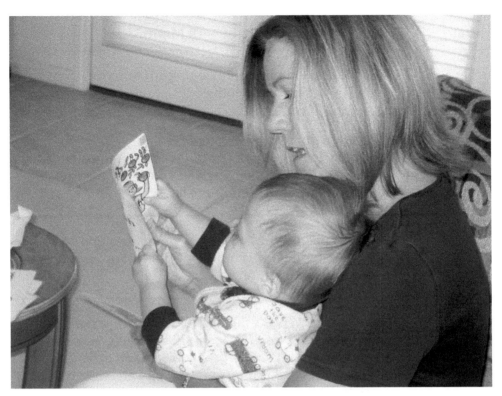

Photo 7.7: By 12 months, words are often heard along with hand and body movement.

Between 12 and 15 months, your child will try to sing along with music or sing when playing on his own. You will also hear changes in pitch, loudness, rate, stress, and intonation when he is vocalizing. For example, his pitch may go up to express a request, express curiosity, or get attention. Pitch is likely to go down when he expresses a greeting, a surprise, persistence, or an attempt to be recognized.

Date	Age: 15–18 Months
	Respiration continues to mature
	Bottom cuspids come in (16–18 months)
	Significant lip and tongue growth occurs (12–24 months)
	Stable jaw closing pattern appears; teeth meet with jaw closure (16 months)[369]

Date	Age: 15–18 Months
	Jaw, lips, and tongue continue to learn to move independently of one another
	Different parts of each structure continue to learn to move separately (eg, the tip of the tongue moves independently of the rest of the tongue, each lip corner contracts independently of the rest of the lips)
	Baby can use at least two words without gestures to make a request or protest (eg, "more," "cookie," "no"); prefers to talk rather than gesture only
	Baby labels or repeats the names of objects, actions, and events most frequently; requests objects, actions, and information; comments on objects and actions; acknowledges and protests events; answers; calls; greets; practices[370–371]
	Baby gestures and vocalizes while looking at another person in conversation (eg, points and says the word approximation for "that" or "there")
	Baby can ask, "What's that?"; uses these words together like a single word
	Baby uses rising pitch when anticipating an event; uses rising then falling pitch for emphasis[372]
	Baby can imitate unfamiliar words with new sounds or sound combinations heard in conversation
	Baby learns many new words slowly but constantly over time (about 10 new words per month)
	Baby can say at least 15–20 words with meaning by 18 months, name five to seven items when asked, and use words to identify objects and events

Date	Age: 15–18 Months
	Words consist primarily of consonant-vowel (eg, "me") and consonant-vowel-consonant-vowel (eg, "puppy")[373–374]
	Baby uses many consonant sounds in words, including lip sounds "p," "b," "m," and "w;" teeth-to-lip sounds "f" and "v;" tongue-tip sounds "t," "d," "l," and "n;" and back-of-the-mouth sounds "g," "k," and "h" by 18 months
	Baby shakes head up and down for "yes" and back and forth for "no"

The growth of your child's mouth and vocal structures continues during the 15- to 18-month period. With breathing patterns maturing, continued lip and tongue growth, and increasing jaw stability, your child is beginning to say more words and speech sounds. The mouth structures have good dissociation of movement (ie, separation), direction of movement (ie, moving in the right direction for the speech task), and grading of movement (ie, moving just enough for the speech task). As we will discuss, many lip sounds, teeth-to-lip sounds, tongue-tip sounds, and back-of-the-mouth sounds are heard. Your child can say most vowel sounds well. Remember, most vowels were heard in your child's first year.

Your 15- to 18-month-old child can now say 15 to 20 meaningful words and name five to seven items when asked. He will label or repeat names of objects, actions, or events frequently. Your child can request objects, actions, or information and can comment on objects or actions. He can acknowledge or protest an event, answer you, call to you, and greet you. You will hear him practicing speech.

Your child can also shake his head up and down for "yes" and back and forth for "no." He can use at least two words without gestures to make a request or to protest (eg, "more," "cookie," "no") and seems to prefer to talk rather than gesture only. He will gesture and talk while looking at you (eg, pointing to an object and saying a word that sounds like "that" or "there" while looking at you). He can ask, "What's that?" by using these words like a single word. You will hear his pitch going up when he is anticipating an event (eg, "outside↑"). You will hear his pitch rising, then falling, if he wants to emphasize something he says ("out↑side↓").

Your child can also imitate or repeat unfamiliar words heard in conversation with new sounds and new sound combinations. He will learn new words slowly but constantly over time (about 10 new words per month). Your child's words will primarily consist of consonant-vowel combinations (eg, "me"); however, you will also hear consonant-vowel-consonant-vowel words (eg, "puppy"). In addition to vowel sounds, you will hear many consonant sounds in words, including the lip sounds "*p*," "*b*," "*m*," and "*w*;" teeth-to-lip sounds "*f*" and "*v*;" tongue-tip sounds "*t*," "*d*," "*l*," and "*n*;" as well as back-of-the-mouth sounds "*k*," "*g*," and "*h*" by 18 months.

Date	Age: 18–21 Months
	Respiration continues to mature
	Top cuspids come in (18–20 months)
	Jaw stability increases significantly (16–24 months)
	Significant lip and tongue growth occurs (12–24 months)
	Jaw, lips, and tongue continue to learn to move independently of one another
	Different parts of each structure continue to learn to move separately (eg, tip of the tongue moves independently of the rest of the tongue; each lip corner contracts independently of the rest of the lips)
	Baby moves jaw, lips, and tongue easily during speech
	Two-word stage begins; baby imitates two- to three-word sentences by using appropriate intonation but primarily speaks in single words
	Baby uses falling then rising pitch to convey a warning; uses rising then falling pitch to convey playfulness[375]
	Baby imitates car, animal, or other sounds (eg, tongue click) during pretend play
	Baby can clearly and appropriately use 10–20 words

The Secrets to Good Speech Development

Date	Age: 18–21 Months
	Baby can name six body parts
	Baby begins using consonant-vowel-consonant (eg, "cat") words around 18 months
	Baby names one familiar object or picture upon request
	Baby says "hi" and "bye" appropriately
	Baby asks simple questions (eg, "What's that?" or "Where's Mommy?")
	Baby answers questions, including those presented while reading books
	Baby begins using different types of phrases to make statements or ask questions (eg, "da ball," "kick ball," "baby sleeping," "pick up," "my cookie?")[376]
	Baby participates in conversation with adults
	Baby uses many consonant sounds in words, including lip sounds "p," "b," "m," and "w;" teeth-to-lip sounds "f" and "v;" tongue-tip sounds "t," "d," "l," and "n;" as well as back-of-the-mouth sounds "g," "k," and "h" by 18 months
	Vowels sounds developed early and are generally accurate; greatest difficulties occur with short "e" and "i"[377]
	Recognizes mistakes or changes when read or told a familiar story[378]

Between 16 and 24 months, your child's jaw stability increases significantly. Notice that your child will have the majority of his primary teeth by 24 months. The two-word stage begins at 18 to 21 months. Your child will imitate two- to three-word sentences by using appropriate intonation. However, he will primarily speak in single words, using 10 to 20 single words clearly and appropriately. He can name six body parts and one familiar object or picture when you ask him. Around 18 months, your child will begin to say more consonant-vowel-consonant words, such as "cat."

Your child now actively participates in conversation with adults. You will hear falling then rising pitch for a warning (eg, "n↓o↑") and rising then falling pitch for playfulness ("O↑K↓"). Your child will say "hi" and "bye" appropriately and will ask simple questions (such as, "What's that?" and "Where's Daddy?"). He can also answer questions, including those presented while reading a book. If you make a change or a mistake in a story, your child will recognize this. Your child will use different types of phrases to make statements and to ask questions (eg, "da ball," "kick ball," "baby sleeping," "pick up," and "my cookie?").[379]

You will hear him imitate car, animal, and other sounds during pretend play. He will use many consonant sounds in words, including lip sounds "*p*," "*b*," "*m*," and "*w*;" teeth-to-lip sounds "*f*" and "*v*;" tongue-tip sounds "*t*," "*d*," "*l*," and "*n*," as well as back-of-the-mouth sounds "*k*," "*g*," and "*h*." His vowel sounds developed early (ie, between 1 and 6 months); however, he may still have some difficulty pronouncing short "*e*" as in Ed and short "*i*" as in "it."

Date	Age: 21–24 Months
	Respiration continues to mature
	Bottom second molars come in (20–24 months)
	Top second molars come in (24–30 months)
	Jaw stability increases significantly (16–24 months)
	Significant lip and tongue growth occurs (12–24 months)
	Jaw, lips, and tongue continue to learn to move independently of one another
	Different parts of each structure continue to learn to move separately (eg, the tip of the tongue moves independently of the rest of the tongue, each lip corner contracts independently of the rest of the lips)

Date	Age: 21–24 Months
	All first (primary) teeth come in by 24–30 months
	Baby moves jaw, lips, and tongue easily during speech
	Baby says two or more words in simple sentences (eg, "go bye-bye;" "no cookie")
	Baby clearly and appropriately uses at least 20 words
	Baby tries to talk about experiences or events by using words and jargon
	Baby is more likely to imitate speech when a variety of interesting toys and materials are present[380]
	Baby names at least two familiar objects upon request
	Baby points to at least five familiar pictures when asked
	Baby can name at least three pictures when asked
	Baby can name familiar people or characters on TV
	Baby may use one word for similar items (eg, may call all animals with four legs a "dog")
	Baby uses "please" and "thank you" appropriately
	Baby can increase the sound of his voice from a whisper to a louder voice
	Baby can talk on the telephone

Date	Age: 21–24 Months
	Baby begins to use pronouns (eg, "me," "my," "mine") and refers to himself by his own name
	Baby can say between 50 and 270 words (mostly nouns with some verbs, adjectives, adverbs, and pronouns)
	Baby begins using plurals and subject-verb agreement
	Baby primarily uses speech to express himself and is understood by an unfamiliar person 50% of the time (22 months)[381]
	Baby uses full range of vowel, diphthong, and consonant sounds in speech[382]
	By 24 months, the following sounds are heard at the beginning of words: lip sounds "b," "p," "m," and "w;" tongue-tip sounds "t," "d," and "n;" back-of-the-mouth sounds "k," "g," and "h;" teeth-to-lip sounds "f" and "v;" and the noisy sound "s"[383–385]
	By 24 months, the following sounds are heard at the end of words: lip sound "p;" tongue-tip sounds "t" and "n;" back-of-the-mouth sounds "k" and "r;" and the noisy sound "s"[386–388]
	Baby may leave final sounds out of words (eg, "ca" instead of "cat"), may simplify words (eg, "cown" instead of "clown"), may say "t" or "d" in place of "k" or "g" (eg, "tat" instead of "cat"), may say "w" for "r" ("wed" instead of "red")
	Echolalia (parroting) decreases
	Speech begins to "stay on topic"[389]
	Baby can answer simple questions (eg, "What does the doggie say?")

Your child's jaw, lips, and tongue now move easily during speech production. By 24 months of age, your child has developed:

- Dynamic stability (ie, one part of a structure stabilizes while another part moves); for example, the sides of your child's tongue stabilize on the sides of his hard palate while the tip of the tongue rises to produce the "*t*," "*d*," and "*n*" sounds

- Dissociation of movement (ie, one structure moves independently of another); for example, your child holds his jaw still in an appropriate open position as the back of his tongue rises to produce the "*k*" and "*g*" sounds

- Direction of movement (ie, structure moving in the right direction for the speech task); for example, your child's tongue retracts (moves back) during what speech-language pathologists call co-articulated speech (a fancy word for putting sounds together into connected speech)

- Grading of movement (ie, structure moving just enough for the speech task); for example, your child's jaw only opens enough for the speech sound he is saying—his jaw opens wider for "*k*" and "*g*" than "*t*" and "*d*;" you already know from our earlier discussion about speech intelligibility that vowels require many different jaw positions

These characteristics allow your child's speech skills to increase rapidly around the age of 2. He now primarily uses speech to express himself. An unfamiliar listener will understand your child at least 50% of the time. You will hear two or more words in simple sentences (eg, "go bye-bye") on a regular basis. He will clearly and appropriately say 20 or more words, and he will try to tell you about experiences and events by using a combination of words and jargon. Echolalia (parroting) is decreasing, and your child's speech begins to "stay on topic."[390]

During this period, your child will say between 50 and 270 different words. Most of these will be nouns, but you will also hear some verbs, adjectives, adverbs, and pronouns. He will say "please" and "thank you" appropriately. You will begin to hear pronouns in your child's speech (eg, "me," "my," "mine"). You will also hear your child use plurals (eg, dog, dogs) and subject-verb agreement (eg, "I see...").

In the 21- to 24-month period, your child will name at least two familiar objects, three familiar pictures, and familiar people and characters on TV when you ask him. He may use one word for similar items (eg, he may call all animals with four legs a "dog"). Your child can now point to at least five familiar pictures upon request (eg, "Anthony, where is the doggy?"). He can answer simple questions with ease. He can change his voice from a whisper to a loud voice and can talk on the telephone.

Your child will use a full range of vowel, diphthong (a complex speech sound that begins with one vowel and gradually changes to another vowel within the same syllable, such as "oi" in "boil"), and consonant sounds in speech. By

24 months, at the beginning of words you will hear the lip sounds "*b*," "*p*," "*m*," and "*w*;" the tongue-tip sounds "*t*," "*d*," and "*n*;" the back-of-the-mouth sounds "*k*," "*g*," and "*h*;" the teeth-to-lip sounds "*f*" and "*v*," as well as the noisy sound "*s*." At the end of words, you will hear the lip sound "*p*;" the tongue-tip sounds "*t*" and "*n*;" the back-of-the-mouth sounds "*k*" and "*r*;" and the noisy sound "*s*." It is typical for children at this age to leave final sounds out of words (eg, saying "ca" instead of "cat"). They may also simplify words by leaving sounds out of blends in words (eg, saying "cown" instead of "clown"). You may also hear some sound substitutions in children this age (eg, "*t*" or "*d*" in place of "*k*" or "*g*," or "*w*" in place of "*r*"). For example, you may hear your child say "tat" instead of "cat" or "wed" instead of "red."

Date	Age: 24–27 Months
	Respiration continues to mature
	Top second molars come in (24–30 months)
	All first (primary) teeth come in by 24–30 months
	Dissociation, grading, and direction of movement of structures used for speech continue to develop
	Child moves jaw, lips, and tongue easily during speech
	Speech sound development continues–see previous "Speech Sound Skills" checklist in this chapter
	Child talks in simple two- to three-word sentences in conversation
	Conversational turn-taking and staying on topic increases over time (24–36 months)
	Child talks about experiences that just occurred
	Child asks for help with activities (eg, eating, using the toilet, opening a container lid)

Date	Age: 24–27 Months
	Social interaction with peers begins (24–36 months)[391]
	Child repeats two numbers or unrelated words in a row (eg, "five, three" or "hat, doggie")
	Child uses personal pronouns, such as "I," "you," "he," and "it"
	Child uses verbs[392]
	Child names pictures of familiar objects

Between 24 and 27 months of age, your child continues to move his jaw, lips, and tongue easily when producing speech (ie, structures are dynamically stable; they move independently, just enough, and in the right direction, with proper coordination for the speech task). Your child has the breath control to say two- and three-word sentences. Most of his primary teeth have come in, and his jaw is stable enough to support speech production. Speech sound development continues, as detailed in the checklist in the earlier part of this chapter.

Your child speaks in simple two- and three-word sentences and can tell you about things that just happened (eg, spilled juice). He can carry a short conversation with you by taking turns talking about a single topic. Your child will also ask you for help with daily activities, such as going to the toilet or opening a container lid. He will also begin to play and interact with his peers when given the opportunity.

Your 24- to 27-month-old child can repeat two numbers or unrelated words if you ask him to. His sentences will contain both action words (verbs) and some personal pronouns (eg, "I," "you," "he," and "it"). Your child can tell you the names of familiar objects in pictures and books (eg, "ball," "doggie").

Date	Age: 27–30 Months
	Dissociation, grading, and direction of movement of structures used for speech continue to develop
	Child moves jaw, lips, and tongue easily during speech

Date	Age: 27–30 Months
	Child says words clearly; speech is understandable
	Speech sound development continues–see previous "Speech Sound Skills" checklist in this chapter
	Child speaks in simple two- and three-word sentences
	Child uses two types of sentences (eg, statements, questions)
	Child sings songs (eg, "happy birthday" song) from memory
	Social interaction with peers begins (24–36 months)[393]
	Conversational turn-taking and staying on topic increase over time (24–36 months)
	Child answers simple questions (eg, "What is that?")
	Child asks questions, beginning with the words "what" and "where"
	Child responds to "hello" and "goodbye" consistently
	Child can name a single color[394]
	Child repeats phrases and short sentences (eg, "Nice kitty," "Give me the ball.")
	Child says sentences with the pronoun "you," refers to himself with a pronoun (eg, "I")
	Child uses words such as "no" and "not" (the use of negation is an important part of your child's language development)

Between 27 and 30 months, your child can say words clearly, and you can understand his speech. The dissociation (ie, separation), grading (ie, moving just enough), and direction (ie, moving in the right direction) of mouth movements for speech support the increased clarity of your child's speech. He continues to speak in two- to three-word sentences, but you will hear different types of sentences (eg, statements and questions). Your child converses with you by using personal pronouns, such as "you" and "I," as well as words of negotiation, such as "no" and "not."

Your child can sing songs like "happy birthday" from memory, as well as ask and answer simple questions. He consistently says "hello" and "goodbye" at appropriate times and can name at least one color. He can also repeat meaningful phrases and short sentences (eg, "Nice kitty," "Give me the ball.").

Date	Age: 30–33 Months
	Dissociation, grading, and direction of movement of structures used for speech continue to develop
	Child moves jaw, lips, and tongue easily during speech
	Speech sound development continues–see previous "Speech Sound Skills" checklist in this chapter
	Child speaks in simple two- to three-word sentences
	Social interactions with peers occur (24–36 months)[395]
	Conversational turn-taking and staying on topic increase over time (24–36 months)
	Child can tell a story, share ideas, express feelings, and talk about experiences[396]
	Child retells simple ideas and events from a short story
	Child talks about a picture or shape he has drawn
	Child answers "yes" and "no" questions

Date	Age: 30–33 Months
	Child answers "where" questions by using words "in," "on," and "under"
	Child tells first and last name when asked
	Child tells whether he or she is a "boy" or "girl" when asked
	Child counts to three
	Child repeats three numbers or unrelated words in a row (eg, "kitty, hat, boy")
	Child can use plural nouns[397] (eg, "hats," "spoons")

Your 30- to 33-month-old child continues to speak in two- and three-word sentences, and his speech continues to become more precise. Now your child can express a simple story, an idea, and his feelings. He can talk about a picture he has drawn and things that have happened. He can answer "yes" and "no" questions. He can also answer "where" questions by using the prepositions "in," "on," and "under."

Your child can tell you his first and last name and whether he is a boy or girl, provided you have taught him this information. He can count to three and repeat three unrelated words in a row (eg, "kitty, hat, boy"). He also uses plurals when talking about more than one item (eg, "one hat," "two hats").

Date	Age: 33–36 Months
	Dissociation, grading, and direction of movement of structures used for speech continue to develop
	Child moves jaw, lips, and tongue easily during speech
	Speech sound development continues–see previous "Speech Sound Skills" checklist in this chapter

Date	Age: 33–36 Months
	Social interactions with peers occur (24–36 months)[398]
	Conversational turn-taking and staying on topic increase over time (24–36 months)
	Child uses two- to three-word sentences to talk about experiences, feelings, etc
	Child talks about events and experiences 2 to 3 days in the past
	Child talks about taking turns
	Child has a vocabulary of 500–1000 words, including nouns, verbs, adjectives, adverbs, pronouns, prepositions, and articles
	Child uses the words "a" and "the" at times in sentences
	Child uses the words "and" and/or "but" to combine simple sentences
	Child asks questions by using the words "when," "why," and "who"
	Child uses many verbs and several of their forms correctly (eg, "eats," "eating," "sits," "sitting")
	Child uses plural pronouns (eg, "we," "you," "they," "them," "us")
	Child uses the words "fast" and "slow" in sentences
	Child counts to five
	Child tells you his age

Your 33- to 36-month-old child continues to use two- to three-word sentences to talk about experiences and feelings. He can now tell you about something that happened 2 or 3 days ago. He also talks about taking turns during activities and has a vocabulary of 500 to 1000 words.

Your child's sentences contain nouns, different verb forms (eg, "eats," "eating"), adjectives, adverbs (eg, "fast" and "slow"), plural pronouns (eg, "we," "you," "they," "them," "us"), prepositions, and articles (eg, "a" and "the"). He will connect sentences with the conjunctions "and" and/or "but" to make compound sentences. Your child asks questions by using the words "when," "why," and "who." He can also count to five and tell you his age.

What to Do If Your Child Is Not on Track with Speech and Communication Development

Remember, the checklists provided in this book are a guide to normal or typical development. Each child has his own unique developmental process, so your child's process may be slightly different from that of another child. I have focused on speech development and expressive language in this chapter, because it can be difficult for parents, pediatricians, and others to find this information in one location. There are also other aspects of language (eg, your child's receptive understanding of language and his social use of language). This information is readily available from many other sources.

If you have a concern about any aspect of your child's development, it is critical that you ask your child's pediatrician for a referral to an appropriate professional. A speech-language pathologist is the person to see if your child has speech and/or language problems. See chapter 9 for further information.

If your child's speech and communication are not on track, your child's pediatrician will most likely refer you to a speech-language pathologist or other early intervention specialist who can evaluate these areas. Most school systems, state departments of education, and/or boards of health have early intervention teams that can evaluate your child's speech and communication skills, as well as other areas of development. If your child is not on track in speech and communication, it's a good idea to have his other areas of development screened. This will help you to know whether your child has a general developmental delay or just a delay in one or more specific areas.

In my opinion, as a speech-language pathologist who has worked on many early intervention teams and in private practice, children should be treated if a delay is found. It is not a good idea to see if your child will outgrow the delay. We know the importance of critical learning periods (ie, periods of time when certain skills develop best). Birth to age 2 appears to be the critical learning period for feeding, eating, and drinking development. Birth to age 3 appears to be the critical learning period for speech sound development. While speech sounds may continue to become refined until your child is in early elementary school, a 3-year-old child should speak in intelligible sentences. Vast bodies of research support the effectiveness of early intervention, which capitalizes on critical learning periods.

While we really do not know the specific causes of speech development concerns, I have seen three apparent problems in the children I treat:

1. A muscle function problem
2. A motor planning problem
3. An auditory problem

A muscle function problem means that the child's muscles are not working the way they need to work for speech. These children often have very slow speech movements, causing speech to sound distorted. A motor planning problem means the child has difficulty making and sequencing speech sounds. These children sometimes sound as if they are speaking another language. Their speech often sounds like a lot of consonants being put together. They frequently have difficulty coordinating respiration with speech production. An auditory problem has to do with hearing and listening. For example, children with a history of ear infections often have trouble hearing sounds in words and, therefore, producing them. In my practice, I frequently treat clients with a combination of these three problems. However, one problem is usually more apparent than the others.

Another term you may hear regarding speech problems in children is *phonological disorder*. While the term *speech delay* or *speech sound disorder* is said to be preferred, you may hear a speech-language pathologist use this term. Kamhi discusses this in his book on phonological disorders in children. According to Kamhi, "the term *phonological disorder* has not worked as a broad-based term that includes speech production" problems because "it is too closely linked with language and reading." You may also hear the term *articulation disorder*. This is an older term in the field of speech-language pathology and is most appropriately used with school-aged children who continue to have speech sound errors.[399]

Some recent resources for parents on this topic include:

- *Teach Me to Say It Right: Helping Your Child with Articulation Problems* by Dorothy R. Dougherty, MA, CCC-SLP[400]

- *Becoming Verbal with Childhood Apraxia: New Insights on Piaget for Today's Therapy* by Pam Marshalla, MA, CCC-SLP[401]

- *Does My Child Have a Speech Problem?* by Katherine L. Martin, CCC-SLP[402]

- *The Late Talker: What to Do If Your Child Isn't Talking Yet* by Marilyn C. Agin, MD, Lisa F. Geng, and Malcolm Nicholl

A Combination of Specific Treatment Ideas for Young Children with Speech and Communication Problems

As a speech-language pathologist specializing in early intervention, I like to begin treatment with a child as soon as a problem or the risk of a problem is recognized. Therefore, I work with children who are at risk for communication problems from birth (eg, children with Down syndrome or cerebral palsy). Many children are born without any obvious problems but do not attain expected development milestones. I prefer to begin working with a child as soon as a problem becomes apparent.

As a parent, you will work with your child's pediatrician regarding the range of time when skills typically appear. Do not panic if your child does not develop a skill at the beginning of a suggested time frame, but do pay attention to developmental time frames. You know that your child will have his own unique developmental process.

When a child has difficulties in the development of feeding, I work on the processes discussed in chapters 2 and 6 as soon as appropriate to keep the child on track as much as possible in feeding. When a child has problems with speech and communication development, I work on the processes discussed in this chapter as soon as appropriate. We will now talk about some of my favorite treatment ideas for babies and small children. Please note that this information applies to full-term or near-term babies. Premature babies require special handling techniques at birth and may benefit from the techniques discussed in this book when they are ready.

Massage and facilitation techniques discussed in chapter 5 can begin as early as birth to improve awareness within the mouth. The specific jaw work presented in chapter 5 can also begin at birth if needed. Other graded jaw, lip, and tongue techniques and respiratory work would be introduced as the child becomes ready for specific activities (eg, appropriate use of mouth toys, horns, bubbles, and straws). These activities help the child develop appropriate awareness and dynamic stability in the mouth, as well as dissociation, grading, and direction of movement, in a fun manner.

However, if a child has a speech and communication concern, it is critical to focus treatment on speech and communication. The only way to help a child learn the motor plans for speech is to work on speech. Now, I will tell you some of my favorite ideas for doing this.

As a therapist, I frequently use The Kaufman Speech Praxis Treatment Kit for Children[403] as a basis for speech treatment with young children. I usually begin with the "Basic Level" cards by using the consonant-vowel-consonant-vowel (such as "mama," "dada," "moomoo") and consonant-vowel (such as "me," "pea," "bee") sets with children as young as 6 months of age for receptive language and early literacy activities.

I have parents look at these pictures with the young child while simultaneously naming and talking about the pictures. Once the parent and child have done this for a while, I have the parent hold two pictures in front of the child and ask him for one of the pictures (eg, "Where is Mama?"). Many parents of 6-month-old children have been surprised when their child looks at the requested picture after being taught what the picture represented. This activity develops both receptive language and listening skills. As the child becomes skilled with this activity, the parent can help him to further develop his listening skills by showing him two pictures with similar-sounding words. For example, the words "pea" and "bee" sound and look similar when pronounced. Then I have the parent ask the child for one of the pictures. The 6-month-old child may only look at the requested picture. However, as the child matures, he will reach, point to, or grasp the appropriate picture. See previous communication development checklists.

Note Regarding the Kaufman Speech Praxis Treatment Kits: These kits were designed to help children with speech motor-planning problems to say word approximations that get closer and closer to the real word. They build speech from the bottom up. The kits help the speech-language pathologist and others to systematically cue speech and fade that cueing over time as the child develops speech. For more information on the work of Nancy Kaufman, speech-language pathologist, go to *www.kidspeech.com.*

While the Kaufman Speech Praxis Treatment Kits were meant for children with late-developing or absent speech, I find the "Basic Level" kit to work wonderfully to help at-risk children (eg, children with Down syndrome or children with characteristics of autism) to stay on track as much as possible with speech development.

As you know, I have parents look at and talk about these materials with their children as early as 6 months of age. However, I begin the actual work on speech production around 12 months of age, when first true words are supposed to emerge. I use a variety of treatment methods for this process.

When a child is 12 months old and ready to say his first words, I use a form of what I call "hands-on" speech facilitation to teach the child to begin to speak. I actually show the child how to move his jaw, lips, cheeks, and tongue by moving my gloved hand on these structures. Prompts for Restructuring Oral Muscular Phonetic Targets, or PROMPT, is one form of "hands-on" speech facilitation I use. I find it to be a very powerful method (ie, one that I could not do without). It was developed by a speech-language pathologist named Deborah Hayden. PROMPT uses "Dynamic Systems Theory" to shape, guide, and educate muscle movement for speech.[404–405] Appropriately trained speech-language pathologists can teach parents to use some of these techniques as a part of their child's speech-learning process. For more information about PROMPT, go to *www. promptinstitute.com.*

There is another, older form of hands-on speech facilitation called *motokinesthetics*. A listing of "Motokinesthetic Cueing" can be found in "Appendix C" of *Oral Motor Assessment and Treatment: Ages and Stages* by Diane Bahr (yours truly). The three motokinesthetics videos and DVDs by Merry Meek (speech-language pathologist) from Clinician's View are also important resources for therapists or parents who want to learn motokinesthetics.[406]

In addition to hands-on speech facilitation techniques, I use other forms of speech facilitation (eg, cues at the place of articulation and pacing) as the child is ready for these. Judy Michels Jelm, speech-language pathologist, created a list of cues at the place of articulation for parents and others to use. These are found in a book entitled, *A Parent Guide to Verbal Dyspraxia*.[407] The technique brings the child's attention to the part of the parent's mouth where the speech sound is produced. These cues are easy for parents and others to learn. The child can also learn to perform these cues on his own mouth. I have found these cues to work well with sign language for speech facilitation.

Some therapists use sign language to help children produce words and eventually phrases and sentences. Many parents have asked whether cueing at the mouth will become confused with signs. I have taught many children to use both signs and cues. I have never seen this confusion occur.

In addition, some parents become concerned that their children will choose to use the sign language or cueing instead of speech. Let me put your mind at ease. Speech is the most efficient and effective means of communication for hearing individuals. Your child will choose to use speech over any other method if he has the ability to do this, unless he is an elective or selective mute. Elective and/or selective mutism is a rare disorder related to emotional or psychological concerns, where the child is choosing not to speak.

Pacing is another form of cueing I use with children who are having speech difficulties. This is a simple technique anyone can use to facilitate speech and improve speech intelligibility. Place circles (for consonants) and lines (for vowels) on cards to represent the speech sound combinations you are teaching. For consonant-vowel-consonant-vowel words (such as "mama," "dada," "papa"), I use a card with ●— ●—. I have the child move his hand or finger with mine from the circle along each line while saying or attempting to say words such as "mama," "papa," or "boo-boo." For consonant-vowel words (such as "bee" and "pea"), I have the child move his finger from the circle and along the line while saying or attempting to say the words. The card for consonant-vowel words would look like ●—. Get the idea?

As you can tell, the circles represent the consonant sounds and the lines represent the vowel sounds. Remember, vowels carry an important part of the message for speech. They also require a great amount of jaw grading and respiratory control. Children need to produce both vowels and consonants well to be intelligible. Notice that the lines are relatively long, so that the child can extend the vowel sound. Slowing down speech and elongating vowel sounds are two of the best methods known to increase speech intelligibility.

Sign language, using cues at the mouth (ie, place of articulation), and pacing also make use of the hand-mouth connection we discussed in chapter 4. Remember, our hands and mouth work together from birth. As a therapist, I have consistently found that children begin to say words when using these methods. It seems like magic, but we are actually seeing connections being made within the child's brain between the hands and the mouth.

In addition to the Kaufman Speech Praxis Treatment Kit, I like to use Silly Songs from Thinking Publications[408] and Noisy Stories from Mayer-Johnson, Inc.[409] These materials contain many of the first words children tend to produce and match many of the words presented in the Kaufman Speech Praxis Treatment Kit. I also use the Mayer-Johnson Boardmaker to create pictures for early phrases and sentences (ie, picture reading, early literacy activity) when my little clients are ready for this.

As you can tell, I like to build speech from the bottom up, beginning with vowels, then combining consonants and vowels, then vowels with consonants, and so on. However, there is another way to work with children who are having difficulty developing speech. This method is used by speech-language pathologists such as Judy Michels Jelm, Deborah Hayden, and David Hammer (contributor to the production of the children's CD *Time to Sing,* the introduction to the apraxia DVD *Hope Speaks*, and the recently released DVD on *Treatment Strategies for Childhood Apraxia of Speech*). These therapists expand the child's speech from the sounds the child can already make. In my treatment, I use this method in combination with the bottom-up approach for a well-rounded program.

Children develop the motor plans in the brain for speech through consistent speech practice. This is the reason you hear young children say words over and over while they are developing speech. To get young children to practice speech, I work in unison with them at the beginning of treatment. This helps the child feel that he is not alone in this process. We make it fun. For example, we might say the word "mama" together a number of times while looking at the picture, looking at the word (believe it or not, 2-year-olds can recognize some words), moving our finger or hand on the pacing board, making the sign, beating on a drum, and stomping our feet. Imitation of words comes later in the treatment process, when the child is ready for this. The approach incorporates the work of Dr Jay Rosenbeck and his associates (originally developed for working with adults, but also found to work with children).[410–411]

In addition to structured treatment methods, I incorporate as much natural language as possible into my treatment. We discussed some of this information in the section of this chapter entitled, "Tips to Encourage Good Vocal Development from Birth." Information on a child-led, natural approach to language and communication development can be found on The Hanen Centre Web site *(www.hanen.org)*. "It Takes Two to Talk—The Hanen Program" has long been a popular program for helping parents learn to communicate naturally with their children. It teaches parents to follow their child's lead, which allows the child to feel empowered when communicating. There is a book available for parents with the same title, *It Takes Two to Talk: A Practical Guide for Parents of Children with Language Delays* by Jan Pepper and Elaine Weitzman.

In summary, my goal is to keep an "at-risk" child on track as much as possible with speech. While I believe that it may be important to get the mouth in shape and ready for speech production with appropriate oral massage and exercise (when needed), I spend most of my treatment time on speech work if the child has a speech delay. I carefully and systematically incorporate the work discussed in chapters 4 and 5 into my sessions as short fun breaks during therapy and as a home program. To get a child on track with speech, the child needs to practice speech over and over again. This is not always easy for a small child.[412–413] **Therefore, it is crucial to work with a speech-language pathologist if your child has a significant speech delay or is at risk for a speech delay.**

8

Your Child's Best Natural Appearance

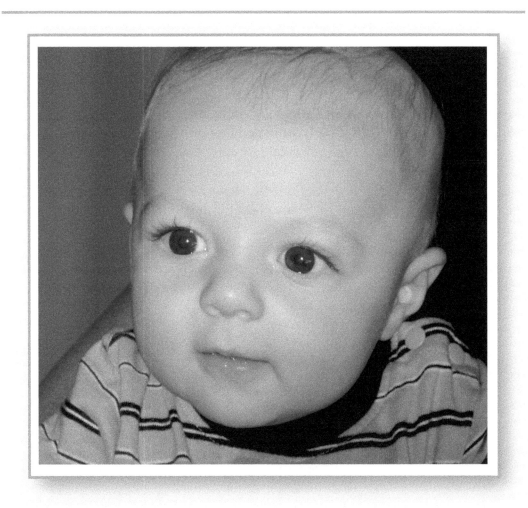

Key Topics in This Chapter

■ What Your Child's Face and Mouth Should Look Like

■ Treatments Offered by Dental and Other Professionals

■ Face, Mouth, and Vocal Development through Adolescence and Early Adulthood

We have discussed many techniques that naturally encourage good mouth development in previous chapters. In this chapter, we will discuss your child's best natural appearance as this relates to face and mouth development. Parents want their children to be as successful as possible and are told daily on news and talk shows how appearance can affect success. We also know from experience how appearance can affect self-esteem.

Raymond D. Kent, an important researcher in the field of speech-language pathology, stated that, "it has been estimated that only about half of young people in the United States have normal jaw and dental relationships, with about 15% having severe malocclusions."[414–416] Orthodontic treatment is important when dental development has gone wrong. However, it has now become the rule rather than the exception for many children. Just think of all the children you know who wear braces. The techniques and ideas already presented in this book, as well as the ideas introduced in this chapter, may help your child avoid extensive orthodontic treatment. The chapter concludes with a chart and description of face, mouth, and vocal development through adolescence and early adulthood for your reference.

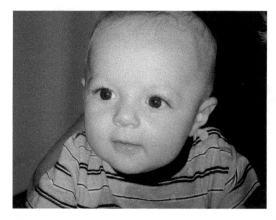 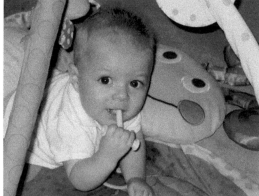

Photo 8.1a and 8.1b: At 4 and 6 months, Anthony's mouth and facial features are already changing significantly.

What Your Child's Face and Mouth Should Look Like

Your child will go through a pronounced period of jaw growth in the first year of life. You will notice how adultlike your child begins to look around 1 year of age. By the age of 2, your child is well on her way to mature face and mouth development. Your child looks less like a baby and more like an adult. By age 6, your child will have achieved most of her skull growth and approximately 80% of her jaw growth.

Activity 8.1 provides some guidelines for what to expect as a child progresses through the face and mouth development process. These guidelines represent good development. I will also explain some of the possible ramifications of structural differences that may occur. This will guide you in getting help from your child's pediatrician, dentist, orthodontist, and others if your child has any of these problems. The measurements found here are from the work of Char Boshart,[417] a speech-language pathologist and orofacial myologist, along with some of my observations as a therapist. Place a date next to what you observe.

ACTIVITY 8.1: APPEARANCE AS THE FACE AND MOUTH DEVELOP[418–419]

Date	What You Want When Looking at Your Child (Front View)	Date	What You Don't Want
	Horizontal width across the eye area of the face is approximately the width of one eye times five		Face too narrow at level of eyes
	Center corners of eyes line up with widest part of nose		Narrow nose
	Imaginary lines drawn at hairline, eyebrow, bottom of nose, and bottom of chin give face appearance of equal thirds		High forehead; small, pulled-back chin

ACTIVITY 8.1: (cont.)[418–419]

Date	What You Want When Looking at Your Child (Front View)	Date	What You Don't Want
	Top and bottom jaws should be aligned, with top teeth slightly over the bottom teeth and molars meeting properly in the back of the mouth		Overbite, overjet, underbite, closed bite, cross-bite
	Lip line straight across horizontally at rest		Mouth turned down in frown at rest

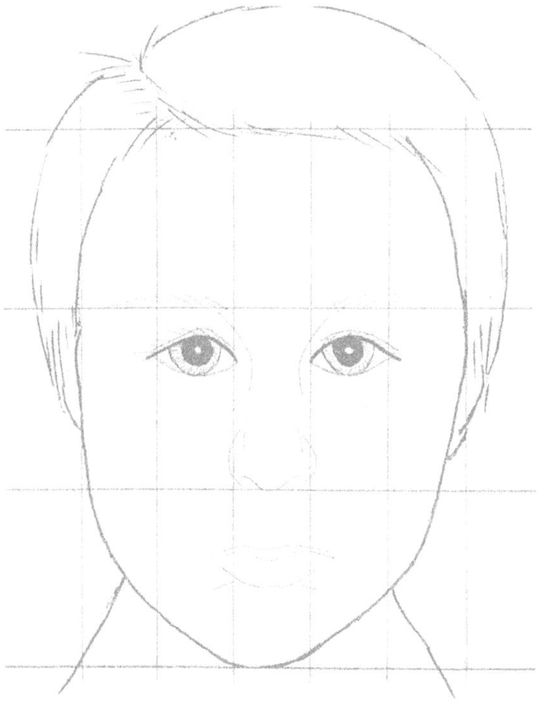

Figure 8.1: Appearance of the face from the front, as suggested by Char Boshart in her book *Oral-Facial Illustrations and Reference Guide.* Original artwork by Anthony Fotia.

Date	What You Want When Looking at Your Child (Side View)	Date	What You Don't Want
	Imaginary straight line can be drawn from the bridge of the nose to the philtrum (area above the upper lip) and to the front of the chin		Convex or concave facial appearance; the jaw is too far forward or too far back
	The angle of the nose and philtrum (area of the upper lip) is 90°–110°		The angle of the nose and philtrum is more than 110°, indicating possible overbite
	The top teeth and jaw should only be slightly in front of the bottom teeth and jaw		Overbite, underbite, closed bite

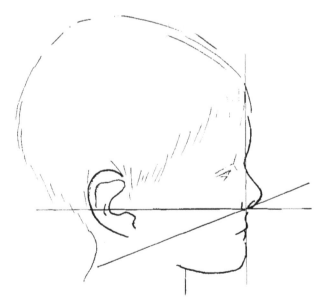

Figure 8.2: Appearance of the face from the side, as suggested by Char Boshart in her book *Oral-Facial Illustrations and Reference Guide.* Original artwork by Anthony Fotia.

DIRECTIONS AND DISCUSSION FOR ACTIVITY 8.1

1. Look at your child from the front. It is a good idea to take a photo. You can draw suggested lines on a photo.

2. Does your child have a width across the eye area of approximately one eye times five? Your child should have a fairly wide appearance across the eye area. If this area is too narrow, your child may have a high, narrow palate (roof of the mouth). Remember that a high, narrow palate also changes the size and shape of the nasal and sinus areas.

Reduced or distorted nasal and sinus areas affect the way your child breathes. They can also affect your child's overall health if your child tends to get sinus infections. Sinus infections seem to be underdiagnosed in young children. A high, narrow palate can affect dental development and tongue placement for eating, drinking, and speech production because of the narrow dental arch that results. See chapter 3 for more information on health.

3. Do the center corners of your child's eyes line up with the widest part of her nose? A narrow nose can affect your child's breathing and can also be related to a high, narrow palate.

4. If you draw an imaginary line (or real line on a photo) across your child's hairline, across your child's eyebrows, across the bottom of your child's nose, and across the bottom of your child's chin, does her face give the appearance of equal thirds? If not, there may be differences in your child's jaw and hard palate growth or position, which then affects tongue position and movement. Therapists often see older children with feeding and speech problems who have high foreheads and small, pulled-back chins.

5. Do your child's top and bottom jaws line up? Do your child's top teeth fit slightly over her bottom teeth when taking a bite or smiling? Do your child's back teeth come together properly? You may need your dentist to help you decide on the last question.

If your child's top front teeth are too far in front of the bottom teeth, this is called an *overbite* or *overjet*, depending on whether the top teeth are pushed forward or the whole top jaw is forward. If your child's bottom teeth and jaw are in front of the top teeth, this is called an *underbite*. If your child's top and bottom teeth meet in the front (edge to edge) but not in the back, this could be a closed bite or posterior open bite. If your child's bottom teeth and/or jaw are shifted to one side compared to the top teeth and/or jaw, this is a cross-bite. Speak with your dentist or orthodontist for more information, as there is differing terminology for specific types of problematic bite patterns.

6. Do your child's lips appear straight across the horizon when she is not smiling or frowning? Your child should also have a nice, broad smile. If your child's mouth is turned down (like a frown) when she is resting or relaxed, the mouth is often mirroring a high, narrow palate and narrow dental arch.

7. Look at your child from the side. It is a good idea to take a photo.

8. Can an imaginary line be drawn from the bridge of the nose to the philtrum (the area above the upper lip), to the front of the chin? You can draw a real line on a photo if you like. This is a measurement of jaw alignment and facial development. Some children have faces that appear convex or concave in shape, reflecting a problem in facial development. Some children have jaws that are too far forward or too far back, reflecting a problem with jaw alignment.

9. Is the angle of your child's nose to her philtrum (the area just above the upper lip) 90° to 110°? An angle greater than 110° may reflect an overbite. There may also be problems with midface growth and lip closure. You can use a protractor to measure the number of degrees when looking at a photo. I use a small device called a *goniometer* (typically used by occupational therapists). One source for the purchase of a goniometer is Therapro, Inc *(www.theraproducts.com)*.

10. Are your child's top teeth and/or jaw only slightly in front of her bottom teeth and/or jaw? If your child's top teeth are too far in front of the bottom teeth, this is called an *overbite* or *overjet*, depending on whether the top teeth are pushed forward or the whole top jaw is forward. If your child's bottom teeth and jaw are in front of the top teeth, this is called an *underbite*. If your child's top and bottom teeth meet in the front (edge to edge) but not in the back, this may be a closed bite or posterior open bite. If your child's bottom teeth and/or jaw are shifted to one side compared to the top teeth and/or jaw, this is a cross-bite. Again, speak with your dentist or orthodontist for more information, as there is differing terminology for specific types of problematic bite patterns.

We will discuss what to do about these structural changes or differences in the next section. Many parents assume that structural differences are purely genetic and inherited. While your child does inherit her structures from you and your ancestors, you will see that a number of these concerns are related to problems with jaw function and tongue movement (such as the tongue-thrust swallow, or immature swallow).

Treatments Offered by Dental and Other Professionals

Let's talk about treatments offered by dental and other professionals who work specifically with mouth development problems. A significant amount of research on these problems and their treatments can be found in the dental and orthodontic literature. The research behind chosen treatments is very important. When working with professionals, be sure to ask questions and discuss the evidence for the treatments being suggested. Evidence includes research being completed in a particular field with control groups, research completed with individual and multiple cases, as well as the individual professional's experience with treatments used. As a parent, it is very important for you to have a full understanding of any treatment your child is undergoing. Here is a list to guide you in finding appropriate professionals and possible treatments if your child has any of the problems listed.

MOUTH DEVELOPMENT PROBLEMS			
Problem	Date (Note Date When Problem Is Seen and When Treatment Begins)	Person to See	Possible Treatments
High, narrow palate (roof of the mouth)		Pediatric dentist, orthodontist, craniosacral and/ or myofascial therapist	Functional jaw orthopedics, orthodontics (eg, palatal expander), craniosacral and/ or myofascial therapy

Problem	Date (Note Date When Problem Is Seen and When Treatment Begins)	Person to See	Possible Treatments
Underbite, cross-bite, closed bite		Orofacial myologist, speech-language pathologist, occupational therapist, physical therapist (properly trained in oral motor treatment), pediatric dentist, orthodontist, craniosacral and/ or myofascial therapist	Orofacial myofunctional therapy; oral motor treatment by a properly trained speech-language pathologist, occupational therapist, or physical therapist; functional jaw orthopedics; orthodontics; craniosacral and/or myofascial therapy
Overbite, overjet, or anterior open bite (open gap in the front teeth when child is smiling)		Orofacial myologist, speech-language pathologist, occupational therapist, physical therapist (properly trained in oral motor treatment), pediatric dentist, orthodontist, craniosacral and/ or myofascial therapist	Orofacial myofunctional therapy; oral motor treatment by a properly trained speech-language pathologist, occupational therapist, or physical therapist; functional jaw orthopedics; orthodontics; craniosacral and/or myofascial therapy

General dentists begin seeing children around 1 year of age. If your child's teeth are not coming in on time, you might want to see a dentist or other appropriate professional earlier. It is good to find a dentist who works with infants, toddlers, and young children. There are dentists who specialize in pediatrics. Good dental care is important for your child throughout her life. There are many illnesses related to problems with the teeth, jaw, and airway.[420]

Some dentists practice functional jaw orthopedics. These dentists know a lot about the development of the mouth and face. They can provide noninvasive treatments to children from a very young age. Noninvasive treatments are important because the mouth is such a vulnerable and sensitive area. Many people do not like going to the dentist for this reason. The oral massage presented in chapter 5 is an excellent way to prepare your child to see the dentist. See *www. smilepage.com* for more information on functional jaw orthopedics.

An appropriately trained pediatric dentist or an orthodontist can help if your child's mouth structure has undergone an inappropriate change (eg, a high, narrow palate; overbite; or underbite). There are many tools that dentists and orthodontists use to correct problems with structure and function (eg, palatal expanders, braces, and other corrective devices).

Orthodontists will often use an appliance called an *expander* to broaden the hard palate when the child is old enough to correct a high, narrow palate. This is usually done prior to the placement of braces and allows most children to keep their permanent teeth. Without palatal expansion, teeth may be removed as part of the orthodontic process. The teeth help to maintain the integrity of the dental arches. The dental arches need to be in good shape for taking food bites, chewing foods, efficient swallowing, effective and efficient speech production, and to have a nice smile. I am not in favor of removal of permanent teeth for these reasons.

It is interesting to me that almost every child, whose parents can afford it, sees an orthodontist. I don't want to put these professionals out of business, but many orthodontic problems and changes in facial appearance can result from improper use of the mouth during early feeding processes and other mouth activities. Parents often assume that their children will need orthodontics. Currently, orthodontic treatment has become the rule rather than the exception. However, this does not need to be the case if a child's mouth is kept in good shape from birth through appropriate mouth experiences.

Having said this, I don't want you, as a parent, to feel the least bit guilty if your child needs functional jaw orthopedics or orthodontics. Remember, this is a no-guilt book. As a parent, you are doing the best job possible to promote your child's development.

Parents need accurate information about ways to circumvent or find appropriate treatment for oral structural issues. Parents also need to know about treatment techniques that go beyond the use of corrective devices (eg, oral motor treatment, orofacial myofunctional therapy, and craniosacral and/or myofascial treatment). These treatment techniques are often effective when used along with the work being done by an orthodontist or pediatric dentist to help avoid repeated orthodontic work.

It is frustrating for a dentist or orthodontist to place braces or other appliances into a child's mouth and see the same problem(s) reappear. This can occur when other appropriate treatments (eg, oral motor, orofacial myofunctional) do not occur before or simultaneously with dental or orthodontic work. I have had clients who were in their third set of braces before they were referred to me for treatment. This tends to happen because the child's movement patterns in the mouth have not changed, even though the structure has been changed. I helped many clients avoid repeated orthodontic work through systematic oral motor and orofacial myofunctional treatment.

Before discussing oral motor treatment and orofacial myology, let's briefly talk about two other related forms of hands-on treatment for structural and functional differences in the mouth. These are craniosacral treatment and myofascial release. Dr John Upledger developed craniosacral treatment, and physical therapist John Barnes developed an advanced form of myofascial release. These methods are often used by physical therapists, occupational therapists, speech language pathologists, dentists, and massage therapists. You can learn more about these techniques by visiting *www.upledger.com* and *www.myofascialrelease.com*.

While I am trained in myofascial release and craniosacral therapies, I tend to focus on oral motor and orofacial myofunctional treatment to address many of the problems listed in the previous charts. Oral motor treatment can include:

- Oral awareness and/or discrimination
- Oral activities and/or exercises
- Feeding
- Orofacial myofunctional treatment (done by a properly trained speech-language pathologist)
- Motor speech treatment (done by a properly trained speech-language pathologist)

We have talked about oral awareness and discrimination throughout this book and specifically in chapter 4. We talked about oral activities and exercises in chapter 5. We covered feeding in chapters 2 and 6. We discussed motor speech treatment in chapter 7. We are now going to talk about orofacial myofunctional therapy.

Orofacial myofunctional therapy has historically been called *tongue-thrust swallow therapy*. However, orofacial myologists also treat jaw and tongue resting posture, lip closure, thumb- and finger-sucking, tooth-grinding, and inappropriate biting and chewing habits.[421] Your child will need orofacial myofunctional treatment if she has failed to develop a mature swallowing pattern or has any of the other problems listed. In chapter 2, we discussed the importance of breathing through the nose. In chapter 3, we addressed pacifier use and thumb- and finger-sucking. In chapter 5, we talked about appropriate chewing and biting activities and the problem of tooth-grinding (technically called *bruxism*). Now, we will focus on the mature swallow and the appropriate rest position of the tongue.

While elements of the mature swallowing pattern emerge in the first year of life (eg, three-dimensional sucking begins at 3 to 4 months of age), the pattern becomes apparent around 12 months of age. This is when your child begins to raise the tip of the tongue to the ridge behind the top front teeth to initiate the mature swallow. The mature swallowing pattern is well established by 2 years of age. Your child's swallow is adultlike by 3 years of age.

The mature swallow consists of the tongue cupping to hold the food or liquid for swallowing (sides of the tongue sealing against the sides of the hard palate), the tip of the tongue rising to the ridge behind the top front teeth to begin the swallow, and the rest of the tongue then squeezing upward (in a front-to-back motion) to move the food to the throat for swallowing. In my experience as a speech-language pathologist, I have seen many children who have not developed a mature swallowing pattern. This seems to be related to some of the early feeding techniques that were used with these children and is one reason that I have written this book.

ACTIVITY 8.2: HOW DO YOU SWALLOW?

1. Take a sip of water from a cup. Notice how you swallow. Take one sip at a time. You may need to do this over and over before you can feel what you are doing. Now take a bite of cracker, chew it, and notice how you swallow.

2. Does your tongue gather the water and/or chewed cracker into the center? Is your tongue cupped with the sides of the tongue sealing against the sides of the hard palate? Does the tip of your tongue go to the ridge behind your top front teeth to start the swallow? Does the rest of your tongue squeeze upward and move the water and/or chewed cracker back to the throat for the swallow?

3. If you are not doing the sequence listed in step 2, try it. This is a mature swallowing pattern.

4. If you don't automatically have this mature swallowing pattern, you may have a form of tongue-thrust swallow. Do not worry too much about this. I have seen many adults with tongue-thrust swallow. However, if you are one of these individuals, it is a good idea to work with a properly trained speech-language pathologist to retrain your swallow. As an adult, an immature swallow may affect your oral hygiene and possibly swallowing control as you age. Speech-language pathologists work with many patients who are elderly and have lost the ability to use the swallowing pattern described here.

A number of terms have been used to describe an immature or unsophisticated swallowing pattern. These include "tongue-thrust swallow," "exaggerated tongue protrusion" (Morris and Klein),[422] and "reverse swallow." While exaggerated tongue protrusion best describes the pattern seen in most typically developing children, the common term used by many speech-language pathologists and others is *tongue-thrust swallow*. The International Association of Orofacial Myology *(www.iaom.com)* is working toward the use of the term *orofacial myofunctional disorder*, because the disorder goes well beyond the thrusting of the tongue.

If a child uses an immature swallowing pattern (a tongue-thrust swallow), she does not efficiently clear the mouth of food, liquid, and saliva. This may lead to oral hygiene problems. Tongue-thrust swallow is also associated with overbite and open bite (ie, an open space between the top and bottom teeth). I have seen open bites in the front teeth and the side teeth. Some individuals actually thrust the side(s) of their tongues toward one or both side tooth surfaces on the swallow. A tongue thrust can be forward, sideways, or both.

Many orthodontists refer their patients to speech-language pathologists to correct the swallow, as well as the other mouth patterns that often occur with the immature swallow (open-mouth resting posture, low and forward tongue-resting position, poor lip closure, thumb- and finger-sucking, tooth-grinding, and inappropriate biting and chewing habits[423]). These patterns, if continued, can undo what braces have done. As I mentioned previously, I have treated some adolescents who were in their third set of braces. This is a great expense for the family and a frustration for the orthodontist.

Another potential result of a tongue-thrust swallow is a speech problem. Lisps (frontal and lateral) are the most common problem. These affect the production of the speech sounds "*s*," "*z*," "*sh*," "*ch*," and "*j*." However, I have seen many individuals with stubborn "*r*" and "*l*" distortions who have tongue-thrust swallow. There are also other problem mouth patterns that tend to occur with tongue-thrust swallow.

So, how do you know if your child has tongue-thrust swallow?

1. Can you see your child's tongue come forward between her gums and teeth when she swallows?

2. If you gently pull your child's cheek out to the side, can you see her tongue coming out between the molars just a little bit?[424]

3. Is there food left on your child's tongue or in her mouth after she swallows one time? Try this with a cracker.

4. Does your child tense her lips when she swallows?

5. Does your child have good movement of the masseter and mylohyoid muscles? Place your fingers in front of your child's ears below the temporomandibular joint (masseter muscles) and central to her lower jawbone on the soft tissue (mylohyoid muscles). These muscles are supposed to contract when we swallow. Your child's dentist can help you with this.

6. Does your child tend to place too much food in her mouth?

7. Does your child want sauces on most of her foods, or does she insist on dipping foods in sauces?

8. Does your child have persistent detrimental oral habits? These include thumb-sucking, pacifier use, and chronic sucking or chewing on fingers, fingernails, straws, pens or pencils, the tongue, clothing, and other inappropriate items.

9. Does your child breathe through her mouth?

If you can actually see your child's tongue coming forward between her teeth and lips when she swallows, you are seeing a tongue-thrust swallow. If you do not see your child's tongue coming forward, there are other ways to tell if she has a tongue-thrust swallow. You can gently pull your child's cheek out to the side and see if her tongue is coming out between her molars when she swallows. You may also give your child a cracker to eat, and ask her to open her mouth or stick out her tongue after one swallow. If you still see pieces of the cracker on your child's tongue, your child is not clearing the mouth of food during the swallow. Once again, this can lead to oral hygiene problems.

When your child swallows, look to see if there is a lot of tension around her lips. If this happens, your child is using the lips and cheeks to generate intraoral pressure for the swallow. Your child should be using skilled tongue movements to initiate and complete the swallow. You should feel movement in your child's masseter (in front of the ears under the temporomandibular joint) and mylohyoid muscles (central to the lower jawbone in the soft tissue under the jaw) when she swallows. Your child's dentist can help you find these muscles.

Children who place too much food into their mouths are often forced to use an immature swallowing pattern. They usually do not chew their food well enough to moisten it with saliva. Poorly chewed food does not mix with saliva to begin digestion. Remember, digestion begins in the mouth with the mixture of food with saliva. In addition, children who insist on eating foods with sauces or gravies may be using them to moisten and bring the food together for an easier swallow. Some medications have a side effect of reduced saliva production. Check with your child's pediatrician if you think this may be a problem for your child.

Many children with immature swallowing patterns also have upper respiratory problems (eg, allergies and sinus problems). This forces the child to breathe through the mouth. We discussed the importance of breathing through the nose, as well as upper respiratory health problems and possible treatments, in chapter 3. Breathing through the mouth is not only unhealthy, but it also leads to a low and forward tongue-resting posture. The tongue is supposed to rest in the closed mouth with the front surface of the tongue (including the tip) touching the ridge behind the top front teeth. Oral habits such as low and forward tongue-resting position, thumb-sucking, pacifier use, and chronic sucking or chewing on fingers, fingernails, straws, pens or pencils, and clothing can perpetuate an immature swallowing pattern.

ACTIVITY 8.3: WHERE DOES YOUR TONGUE REST?

1. Notice where your tongue rests when your mouth is still and not moving. Hopefully, your lips are together at rest. If your lips are not together, it is impossible for you to have a normal tongue-resting position.

2. If your lips are closed, does the front surface of your tongue (including the tip) rest against the ridge behind your top front teeth? If not, where does your tongue rest? You should also notice a small space (about 2 mm) between your top and bottom back molars when your mouth is at rest.

3. The front surface of your tongue (including the tip) is supposed to rest against the ridge behind your top front teeth. If your tongue rests at any other location (such as on the front teeth or in the bottom of the mouth), you do not have a typical tongue-resting posture.

4. You can train the front surface of your tongue (including the tip) to rest on the ridge behind your top front teeth if you don't already do this. Practice keeping the front surface of your tongue on the ridge behind your top front teeth for longer and longer periods of time. Begin with 10 seconds, then 30 seconds, then 1 minute, then 10 minutes, then 30 minutes, and so on. You can practice while watching TV, reading, or walking. Retraining the tongue's resting position is the first step in retraining the swallow. This is probably where your child will begin if she needs orofacial myofunctional treatment.

If your child is demonstrating the characteristics discussed in this section of the chapter, talk to your child's dentist and/or orthodontist. Dentists and orthodontists usually know the speech-language pathologists who specialize in orofacial myofunctional treatment to retrain your child's swallowing pattern. The International Association of Orofacial Myology also has a "Parent's Page" for more information on this topic. See *www.iaom.com.*

Face, Mouth, and Vocal Development through Adolescence and Early Adulthood

It is difficult to talk about face and mouth development without at least mentioning vocal development. These structures develop and work together for eating, drinking, and speaking. As your child grows, she will experience changes in the size, shape, and position of the mouth relative to the vocal structure (ie, the voice box, throat, and windpipe). Movements for eating, drinking, and speaking develop as your child's mouth and vocal structures grow. These structures are also shaped by the movements of eating, drinking, and speaking.[425]

While human development may seem slow compared with other species,[426] there are important periods of time where growth spurts occur. The first one is birth to 12 months of age. The following chart will help you track your child's face, mouth, and vocal development from birth though adolescence and early adulthood. Remember, your child has her own unique developmental process. The information in this book provides guidelines for you, to help you know when to ask your child's pediatrician, dentist, and others about your child's development. Place a date next to characteristics you see. You may not be able to see all of them, because some are difficult to observe.

ACTIVITY 8.4: FACE, MOUTH, AND VOCAL DEVELOPMENT[427-445]

Date	Characteristics of a Full-Term Newborn[446-448]
	Mouth contains small open space
	Lower jaw is small and somewhat retracted (approximately 30% of adult size at birth)[449]
	Sucking pads in cheeks assist in feeding
	Tongue fills mouth
	Baby prefers breathing through the nose
	Baby makes nasal-sounding vowels when vocalizing
	The epiglottis and soft palate are close together
	The voice box is high in the neck
	Rooting, suckling, tongue, swallowing, bite, transverse-tongue, and gag reflexes are present
	Eustachian tube is horizontal

You may remember from chapter 1 that your newborn baby's mouth is very different from your mouth. Your full-term, newborn baby has little open space inside her mouth because:

- The bottom jaw is small and a little pulled back (retracted).
- The sucking pads (fat pads in the cheeks) take up a lot of space within the mouth from the sides.
- The tongue fills most of the remainder of the space within the mouth.

The small open space, along with suckling and sucking, help your baby achieve adequate pressure inside the mouth to move breast milk or formula back to the throat for effective, efficient, and safe swallowing.

Your newborn baby also prefers to breathe through the nose (remember the importance of breathing through the nose, as discussed in chapter 3). When your baby makes vocal sounds, they may come through your baby's nose (eg, nasal-sounding vowels) and mouth (eg, crying sounds).

Your baby was also born with reflexes that assist in feeding and mouth development. These are the rooting, suckling, tongue, swallowing, bite, transverse-tongue, and gag reflexes. See chapter 1 for details about these processes.

In addition to the differences in your newborn baby's mouth structure (compared with your mouth structure), there are also differences in the structure of her throat:

- The epiglottis and soft palate (two throat structures) are close together.
- The voice box is high in the neck.

These characteristics help protect your newborn baby from choking on liquid when swallowing. Again, see chapter 1 for more detail.

We discussed the importance of healthy Eustachian-tube function in the section entitled, "The Best Positioning for Feeding and Why," in chapter 2. Eustachian-tube problems can cause ear problems (eg, ear infections). Remember, your newborn baby's Eustachian tube is horizontal, while yours is more vertical. This tube connects the nasopharynx (the place where the nasal area and throat meet) to the middle-ear space. The middle-ear space is behind the eardrum and has three little bones that send sound from the outer ear to the inner ear and brain.

It is important for the middle-ear space to remain free from excessive mucus. Excessive mucus can become trapped in the middle-ear space and become infected if the Eustachian tube is not working properly. This is how ear infections occur. You will remember that we talked about feeding your baby with her ear above her mouth to keep liquid from entering the Eustachian tube (particularly after 2 to 3 months of age). If your child is bottle-fed, you can use this feeding position from birth. See chapter 2 for more information on this topic.

Date	Characteristics of a 1-Month-Old Baby
	Significant jaw growth occurs (birth to 1 year)[450–452]
	Jaw stability is developing; lip and tongue stability follows (birth to 1 year)[453–454]
	Significant lip and tongue growth occurs (birth to 2 years)
	Significant growth of the sphenoid sinus occurs (birth to 5 years)
	Control of the rooting reflex is developing
	Baby can match pitch and duration of care provider's voice[455]

At 1 month of age, your baby's jaw is growing, and the process of jaw stability has begun. The lower jaw needs to be dynamically stable (ie, be still but adjust in different positions) for feeding. For example, the lower jaw opens just enough for the bottle or breast and makes small adjustments or movements to maintain the latch and extract the liquid.

Lip and tongue stability develop slightly behind and in conjunction with jaw stability. If the jaw is not working properly, then it is difficult for the lips and tongue to work properly. Your 1-month-old baby's lips, tongue, and sphenoid sinus are also growing.

At 1 month of age, your baby is already starting to control the rooting reflex. You will see the rooting reflex less often in bottle-fed babies than in breast-fed babies because bottle-fed babies do not need it. Vocally, your baby will begin to match your voice pitch (a high or low sound) and duration (a long or short sound). Vocal sound can be heard coming through your baby's nose and mouth.

Date	Characteristics of a 2–3-Month-Old Baby
	Jaw growth is most pronounced in the first year of life[456–458]
	Significant lip and tongue growth occurs (birth to 2 years)

Date	Characteristics of a 2–3-Month-Old Baby
	Jaw stability is developing; lip and tongue stability follows (birth to 1 year)[459–460]
	The mouth begins to change shape, and the tongue begins to move more within the mouth
	Baby learns to send air through the mouth when cooing
	Baby learns to control the flow of air across the vocal cords in the voice box
	Control of the suckling reflex is developing

By 2 to 3 months of age, your baby's mouth is beginning to change shape. Your baby's jaw, lips, and tongue continue to grow. There is now more space within the mouth, the tongue can move more, and your baby can begin to direct air through the mouth when cooing. More space within the mouth allows the development of more control over the movement of mouth structures. Your baby is also learning to control the air as it moves across the vocal cords in the voice box. Her voice is mostly used for cooing and crying at this time, but will eventually be used for speech.

When feeding, your baby is starting to control the suckling reflex. She may be sucking more than suckling. Sucking involves more active use of the lips and elevation of the tongue than suckling. Control over the reflexes reflects brain development and purposeful control. This means your baby is beginning to control her own mouth movements. Chapter 1 details when babies begin to demonstrate control over oral reflexes and when these reflexes seem to disappear.

Date	Characteristics of a 3–4-Month-Old Baby
	Baby adapts to more space developing between the structures in the throat (the soft palate, epiglottis, and larynx); jaw, lip, tongue, and sinus growth continues
	Jaw stability is developing; lip and tongue stability follows (birth to 1 year)[461–462]

Date	Characteristics of a 3–4-Month-Old Baby
	The tongue seals toward the front third of the mouth, leading to a three-dimensional suck by 4 months (the tip of the tongue and sides come up, the lips pucker, the fat pads get smaller, and cheek and jaw muscles are developing)
	Suck-swallow-breathe coordination increases
	Baby demonstrates increase in vocalizations (ie, laughing, cooing)

At 3 to 4 months of age, your baby needs more control of the suck-swallow-breathe sequence when feeding. There is now even more space between the structures in the mouth and throat. Remember that sudden infant death syndrome, or SIDS, is most common between 2 and 4 months of age, when the mouth and throat structures are changing significantly. By 4 months, the three-dimensional suck is established, with the tongue sealing toward the front third of the mouth. At the same time, the fat pads in the cheeks are getting smaller, the cheek and jaw muscles are developing, and the lips are becoming more active. Your baby will also become increasingly vocal (ie, laughing, cooing, and starting to babble).

Date	Characteristics of a 4–6-Month-Old Baby
	Jaw growth is most pronounced in the first year of life[463–465]
	Teeth begin to come in with increased chewing and biting experiences (5–6 months)
	Significant lip and tongue growth occurs (birth to 2 years)
	Jaw stability is developing; lip and tongue stability follows (birth to 1 year)[466–467]
	Open space in the mouth continues to increase through jaw growth and the sucking pads getting smaller (4–6 months)
	Significant growth of sphenoid sinus occurs (birth to 5 years)

Date	Characteristics of a 4–6-Month-Old Baby
	Space between the mouth and nasal area is increasing (4–6 months)
	Baby begins to learn to use jaw, lip, and tongue muscles independently of one another
	Third lips disappear (3–6 months)
	Tongue moves up-down and front-to-back with a little less cupping (4–6 months)
	Gag reflex is coming under control (4–6 months)
	Rooting reflex is seen less and less; seems to be disappearing (3–6 months)
	Lip movement and control is developing (4–6 months)
	Appropriate intraoral air pressure, changes in voice pitch (the voice box is lower in the neck), and babbling are developing (4–6 months)
	The voice becomes louder as coordination improves between breathing and the voice box (4–6 months)

Between 4 and 6 months, your baby's sinuses, jaw, lips, and tongue continue to grow. Her vocal and swallowing mechanisms are developing. The open space within your baby's mouth increases with jaw growth and the decreasing size of the sucking pads. The space between your baby's mouth and nose increases. Your baby's jaw, lip, and tongue muscles begin to work independently of one another.

The swelling of the gums with feeding (called *the third lips*) disappears. Your baby's actual lips are now more active. The tongue can move front and back, side to side, and up and down inside the mouth. You will also notice that your baby's tongue is less cupped than before (ie, the sides of the tongue are not lifted as far). Tongue movement is more graded (ie, moving just enough for the activity). By 5 to 6 months, your baby's teeth will usually begin to emerge from an increase in chewing and biting activities.

Between 4 and 6 months, your baby has more control of the gag reflex. She can tolerate increasing stimulation to a larger area of the tongue without gagging. Your baby's rooting reflex is seen less, even if you are nursing. When your baby makes vocal sounds, most sound will now be coming through the mouth. Your baby's voice will become louder because your baby's voice box and breathing are maturing. The voice box is lower in the neck and increased control over the suck-swallow-breathe sequence during feeding is needed.

Date	Characteristics of a 6–9-Month-Old Baby
	Jaw, lip, tongue, and sinus growth continues
	Jaw stability is developing; lip and tongue stability follows (birth to 1 year)[468-469]
	Bottom two front teeth (central incisors) come in (5–9 months)
	Top two front teeth (central incisors) come in (6–10 months)
	Bottom lateral incisors come in (7–20 months)
	Top lateral incisors come in (8–10 months)
	Control develops over the bite reflex; more diagonal rotary jaw movement can be seen with feeding (5–9 months)
	Control develops over the transverse (side) tongue reflex (6–8 months)
	Around 7 months, the tongue moves toward food placed on the side of the gum area with a rolling, shifting motion
	Involuntary suckling reflex is seen less and less; seems to be disappearing (6–12 months)
	Most pronounced period of mouthing occurs (5–7 months)
	Gag reflex is found on the back third of the tongue (6–9 months)[470]

Date	Characteristics of a 6–9-Month-Old Baby
	Increased control of air through the throat, mouth, and nose is developing (5–9 months)
	Increased vocalization is noted with mouth play
	Baby vocalizes or raises voice to get attention or protest (7–9 months)

The 6- to 9-month period is another time of significant growth. Your baby's jaw, lips, tongue, sinuses, and other structures continue to grow. She will demonstrate improving stability (ie, holding the structure still but not rigid), grading (ie, moving the structure just enough), dissociation (ie, moving one structure independently of another), and direction (ie, moving the structure in the right direction) of the jaw, lips, and tongue for the processes of feeding and vocal sound production.

Between 5 and 7 months of age, your baby will show an increase in mouthing. This period is called *discriminative mouthing*. Good discrimination in the mouth is important for eating, drinking, and speaking. Your baby will also mouth, bite, and chew on safe toys and appropriate foods to help with the eruption of teeth. See chapters 4 and 5 for more information on the importance of appropriate mouthing experiences.

Teeth emerge with the increase in your baby's biting and chewing activities. Genetics also play a role in tooth eruption. The bottom two front teeth (central incisors) usually come in between 5 and 9 months. The top two front teeth (central incisors) usually come in between 6 and 10 months. The bottom lateral incisors usually come in between 7 and 20 months. The top lateral incisors usually come in between 8 and 10 months. Front teeth are important for taking bites. The top front teeth will also become contact points for later developing speech sounds (ie, "*f*" and "*v*" as early as 15 to 18 months and "th" as late as 7 years).

Your baby will develop control over the bite reflex between 5 and 9 months of age and the transverse (side) tongue reflex between 6 and 12 months of age. The control over the bite reflex means she is gaining control over up-and-down jaw movement used in taking bites of food, chewing food, and speech sound production. The control of the transverse (side) tongue reflex helps with management and manipulation of food within the mouth during chewing. Around 7 months, you will see this control demonstrated when your baby moves her tongue in a rolling, shifting motion toward food placed on a side gum surface.

Between 6 and 9 months of age, your baby's gag reflex should be located on the back third of the tongue. This allows your baby to handle more food textures within the mouth. In addition, your baby is now using more diagonal rotary jaw movements for chewing. This will eventually lead to a mature circular rotary chewing pattern. Effective jaw, lip, and tongue movements support good jaw, lip, and tongue growth and development. See chapter 6 for more detail on feeding development.

Also during the 6- to 9-month period, your baby will have more control over the air going through the throat, mouth, and nose. She will make many more speech sounds as a result. You will hear an increase in vocal sounds during mouth play. Your baby will vocalize or raise her voice to get attention or protest. See chapter 7 for specific information on speech sound and communication development.

Date	Characteristics of a 9–12-Month-Old Baby
	Jaw growth is most pronounced in the first year of life[471–473]
	Jaw stability is developing (birth to 1 year); lip and tongue stability follows[474–475]
	Bottom first molars come in (10–12 months)
	Bite reflex is seen less and less; seems to be disappearing
	Diagonal rotary jaw movement increases during chewing
	Significant lip and tongue growth occurs (birth to 2 years)
	Significant growth of the sphenoid sinus occurs (birth to 5 years)
	From 9–24 months, the transverse (side) tongue reflex is seen less and less; seems to be disappearing
	Involuntary suckling reflex is seen less and less; seems to be disappearing (6–12 months)
	Baby practices changes in speech volume, intonation, timing patterns, and rate when playing by herself and begins to use these when vocalizing with others

During the 9- to 12-month period, your baby is completing her first very important period of jaw growth (ie, birth to 12 months of age). Through feeding and other appropriate mouth activities, she develops a significant amount of jaw stability during this first year. A stable jaw is important for eating, drinking, and speaking (eg, opening the jaw to the right position to admit the spoon or cup and to make speech sounds).

Lip, tongue, and sinus growth also continues during the 9- to 12-month period. Tongue and lip stability have been developing, along with jaw stability. For example, around 12 months, your child's tongue tip begins to stabilize on the ridge behind the top front teeth to initiate the mature swallow. The sides of her tongue stabilize on the side gum ridges, so the tip of the tongue can move separately to produce the "*t*" and "*d*" sounds. Her lips stabilize along with the jaw on the open cup rim for drinking.

In the 9- to 12-month period, more teeth erupt, oral reflexes are seen less, and more oral control develops. The bottom first molars usually erupt between 10 and 12 months. The bite reflex (between 9 and 12 months), transverse-tongue reflex (between 9 and 24 months), and involuntary suckling reflex (between 6 and 12 months) are seen less. Diagonal rotary chewing is also seen more. While your child's mouth movements for eating and drinking will continue to become refined, she now has good control over mouth movements for eating and drinking.

Your child is also going through a period of significant vocal development between 9 and 12 months. She will practice changes in speech volume (ie, loud, soft, or in-between), changes in speech intonation (ie, changing pitch to match what she is trying to communicate), and changes in speech timing and speech rate when vocalizing. You may hear your baby begin to say approximations that sound like single words (eg, "dada," "mama," "bye-bye," "no," or "go").

Date	Characteristics of a 12–18-Month-Old Baby
	Significant growth of the sphenoid sinus occurs (birth to 5 years)
	Stable jaw-closing pattern appears; the top and bottom teeth meet (16 months)[476]
	Top first molars come in (14–16 months)
	Bottom cuspids come in (16–18 months)
	Significant lip and tongue growth continues (12–24 months)

Date	Characteristics of a 12–18-Month-Old Baby
	Front-to-back tongue reflex is seen less and less; seems to be disappearing
	From 9–24 months, the transverse (side) tongue reflex is seen less and less; seems to be disappearing
	Jaw, lips, and tongue continue to learn to move independently of one another
	Different parts of each structure continue to learn to move separately (eg, the tip of the tongue moves independently of the rest of the tongue, each lip corner contracts independently of the rest of the lips)
	Changes in pitch, loudness, rate, stress, and intonation occur when vocalizing (eg, pitch goes up for request, attention, and curiosity and goes down for greetings, surprise, persistence, and attempts to be recognized), 12–15 months[477]
	Baby uses rising pitch when anticipating an event; uses rising then falling pitch for emphasis (15–18 months)[478]

During the 12- to 18-month period, even more teeth erupt. The top first molars usually come in between 14 and 16 months. Bottom cuspids usually come in between 16 and 18 months. Your baby now has both top and bottom first molars. According to Dr Raymond D. Kent, "occlusal contact" (ie, the top and bottom teeth coming together) around 16 months of age marks "the appearance of a stable jaw-closing pattern."[479] The jaw needs to stabilize dynamically in a variety of positions and remain relatively still in just the right location(s) so we can effectively take bites of food, eat from a spoon, drink from a cup, and produce speech sounds.

Your child's jaw, lips, and tongue continue to grow between 12 and 24 months. She also has more control over tongue movements because the tongue reflexes seem to be disappearing. Jaw, lip, and tongue movements for eating, drinking, and speaking become increasingly dissociated (ie, one structure moves independently of another) and graded (ie, structures move just enough for the activity in the right direction). You will hear even more changes in pitch, loudness, rate, stress, and intonation when your child is vocalizing. These vocal changes help your child make her communication clear. See chapter 7 for more detail.

Date	Characteristics of an 18–24-Month-Old Child
	Significant growth of the sphenoid sinus occurs (birth to 5 years)
	Jaw stability is increasing significantly (16–24 months)
	Top cuspids come in (18–20 months)
	Bottom second molars come in (20–24 months)
	Top second molars come in (24–30 months)
	All first (primary) teeth come in by 24–30 months (See Figure 8.3)
	Significant lip and tongue growth occurs (12–24 months)
	Transverse (side) tongue reflex is seen less and less; seems to have disappeared by 24 months
	Jaw, lips, and tongue continue to learn to move independently of one another
	Different parts of each structure continue to learn to move separately (eg, the tip of the tongue moves independently of the rest of the tongue, each lip corner contracts independently of the rest of the lips)
	Good control of swallowing is achieved by 18 months
	Child moves jaw, lips, and tongue easily during speech
	Child uses falling then rising pitch to convey a warning; uses rising then falling pitch to convey playfulness (18–21 months)[480]
	Child can change voice from a whisper to a louder voice (21–24 months)

The 18- to 24-month period is a time of refinement for your child's eating and drinking skills. These skills will be relatively complete by 24 months of age. However, her speech sound development will continue until around age 8.

During the 18- to 24-month period, your child will continue to experiment and develop the use of vocal pitch to convey meaning (eg, raising then lowering her voice to express playfulness, as in "ut↑oh↓"). Between 21 and 24 months, your child will play with changing her voice from a whisper to a louder voice. Most children love to whisper.

Your child's top cuspids usually erupt around 18 to 20 months. Her bottom second molars usually erupt around 20 to 24 months, and her top second molars usually erupt around 24 to 30 months, completing the eruption of the primary teeth. Figure 8.3 illustrates the difference between the young child's jaw, with a full set of primary (deciduous) teeth, and the adult jaw, with a full set of permanent teeth. Teeth provide important contact points for the tongue and lower lip during speech production. The back of the tongue dynamically stabilizes in the back molar area for smooth, connected speech production. The sides of the tongue stabilize along the side teeth and gums as the tongue tip moves independently for the production of speech sounds such as "*t*," "*d*," and "*n*." The lower lip stabilizes and makes light contact with the top front teeth for the speech sounds "*f*" and "*v*."

Along with tooth development, jaw stability increases significantly between 16 and 24 months. Significant lip and tongue growth continues during this period of time. The transverse (side) tongue reflex seems to have disappeared by 24 months. Your child has good control over jaw, lip, and tongue movement. By 24 months, jaw, lip, and tongue movements are dissociated, graded, and moving in the right direction for eating, drinking, and speaking. This is one reason your child's speech and expressive language skills can increase rapidly after her second birthday.

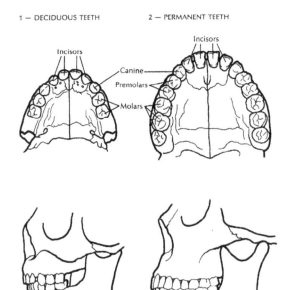

1 — DECIDUOUS TEETH   2 — PERMANENT TEETH

Incisors

Incisors

Canine
Premolars
Molars

Illustration 3-27
Distribution of Deciduous and Permanent Teeth

Figure 8.3: Distribution of deciduous and permanent teeth (tooth, jaw, and palate growth).

Source: Reprinted from Craniosacral Therapy II: Beyond the Dura by John E. Upledger, p. 192, with permission of Eastland Press.

Date	Characteristics of a 3–7-Year-Old Child[481–483]
	Gradual growth of the mouth, face, and head continues
	80% of upper and lower jaw growth is complete (6 years)[484–485]
	Skull is essentially adult sized (6 years)
	Permanent teeth come in (6–14 years, except wisdom teeth); see Figure 8.3
	Permanent top and bottom first molars come in (6–7 years)
	Permanent bottom central incisors come in (6–7 years)
	Significant growth of the sphenoid sinus occurs (birth to 5 years)
	Significant growth of the frontal sinus occurs (3–12 years)
	Adultlike swallow has developed (3 years)
	Adultlike vocal tract has developed; adenoids shrink (4 years)
	Child essentially has an adult vocal tract (5 years)

The gradual growth of your child's mouth, face, and head continues throughout the 3- to 7-year period. Your child has an adultlike swallow by age 3. Her vocal tract (ie, windpipe, voice box, and oral, throat, and nasal areas responsible for resonance) is adultlike by 4 years of age. Her adenoids hopefully begin to shrink at this time. If your child has had a problem with enlarged tonsils and adenoids, this process may help.

Children with chronically enlarged adenoids and tonsils often have what speech-language pathologists call denasal or hyponasal voices. This means that the sounds "m," "n," and "ng" that are supposed to come through the nose do not. It is important to know that enlarged adenoids and tonsils often mean that your child is fighting an infection or has allergies. See chapter 3 for more information on ideas to resolve these types of health problems.

Significant growth of the sphenoid sinus continues until around age 5, and significant growth of the frontal sinus occurs between 3 and 12 years of age. This growth is important for cranial and facial development. Your child's skull is essentially adult sized by age 6, and her upper and lower jaw growth is about 80% complete by age 6. That is when her permanent teeth will begin to erupt (between 6 and 14 years of age, with the exception of wisdom teeth, which erupt later). See Figure 8.3.

The speech sound production system matures between 3 and 8 years of age. See chapter 7 for details. You already know that teeth play an important role in your child's ability to produce speech. This becomes particularly apparent when children lose their top front "baby" teeth. A lisp may be heard until the new front teeth come in.

Date	Characteristics of a 7–10-Year-Old Child[486-487]
	Significant growth of the frontal sinus occurs (3–12 years)
	Noticeable growth spurt in the lower face occurs (7–10 years)[488]
	90% of upper and lower jaw growth is complete (8–10 years)[489-490]
	Permanent teeth come in (6–14 years, except wisdom teeth); see Figure 8.3
	Permanent top central incisors come in (7–8 years)
	Permanent bottom lateral incisors come in (7–8 years)
	Permanent top lateral incisors come in (8–9 years)
	Permanent bottom cuspids come in (9–10 years)
	Jaw moves with adultlike precision[491] (age 8)
	Differences begin to be found in voice tissue between boys and girls (age 8)
	A change in resonance occurs secondary to tonsil shrinkage (age 9)

Between 7 and 10 years of age, the lower face and jaw go through a noticeable growth spurt. Your child's upper and lower jaw development is 90% complete between ages 8 and 10. Jaw development will be somewhat different in boys and girls. By age 8, the jaw moves with adultlike precision.[492] This is the same time your child's speech sound production system matures. Most children produce most speech sounds accurately by age 8. This has been a long process from birth, with the mastery of many different speech sounds occurring over time. See chapter 7 for complete information on speech sound development.

A number of permanent teeth erupt during the 7- to 10-year period. See the previous chart for a schedule of tooth eruption. The frontal sinus continues to grow, and your child's facial appearance will mature. Changes in resonance occur with changes in tonsil tissue, sinus growth, and mouth growth. By age 9, you may begin to hear the change in your child's vocal resonance that results from tonsil atrophy. Around this time, the tonsils begin to shrink. This can change the quality of your child's voice. The tissue in your child's voice box will also begin to change. This is where the voices of boys and girls begin to sound different.

If the tonsils and adenoids had been chronically enlarged prior to this time, your child's voice may actually begin to sound clearer. However, if the tonsils and adenoids shrink and the uvula of the soft palate does not rise properly, your child may sound hypernasal. The soft palate has a structure called the *uvula* that hangs down at the back of the throat and rises for all speech sounds except "*m*," "*n*," and "ng." Hypernasality can also occur with a submucous cleft palate (a hole in the bony center of the hard palate with skin and tissue over it). You know what hypernasal speech sounds like from hearing Fran Drescher portray "The Nanny" on television. If your child has either hyponasality or hypernasality, see an ear, nose, and throat physician.

Date	Characteristics of a 10–16-Year-Old Child[493–494]
	Significant growth of the frontal sinus occurs (3–12 years)
	90% of jaw growth is complete (10–12 years)
	Permanent teeth come in (6–14 years, except wisdom teeth); see Figure 8.3
	Permanent bottom first bicuspids erupt (10–12 years)
	Permanent top first bicuspids erupt (10–11 years)

Date	Characteristics of a 10–16-Year-Old Child[493-494]
	Permanent top second bicuspids erupt (10–12 years)
	Permanent bottom second bicuspids erupt (11–12 years)
	Permanent top cuspids erupt (11–13 years)
	Permanent bottom second molars erupt (11–13 years)
	Permanent top second molars erupt (12–13 years)
	Period of tongue growth occurs (9–16 years)
	Period of lip growth occurs (9–17 years)
	Girls achieve a relatively mature-sounding voice (12 years)
	Girls achieve an adultlike voice (16 years)
	Voice change begins in boys (12½–14½ years)

The 10- to 16-year period is another period of significant growth. Ninety percent of jaw growth is complete between the ages of 10 and 12 years. By the age of 14, your child should have all of her permanent teeth, with the exception of wisdom teeth. See Figure 8.3. Girls have a relatively mature-sounding voice by age 12 and an adultlike voice by age 16. Boys usually experience significant voice changes between 12½ and 14½ years of age. Speech therapists sometimes see children who previously required speech therapy for a checkup and/or tune-up during times of rapid jaw, lip, and tongue growth because they may reexperience imprecise speech or other problems with mouth movement during this time.

Date	Age	Sex	Additional Characteristics[495-497]
	Up to age 16	Females	Jaw, tongue, and lips continue to grow
	Up to age 16	Females	Jaw and face reach adult size (around 15–16 years)
	Up to age 18 or later	Males	Jaw, tongue, and lips continue to grow
	Up to age 18 or later	Males	Jaw and face reach adult size (around 18 years)
	17–25 years	Both	Permanent top and bottom third molars (ie, wisdom teeth) erupt

Your daughter's jaw, tongue, and lips will continue to grow until approximately 16 years of age. Your son's jaw, tongue, and lips may continue to grow until 18 years of age or beyond. The permanent top and bottom third molars (ie, wisdom teeth) usually come in between the ages of 17 and 25 years in both males and females.

9

Working with Professionals

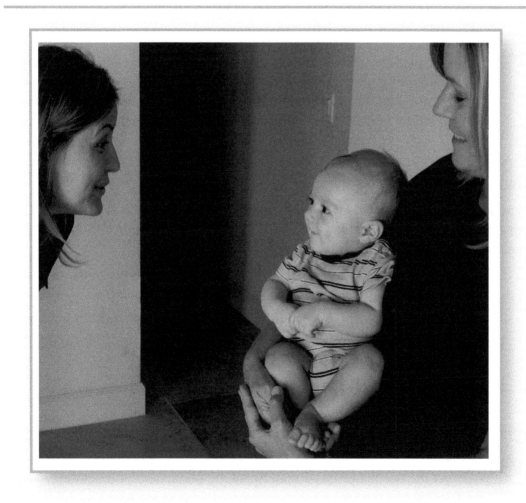

Key Topics in This Chapter

■ Suggestions for Finding and Working with an Appropriate Professional

■ Your Child's Lactation Consultant, Pediatrician, and Other Medical Professionals

■ Speech-Language Pathologists and Audiologists

■ Occupational Therapists

■ Other Professionals You and Your Child May Need or Encounter

■ Teams

T his chapter describes your role and the roles of professionals you may encounter if your child has health or developmental issues. Parents become stressed when their child has a problem. So, choose professionals with whom you and your child can work with comfort and confidence.

Suggestions for Finding and Working with an Appropriate Professional

Here are some suggestions for finding an appropriate referral and working in partnership with professionals your child may need. You will usually begin by speaking with your child's pediatrician.

1. Speak with your child's pediatrician about your concern(s). Ask him or her for a referral to an appropriate professional, if needed.

2. Ask other parents who have children with a similar concern for a referral.

3. Speak with the county or state infant-toddler program about available assessments and resources.

4. Check with your local hospital regarding available assessments and resources.

5. Check with universities in your area with training programs for therapists for available assessments and resources.

6. Contact the needed professional. Speak by phone and/or meet the professional in person to see if this person is a good match for you and your child.

7. When choosing or working with professionals, ask questions and discuss the evidence for the treatments being suggested. Evidence includes research completed with control groups, research completed

with individual and multiple cases, and the professional's experience with specific treatments. As a parent, it is very important for you to have a full understanding of any treatment your child is undergoing.

A Note about Research: In the area of child development, many wonderful studies have been completed in the past 30 years and even prior to that. Research is not necessarily old, unless it was poorly done or there is new research to replace it. I make this point because many people think that old research is not good research.

8. Work with the professional that suits your child's needs. You know your child's needs better than anyone.

9. Be a partner in treatment. You play a key role in any process involving your child. Partnerships require "give and take" by all people who participate in a process. As a partner, you support the work of the professional, and the professional supports your work with your child. This empowers you as a parent. **Please do not be a bystander.** I have met many frustrated and angry parents who were bystanders instead of partners and participants.

10. If you begin to feel that a professional is not meeting your child's needs at any time, speak with the professional about this. I discourage parents from overshopping for professionals if possible (ie, trying one therapist or physician, then another, then another, then another) because the child does not get consistent treatment when this occurs. Sometimes, there is merely a need for clarification and communication between you and the professional to resolve concerns and issues that arise. However, if you and the professional cannot resolve problems after working together on them, go for a second opinion.

11. Know that not all professionals are created equal, and this is perfectly all right. Each of us is more skilled and talented in some areas than in others. It is important for you to locate the professional that suits your needs as a parent and the needs of your child.

Remember, you are your child's best advocate. You know your child better than other people. Many parents seem intimidated by professionals. However, professionals are people too, so try to relax when you are working with them. It is best for you and your child if you can work in partnership with any professional your child may need. Now, let's talk about some of the professionals you may encounter in addition to the dentists and orthodontists we discussed in chapter 8.

Your Child's Lactation Consultant, Pediatrician, and Other Medical Professionals

I have worked with many parents who have been angry with their children's pediatricians for not knowing certain information. You must remember that your child's pediatrician is your child's general physician. In this role, the pediatrician really needs to know details about your child's overall medical needs and something about your child's developmental needs. This is a big job.

One reason for writing this book is to give you, your child's pediatrician, and others an informed, well-researched resource on feeding, speech, and mouth development. Much of this information is known by therapists and other specialists who work with children who have special needs. However, it is not known by the general public. Knowing this information can make your life and your child's life a lot easier.

The information will also help you know when it is appropriate to ask your child's pediatrician about a referral to a specialist. I have tremendous regard for pediatricians and all they need to know. Please help your child's pediatrician provide your child with the best care possible by becoming an informed parent. Use the developmental checklists and information from this book to become a partner with your child's pediatrician in the care of your child.

Let's talk about lactation consultants. International Board Certified Lactation Consultants, or IBCLCs, strategize to protect the mother's milk supply and the breast-feeding relationship (according to Caroline L. Bias, Susan Chick, and Beverly Morgan). They can help Mom to:

- Assist a baby who refuses to breast-feed to go to the breast

- Build and maintain breast milk supply

- Learn about herbs and foods that support breast milk production

- Work with a baby who is sensitive to touch or mother's milk let-down

- Work with latching problems, breast milk pumping, supplemental feeding, syringe-feeding, finger-feeding, nipple shields, and Haberman feeders[498]

Work with IBCLCs in the hospital where you delivered your baby if possible. I suggest working with IBCLCs because they are highly trained. If they are not *readily available* at your hospital, contact other hospitals in your area to find out what lactation services are offered. I accentuate the words *readily available* because mothers of new babies need skilled lactation consultants who can be available when they are needed. This sometimes means nights and weekends.

I had the advantage of working with a wonderful team of IBCLCs from the Greater Baltimore Medical Center in Maryland for a number of years. I learned as much from them as they learned from me. This dedicated group of nurses worked with anyone who needed them. They made home visits and attended evaluation sessions with their young clients and parents. Most of the time, babies were referred to me because there was some unidentified reason they were not breast-feeding efficiently and effectively.

Many of the babies I saw had the subtle difficulties discussed in chapter 2 (eg, small to nonexistent sucking pads, and/or mild problems with jaw, lip, and tongue movement). The lactation consultants and I worked together with parents to resolve the problems. I generally had one consultation with a baby and the baby's parent(s) to diagnose the problem and make some new recommendations. The lactation consultants could usually help the mom and baby from that point on.

I have also had the honor of presenting material at professional meetings for lactation consultants. I found that I had some information from the fields of speech-language pathology and occupation therapy that many lactation consultants had not received in their own training. My work with lactation consultants, families, and babies has been a true highlight of my career and one reason I dedicated this book to them.

Many medical professionals are listed in the "Health Problems and Possible Treatments" section in chapter 3. We will discuss them again here. The pediatric gastroenterologist can evaluate and treat your child's reflux and stomach, bowel, or any other gastrointestinal problems. The pediatric ear, nose, and throat specialist (ie, otolaryngologist) is the physician to see if your child is having chronic middle-ear, sinus, or other upper respiratory problems. The pediatric audiologist can evaluate your child's hearing from birth. Please be sure to have your child's hearing screened on a regular basis. The pediatric allergist can evaluate and treat your child for food and environmental allergies or sensitivities. While it has historically been difficult to test young children for allergies and sensitivities, medical knowledge in this area is now greatly improved. If your child has chronic respiratory problems, your child's physician may suggest you work with a pulmonologist and respiratory therapist.

The pediatric registered dietitian or nutritionist can help you make sure that your child is receiving proper nutrition. Ellyn Satter is a registered dietitian and social worker who wrote some highly recommended books on feeding. These are listed in Appendix A under "Resources for Parents and Care Providers." However, you may need a feeding therapist to help you with feeding your child. We will discuss the work of the feeding therapist in the following sections on speech-language pathology, occupational therapy, and teams.

Speech-Language Pathologists and Audiologists

I have worked as a speech-language pathologist for around 30 years. I have truly been blessed to be part of a wonderful field that is dedicated to help all individuals with eating, drinking, speech, language, and other related difficulties.

Before we discuss the role of the speech-language pathologist, however, I want to talk about the importance of the pediatric audiologist. Audiologists are certified by the American Speech-Language-Hearing Association, or ASHA, and the American Academy of Audiology, or AAA. It is critical that your child have his hearing screened at birth and at regular intervals throughout childhood. See *www.asha.org* (the American Speech-Language-Hearing Association) and *www.aap.org* (the American Academy of Pediatrics) for more information on hearing screening.

Children are particularly susceptible to middle-ear problems that can cause fluctuating hearing loss. This may be a particular concern for children who use a pacifier long-term and who are improperly bottle-fed. Children need good hearing to develop speech, language, and communication skills, as well as subsequent academic skills. If your child has hearing loss and is identified early, he can receive appropriate treatment from an audiologist, speech-language pathologist, or other early intervention specialist.

Now back to speech-language pathologists. This is an area I definitely know something about! Speech-language pathologists work with children who have feeding, speech, language, and other communication problems. Here are some guidelines for you to use when looking for a properly trained speech-language pathologist.

Characteristics of a Properly Trained Speech-Language Pathologist

Age of Your Child	What to Look for
Child born prematurely	Speech-language pathologist working in a neonatal intensive care unit
Newborn	Speech-language pathologist trained in feeding and mouth development
Birth to 6 months	Speech-language pathologist trained in feeding and mouth development
6 to 12 months	Speech-language pathologist trained in feeding, mouth development, and early speech sound and language development
12 to 24 months	Speech-language pathologist trained in feeding, mouth development, and early speech sound and language development
24+ months	Speech-language pathologist with training determined by your child's needs

Let me tell you how a properly trained speech-language pathologist can help you and your child when needed. Remember, we talked about the idea that not all professionals are created equal. This is true in every professional. We all have different interests, specialties, and skills. Speech-language pathologists are trained according to certain standards from the American Speech-Language-Hearing Association, or ASHA. When looking for a speech-language pathologist, it is best to find one who holds a certificate of clinical competence from ASHA. These therapists write "CCC-SLP" as part of their credentials. You will find some therapists who have different types of credentialing. This is particularly true in some school systems. Also, if you live outside the United States, you will find other types of credentialing.

The most important thing is to be well informed and to know what questions to ask when looking for a therapist. I have given you some ideas in the previous chart. Information is power. Don't be afraid of it. Review appropriate sections of this book and ask if the therapist knows about the techniques or information listed in those pages or something comparable. If you think your child needs to see a speech-language pathologist, go over the concerns you have with your child's pediatrician. The pediatrician's office staff can often help you find the therapist or team you need.

If your child was born prematurely, you are likely to find a well-trained speech-language pathologist in the neonatal intensive care unit. If there is not a speech-language pathologist in the unit, you are likely to find an equally well-trained occupational therapist. The therapists found in a particular setting are often based on availability of the therapists and the way that particular team defines the needs of the patients.

If you have a full-term or near-term newborn who is having difficulty with breast- or bottle-feeding, look for a speech-language pathologist trained in infant feeding. Some speech-language pathologists are also trained lactation consultants. There are also occupational therapists who are similarly trained. In addition, there are special feeding teams where speech-language pathologists and occupational therapists work together. Some children who have early feeding difficulties also have later speech concerns. While follow-up is important for these children (ie, periodic developmental checkups), a child with an early feeding problem may not have any later speech concerns. I don't want parents fretting about this.

From birth to 6 months of age, your baby will primarily feed from the bottle or breast. Between 4 and 6 months of age, you will likely introduce baby cereals and other soft solid foods as directed by your child's pediatrician. If your child has difficulties, speak with your child's pediatrician and consider contacting a speech-language pathologist or occupational therapist trained in feeding and mouth development. It is also important to observe your baby's hearing and communication development during this period to be sure these are on track. If

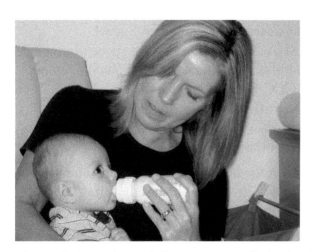
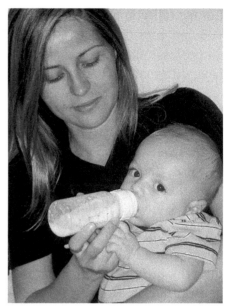

Photo 9.1: a. Speech-language pathologist Diane demonstrates correct bottle-feeding positioning with Anthony. **b.** Anthony's mom Cris practices correct positioning.

your baby is not following the sequences listed in this book, speak with your child's pediatrician, and consider contacting the early intervention program in your state to request an evaluation. Also, be sure your child undergoes regular hearing screenings, as recommended by your child's pediatrician.

Note on Autism: The information presented throughout this book is particularly important for children with a history of autism in the family. Some of the earliest signs of autism include difficulties with social and communicative interaction (eg, responding to the child's own name, smiling, producing speech sounds, and participating in social play). These children often have difficulties with feeding, as well.

From 6 to 12 months of age, your baby will develop many new skills in many areas. In the developmental checklists throughout this book, you can follow your baby's mouth, feeding, and communication development. Again, your child's pediatrician and the early intervention team are often good places to start when looking for a speech-language pathologist (ie, if your child has problems in these areas). Look for a therapist who is skilled in feeding and mouth development and who can specifically assess and treat the development of speech sounds, in addition to language development.

From 12 to 24 months of age, your child is completing a critical learning period for mouth development. Most of his feeding skills will be complete, and speech development is well underway. By 24 months, your child will be putting words together. If your child has difficulty with feeding and speech-language development during this time, you will need a speech-language pathologist trained in mouth development, speech sound development, language development, and feeding.

Beyond 24 months of age, your child should have the feeding skills that he will use throughout life. Your child's speech, language, and communication skills will continue to develop. There are many speech-language pathologists who are well trained to work with children over 24 months of age. However, if your child is having a problem with any of the areas of development discussed in this book before the age of 24 months, have him evaluated and treated by an appropriately trained therapist (if needed). Remember that birth to age 2 is the best time for your child to develop the skills listed in this developmental period. It may be more difficult for your child to learn them later.

Occupational Therapists

Now this is a group with which I truly enjoy working. You may see an occupational therapist instead of a speech-language pathologist if your baby has a feeding problem. Speech-language pathologists and occupational therapists often do similar work. The person with whom you work frequently depends on the team or the special skills of the therapist. When I offer my training course on oral motor treatment (ie, feeding, speech, and mouth function), I often have an equal number of speech-language pathologists and occupational therapists in my courses. This is true for courses I have taught in the United States, Europe, and Asia.

Occupational therapists generally work on activities of daily living and anything that can cause a problem with these. Therefore, feeding, personal care, dressing, and the cognitive skills that go along with these activities are some of the areas addressed by occupational therapists. They have standardized training procedures and are certified through the American Occupational Therapy Association, or AOTA, and the National Board for Certification in Occupational Therapy, or NBCOT.

Occupational therapists are usually part of early intervention teams. In some areas of the United States resources are quite limited, so occupational therapists are often asked to do the work of other disciplines (eg, speech-language pathology and physical therapy). This situation is less than ideal, because each discipline has been trained to look at your child in a somewhat different manner, focusing on different areas of development. This is the reason that early intervention treatment teams usually include speech-language pathology, occupational therapy, physical therapy, education, and others as needed.

Many occupational therapists are trained in the assessment and treatment of sensory processing disorders. We talked a lot about sensory processing in chapters 4 and 5. The understanding of sensory processing helps therapists, teachers, parents, and others better identify the way children learn and function in the world. We are all constantly bombarded with sensory information. How we process and use this information determines how we react in a given situation. All of the sensory systems (eg, senses of movement, touch, taste, smell, sight, and hearing) need to work well together so we can concentrate, participate in our world, and learn. See *www.thesensoryworld.com* for books and information on this topic.

While many occupational therapists tend to have a good understanding of the sensory systems in the body, some occupational therapists are specifically trained in vision work. If you have any questions about your child's vision, you will want to see a pediatric ophthalmologist. However, there are other specialists (eg, behavioral optometrists and low-vision specialists), including many occupational therapists who can help your child better use his vision.

I also want to mention the body of research that the field of occupational therapy has provided for the field of speech-language pathology and others. When I was researching mouth and feeding development for this book, I found a substantial amount of information in the occupational therapy literature.

Other Professionals You and Your Child May Need or Encounter

Here are some other professionals you may encounter. The pediatric physical therapist can help you if your child has orthopedic problems or a developmental motor delay that affects the entire body. There are also physical therapists who work with jaw problems (eg, temporomandibular joint dysfunction) and feeding problems. Some pediatric physical therapists and massage practitioners specialize in craniosacral treatment and myofascial release treatment, which was discussed briefly in chapter 8. Physical therapists are certified through the American Physical Therapy Association, or APTA. There are also pediatric physical therapists, occupational therapists, speech-language pathologists, and certified massage therapists who teach infant massage courses for parents. We discussed the importance of massage in chapter 5.

Note: If your child has an orthopedic and/or motor disorder that affects his or her movement patterns in the body, see a physical therapist. Physical therapists are properly trained to work with these disorders.

If you work with a massage practitioner, make sure he or she is qualified to work with children. When working with a massage practitioner, find out the massage school attended and what additional courses were taken. A qualified massage practitioner should have credentials from the National Certification Board for Therapeutic Massage and Body Work, or NCBTMB, as well as a license from the state. He or she may also be a member of the American Massage Therapy Association, or AMTA. I went to massage school and became credentialed by the NCBTMB because I wanted to know more about hands-on techniques to use with children. I also received additional training in myofascial release and craniosacral treatment. You can refer to *www.upledger.com* for a list of qualified practitioners who do craniosacral work and *www.myofascialrelease.com* for more information on myofascial release. We discussed these treatment modalities very briefly in chapter 8.

Psychologists and social workers are two other professionals you may encounter. Pediatric psychologists can provide testing for cognitive and learning problems. Both psychologists and social workers can provide counseling and can work with families on social and emotional problems. I also want to mention the body of developmental research the field of psychology has provided. When I was researching communication development for this book, I found a substantial amount of information in the psychology literature.

Teams

Your child's pediatrician can usually help you find the early intervention team in your area. Early intervention teams are usually provided by the local school system, state department of education, or health department. However, there are also early intervention teams at hospitals and medical facilities. The team often consists of an early childhood special educator, a speech-language pathologist, an occupational therapist, a physical therapist, and others as appropriate. Other disciplines may include an audiologist, a psychologist, a social worker, and other specialized disciplines as needed.

The early intervention team provided by the local school system, state department of education, or health department usually follows an educational model. The therapists on this type of team may be limited by funding as well as federal, state, and local regulations. A hospital-based early intervention team generally uses a medical model. The medical model usually involves "hands-on" work with your child, while the educational model focuses on training the parent to work with the child. I think there is value in both models. You can work with your child's pediatrician to help you decide which type of team is best for you and your child. I have served on both types of early intervention teams with excellent therapists who had outstanding results.

There are two other teams you may need if your child has oral structural problems (eg, a cleft lip or palate) and/or feeding problems. In chapter 10, you will see that there are a number of disorders in which children are born with cleft lips and/or palates. These children need a specialized team to work with the problems associated with clefts. If your child has a cleft, you may need the early intervention team (discussed previously), as well as the cleft-palate team and the feeding team discussed in this section.

The cleft-palate team usually consists of a speech-language pathologist, a surgeon, a special dentist, and other medical professionals that will follow your child as he goes through surgical intervention. From my experience as a therapist, children who undergo surgery for most types of clefts also require ongoing treatment for feeding and speech. This treatment is usually done by a hospital or other early intervention therapist, not the therapist on the cleft-palate team. There are entire books written on surgical intervention for cleft palate; however, information is just becoming available on specific oral-motor intervention for children with repaired clefts. See "Resources for Parents and Care Providers" in Appendix A for books and resources on this topic.

A feeding team is often found in a specialty hospital for children. These teams work with children who have significant feeding problems and their parents. Some of these teams want children and parents to live at the hospital for a period of time until the parents and children can work effectively on feeding together. Depending on the age and problems demonstrated by the child, team members and team function may vary.

I have worked on several feeding teams in my career. These usually consisted of a speech-language pathologist, an occupational therapist, a physical therapist, the parents and/or care provider(s), and others as appropriate. Other professionals may include an educator, a psychologist, a social worker, a vision specialist, and an audiologist. If you are looking for a feeding team for your child, look for a team that can evaluate and treat your child's mouth movement and sensory processing.

Some feeding teams focus primarily on behavioral concerns, and behavioral problems generally accompany feeding issues. Behavior is a form of communication and often results from problems with sensory and motor function. Treating the communicative behaviors that go along with feeding difficulties is important. However, it is also important to have a team that can evaluate and treat the underlying problems that cause behaviors. Teams that evaluate and treat behavior alone are less than ideal, because most feeding problems go beyond behavioral problems. They usually involve sensory, motor, and behavioral concerns. See information on feeding problems in chapter 6.

Note: When you work with any team, you and your child are part of that team. If you do not feel like you are a team member, discuss this with the team. See "Suggestions for Finding and Working with an Appropriate Professional" at the beginning of this chapter.

10

How Does This Apply to My Child with Particular Special Needs?

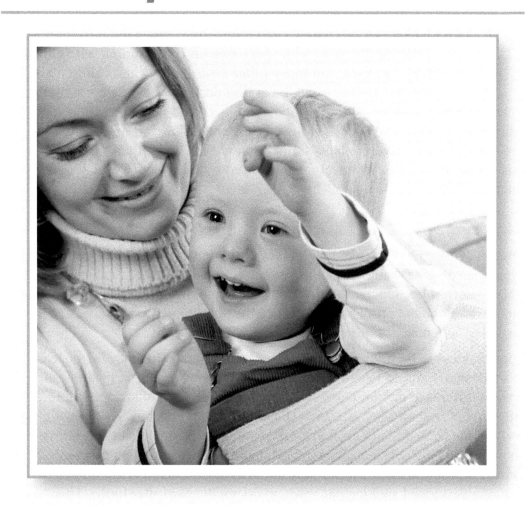

Key Topics in This Chapter

- Children Born Prematurely
- Children with Down Syndrome
- Children with Autism
- Children with Cerebral Palsy
- Children with Hearing Loss
- Children with Other Developmental Delay
- A Few Comments Regarding Treatment of Children with Cleft Lip and Palate

This chapter teaches parents and others how to use the information in this book for the child with special needs (eg, children with Down syndrome, autism, and many other disorders). When children are taught skills during typical learning periods, they are more likely to learn them. Children with developmental disorders may not automatically learn feeding and speech skills on their own. They often require special techniques to develop these skills. Many of the techniques discussed in this book were originally developed and used by therapists working in early intervention.

Children Born Prematurely

Over the years, I have worked with many children who were born prematurely. More than 500,000 babies are born prematurely in the United States each year.[499] This group has been increasing for some time, and they often have feeding and mouth development problems. I have had the opportunity to see advances in medicine help many of these children live more typical lives.

Some babies are born just a little early, or "near term." This may be related to scheduled, induced labors. Even being a couple of weeks premature can make a difference in your baby's development. An article that appeared in *The Washington Post* on May 20, 2006, stated that 350,000 babies are born slightly early in the United States each year (the average U.S. pregnancy has been shortened to 39 weeks), leading to feeding difficulties and other problems.[500] One of the biggest differences I have seen in these children is missing or only partially developed sucking pads (which do not develop after birth). This can significantly affect feeding. See chapters 1 and 2 to read more about the importance of sucking pads.

The structures, movements, and coordination for feeding and swallowing are not well developed in preemies (ie, babies born more than 3 weeks early).[501] We wait until an appropriate developmental age to feed these little ones by mouth. This depends on how early a baby was born and is determined by the neonatal intensive-care unit, or NICU, team. When feeding a preemie, many differences must be taken into consideration. The following chart is a summary of these differences from the book *Pre-Feeding Skills: A Comprehensive Resource for Mealtime Development* (2nd edition) by Suzanne Evans Morris and Marsha Dunn Klein.[502]

ACTIVITY 10.1: DIFFERENCES BETWEEN A FULL-TERM BABY AND A PREMATURE BABY[503]

This activity is meant for parents and care providers of preemies. Place a date next to the characteristics that describe your baby. You will see some characteristics of prematurity. However, you may also see some skills that are more like those of a full-term baby. The NICU staff can help you observe what your child is doing, once your baby is medically stable.

Date	Full-Term Baby	Date	Premature Baby
	Exhibits flexion (bending) in the body		Exhibits extension (stiffening and straightening) in the body
	Exhibits appropriate stability in the body		Exhibits poor stability in the body
	Is ready to suckle		Often is not ready to suckle
	Has a strong suckle		Has a weak suckle
	Has a good lip seal		Has a poor lip seal
	Has developed sucking pads		Has not developed sucking pads
	Has enough jaw stability for suckling		Has poor jaw stability for suckling

ACTIVITY 10.1: (Cont.)

Date	Full-Term Baby	Date	Premature Baby
	Can feel when he or she is hungry or thirsty		Has limited hunger and/or thirst
	Has a rhythmic suck-swallow-breathe pattern		Has a poor suck-swallow-breathe rhythm
	Has complete oral reflexes		Has limited oral reflexes

We do not expect a baby born prematurely to be ready for feeding in the same way as a full-term baby. However, premature babies do have different developmental paths, depending on how early they are born. When assessing readiness for feeding, nurses, therapists, and physicians consider corrected age (ie, the age calculated from the full-term due date rather than the delivery date).

Some babies are ready to begin breast-feeding as early as 28 to 36 weeks gestation or postconception age, or PCA, while bottle-feeding is often started at 34 to 35 weeks.[504] In most of the references reviewed for this chapter, breast-feeding was the preferred method of feeding for premature infants because it required less energy, resulted in fewer breathing complications, provided more appropriate nutrition, and was generally more efficient. However, bottle-feeding may be the method of choice for some babies. Choosing to breast- or bottle-feed is a choice you will make with the help and support of the NICU staff.

You can also explore some other techniques with the NICU staff to improve the results of feeding. Kangaroo care (ie, when the child is fed during skin-to-skin contact) has been shown to improve feeding results. Properly applied infant massage has also been very effective in helping premature infants gain weight and receive clearance to go home.[505]

Note about Massaging Premature Infants: Preemies are more likely to become overwhelmed by too much sensory input (as demonstrated by changes in their vital signs) than full-term infants. There is special full-body massage for preemies. Work with your NICU staff on this, and contact the International Association of Infant Massage Instructors *(www.iaim.ws)* for further information.

The information in this book can be applied as your baby is developmentally ready to do the activities. Your baby's NICU staff will guide you as your child is deemed medically stable by your developmental pediatrician. When your child goes home from the hospital, I recommend that you work with a feeding therapist.

It is important to help your child develop skills at the chronological age when those skills are supposed to be learned, if possible (ie, corrected age is used for a preemie). It is much easier to teach a child a new skill during a critical learning period than after this time period has passed. For many of the skills listed in the developmental checklists in this book, you will see a chronological time period (eg, 3 to 6 months) when skills are usually learned.

One of my greatest frustrations as a therapist is the referral of children after critical learning periods have long passed. For example, I have many children with gastrostomy tubes referred between 18 months and 3 years of age for feeding therapy. Most of these children have had little previous mouth activity and have developed few mouth skills. They have missed many of the learning opportunities discussed in this book, particularly the critical learning period for the development of feeding skills (birth to age 2). They have not even participated in the nonfood mouth activities described in chapters 4 and 5. Consequently, they have a very difficult time learning to eat and drink.

Many children who receive gastrostomy tubes at or near birth can be partially fed by mouth if proper and safe feeding methods are used. Gastrostomy tubes are often placed when a child does not obtain adequate nutrition from oral feeding methods (eg, the breast or bottle). A well-trained feeding therapist can help parents safely feed their baby part-time if the child is not at risk for aspiration.

Here are some resources for parents and professionals:

1. *Pre-Feeding Skills: A Comprehensive Resource for Mealtime Development* (2nd edition), by Suzanne Evans Morris and Marsha Dunn Klein, has a chapter on feeding premature children.[506]

2. *The Nursing Mother's Companion* (4th revised edition), by Kathleen Huggins, has a section on nursing the premature infant.[507]

3. *The Preemie Parents' Companion: The Essential Guide to Caring for Your Premature Baby in the Hospital, at Home, and Through the First Years,* by Susan L. Madden, has sections on feeding.[508]

4. *Preemies: The Essential Guide for Parents of Premature Babies,* by Dana Wechsler Linden, Emma Trenti Paroli, and Mia Wechsler Doron, has information on breast-feeding and bottle-feeding.[509]

Here are some other resources for professionals:

1. *Handbook of Neonatal Intensive Care* (5th edition), by Gerald B. Merenstein and Sandra L. Gardner (Editors), has a chapter on breast-feeding neonates with special needs.[510]

2. *Breastfeeding and Human Lactation* (2nd edition) by Jan Riordan and Kathleen G. Auerbach has a chapter on breast-feeding preterm infants.[511]

Children with Down Syndrome

I have had the good fortune of working with many children with Down syndrome. I had the opportunity to see about 45 children with Down syndrome per week in one clinic where I worked. When a mom or dad asks me when I want to see their new baby, I say, "As soon as you can travel to my office or I can visit your home." Children with Down syndrome have a variety of concerns that affect feeding and mouth development. In my opinion, treatment in these children should begin at birth or as close to birth as possible.

Let's talk about the mouth of a baby with Down syndrome at birth. When you look at babies with Down syndrome, they do not have many structural abnormalities. Their mouths look pretty much like the mouths of other babies. However, their muscles are different. I believe that this difference is what causes many of the structural problems seen in children with Down syndrome.

Here are some of the characteristics seen in children with Down syndrome:[512]

- Poor muscle tone throughout the body
- A flat facial profile (problems with development of the midface)
- Small mouth (may be related to problems with jaw growth)
- Differences in the hard palate (eg, a high, narrow palate)
- Problems with tooth development (eg, underdeveloped teeth, misshapen teeth, poor tooth enamel, teeth emerging in an irregular sequence) and occlusion (ie, problems with teeth coming together for biting and chewing)
- Tooth-grinding (also called *bruxism*)
- Loose ligaments in the jaw joint
- Open mouth posture, mouth breathing, and tongue protrusion
- Abnormal tongue development
- Problems with movements of the jaw, lips, and tongue
- A variety of speech development difficulties, including delay, dysarthria (slurred, distorted speech, related to muscle movement problems), and childhood apraxia of speech (undeveloped or uncoordinated speech related to motor planning or programming problems)

Having said this, I want to expand on why I think many of the items on the list become a problem in the first place. I also want to tell you how therapists have helped parents avoid or reduce the effects of many of these problems.

One problem I cannot help you avoid is the poor muscle tone and the resulting muscle weakness in your child's body. Poor muscle tone is not a problem seen only in children with Down syndrome. In fact, many children have muscle tone that is on the low side of normal. Poor muscle tone is a problem for anyone who has it. One of the biggest problems for children with significantly poor muscle tone is that they often cannot do some of the things on their own that children with good muscle tone can do. Most children with poor muscle tone, or even a low level of normal muscle tone, can use some help with this.

Therefore, it is particularly important for you to work with a physical therapist who can accurately diagnose and treat the poor muscle tone and resulting weakness in your child's body. I highly recommend Patricia C. Winder's book, *Gross Motor Skills in Children with Down Syndrome: A Guide for Parents and Professionals*.[513] I have had far greater success in treating the mouths of children who had good full-body treatment. I have also been lucky enough to work directly with many of Pat Winder's little clients.

I believe that the "flat" facial profile[514] of children with Down syndrome is certainly related to poor muscle tone. The muscles of the face and jaw do not move as they should, and midface development does not occur as it should. I have seen similar facial profiles in other children with significantly poor muscle tone who do not have Down syndrome. However, those children do not have the other facial characteristics of children with Down syndrome.

I have also seen significant changes in a facial profile as a child with Down syndrome begins to actively move the face and jaw muscles or have the facial muscles moved for her (eg, Beckman facilitation techniques, myofascial release techniques). Many babies with Down syndrome cannot adequately move their muscles without some help at first. I treated one little boy whose mother called me to say he had developed a bridge of the nose after she had been performing several of Debra Beckman's techniques around the bridge of the nose with her son for a period of time.

Appropriate active use of the face and mouth muscles improves face and mouth development. Chapters 2, 4, 5, 6, and 7 discuss ways to encourage appropriate face and mouth movement through feeding, mouth, and speech activities.

I also ask the question, "Is it possible some differences in face and mouth development in children with Down syndrome occur because of the lack of jaw and facial growth during the first 6 to 12 months of life?" When I am successful in helping babies with Down syndrome move their face and mouth muscles more appropriately through good feeding and mouth experiences during the first 6 to 12 months, more typical face and mouth develement is apparent. Therefore, why would children with Down syndrome be more susceptible to the problem of decreased jaw and facial growth? Again, I suspect that poor muscle tone and resulting movement problems are major contributing factors. See the developmental checklists in chapter 8 for more information on mouth development.

The differences in the hard palates of children with Down syndrome (eg, high, narrow palates) are not unlike the differences we would see in anyone who does not have the ability to keep the mouth closed. In chapters 3 and 8, we talked about the importance of your baby's mouth being closed at rest and breathing through the nose. When your young baby's tongue rests within a closed mouth, it helps to maintain the palate's shape (ie, the roof of the mouth). When your baby's mouth is open at rest, the hard palate is free to change shape. A change in the shape of the hard palate can affect the development of the nasal and sinus areas. If nasal and sinus areas are not formed properly, sinus and breathing problems can result.

Breast-feeding can also assist in the shaping of the hard palate if done properly. Mom's breast is drawn deeply into the child's mouth to help keep the shape of the palate. It is a myth that babies with Down syndrome cannot breast-feed. In my opinion, breast-feeding is the best way to feed a baby with Down syndrome, or any baby. The tips in chapter 2 will help you to do this. I have helped many moms breast-feed their babies with Down syndrome.

Children with Down syndrome often have problems with tooth development (eg, underdeveloped teeth, misshapen teeth, poor tooth enamel, and teeth emerging in an irregular sequence). In my experience, these problems decrease significantly with early treatment. Treatment includes mouth massage, appropriate biting and chewing activities, appropriate mouthing activities, and appropriate feeding techniques, which are discussed in chapters 2, 4, 5, and 6. While late tooth eruption still occurred in a number of my young clients with Down syndrome, their teeth tended to emerge in a typical sequence and were fully formed.

The problems reported with occlusion, or bite (eg, underbite, overbite, open bite, cross-bite), in children with Down syndrome also seem related to patterns that begin in the first year of life if the mouth is not working well. Underbite (where the bottom jaw slides out beyond the top jaw) and cross-bite (where the bottom jaw slides to one side) are related to jaw weakness and stability problems caused by problems with muscle tone. Overbite or open bite is usually caused by a tongue thrust and persistent oral habits, such as thumb-sucking beyond the first year.

Not all children with Down syndrome automatically develop a tongue thrust. A tongue thrust is a compensatory pattern the child develops as a result of jaw weakness and instability. Babies with Down syndrome are not born with this. Also, children with Down syndrome are not alone in this problem. Many children develop some form of tongue thrust that could be avoided with appropriate feeding techniques and proper mouth development activities.

Tooth-grinding (also called *bruxism*) is a problem for anyone who does it. It can harm the very delicate temporomandibular joint and the teeth. The sound is annoying to others and is socially inappropriate.

Why do so many children with Down syndrome do this? Children with Down syndrome usually have jaw problems. Grinding or clenching the jaw is a way to get deep sensory input into the muscles and joints of the jaw. Clenching is also a way to hold a jaw still or stabilize it, if the muscles cannot do this. We discussed the importance of jaw stability and grading (eg, opening the jaw just enough for the spoon, instead of flinging the jaw open; opening the jaw just enough to produce a particular speech sound) in the feeding and speech chapters.

Some therapists have questioned whether tooth-grinding relieves Eustachian-tube and middle-ear discomfort. Children with Down syndrome tend to have both middle-ear and sinus problems. No matter what the initial reason, tooth-grinding is a problematic habit. See chapter 5 for ideas on how to get rid of this habit.

So far, we have talked about how to possibly change some outcomes for children with Down syndrome by using good feeding techniques and mouth development activities. Like poor muscle tone, loose ligaments in the jaw joints (temporomandibular joints) are something we cannot change. However, we can work with the jaw to keep these joints in the best shape possible. Your child may need to have treatment of the jaw as long as she is growing. See chapter 8 for information on jaw development from birth and chapter 5 for information on appropriate jaw activities. Aligned, up-and-down jaw movement with a jaw exerciser will work the muscles that raise and lower the jaw (ie, jaw elevators and depressors) and can relieve stress on the jaw joints. The jaw needs to open and close in a graded manner for effective eating, drinking, and speaking.

The combination of loose jaw ligaments and poor muscle tone contributes to open-mouth posture, breathing through the mouth, and tongue protrusion.[515] If gravity pushes the bottom jaw open and your child cannot use the jaw muscles and ligaments to close the mouth, you will see these problems and more (eg, drooling). The bottom jawbone is heavy, and becomes heavier with growth. Chapter 3 addresses the importance of breathing through the nose. Chapter 4 addresses drooling. Chapter 5 contains techniques for working with the jaw.

Another concern often reported in children with Down syndrome is abnormal tongue development (eg, abnormally large tongues). I ask, "Do children with Down syndrome have large tongues, or do they have tongues with poor muscle tone and jaws that did not grow properly?" This would give the appearance of a large tongue, wouldn't it? Look at the development of the jaw and tongue in the first 2 years of life in chapter 8.

In my practice, I have seen some children with Down syndrome who underwent surgery to reduce the size of their tongues. This made it even more difficult for the children I treated to move their tongues properly to eat, drink, and speak.

An important area of the tongue had been removed, and scar tissue was present. I prefer to work on tongue movement proactively with a baby from birth. If I cannot do this, I prefer to work with a child who has an intact tongue.

As you can see, the problems seen in the mouths of children with Down syndrome are related to structure (ie, poor muscle tone and loose ligaments in the temporomandibular joints) and resulting movement problems. The information in this book helps you to facilitate more typical movement patterns in your baby with Down syndrome through simple, everyday experiences.

In addition to feeding and other mouth development information presented in chapters 1–6 and 8, chapter 7 provides you with specific information on speech development. The detail of the information presented in chapter 7 is usually not available to parents, pediatricians, and others because it comes from many different sources in the speech-language pathology literature.

Most children with Down syndrome need speech therapy. These children tend to have two types of speech problems: dysarthria and childhood apraxia of speech.

Dysarthria is slurred-sounding, imprecise speech that is caused by the muscles not working well. I am not just talking about muscle weakness. Precise speech production requires separation (or dissociation) of movement (ie, structures moving independently of one another), direction of movement (ie, structures moving in the proper direction), and grading of movement (ie, structures moving just enough for the activity). Strength is just a small part of the picture for speech development, because speech is a "light-touch act"[516] that requires a great deal of precision. The questions really are:

- Does your child use the right amount of strength needed for the activity?
- Is her strength graded and used efficiently?

The other speech problem commonly seen in children with Down syndrome is called *childhood apraxia of speech* in the United States and *dyspraxia of speech* in other parts of the world. As far as we know, it is usually not related to brain damage in most children. Rather, an area of the brain called the *premotor cortex* does not seem to be working well. This area in the frontal lobe of the brain plans the movements for speech and other parts of the body. It helps your child sequence mouth movements for producing speech sounds and speech sound combinations.

Though related to poor muscle tone, childhood apraxia of speech is a very different problem. It is the old story about the chicken and the egg. Children with poor muscle tone do not use the speech muscles adequately to babble and practice movements to establish the motor plans for speech. You know that any activity you want to learn requires practice. For instance, would you expect to learn a tennis serve or golf swing without having practiced this activity over and over? The same is true of every voluntary movement in the body. We need a motor plan for every one of them, particularly speech. Children with poor muscle tone do not move in the same way as children with typical muscle tone. This leads to related motor-planning problems.

Chapter 7 gives you and your therapists some strategies to work on speech problems caused by muscle function and motor-planning concerns. However, speech problems can also be related to hearing problems. Children with Down syndrome tend to have middle-ear problems that may be related to problems with Eustachian-tube function. Therefore, it is crucial for you to have your child's hearing screened on a regular basis. You can find the hearing screening guidelines of the American Academy of Pediatrics (The National Center of Medical Home Initiatives for Children with Special Needs) at *www.aap.org*.[517] See chapter 3 for more information on health problems and possible treatments.

Personality and learning style are also important considerations when working with children with Down syndrome. Children with Down syndrome tend to be very visually and musically oriented. If your child is not participating in or cooperating with a recommended activity, model the activity with your own mouth or make up a song to go with your activity. This will make the activity fun for you and your child. Remember that it is easier to learn something when you are having fun.

Children with Down syndrome can also become very determined individuals as they grow and mature. Some people call this "stubborn." For example, once your child has learned one way to perform an activity (eg, drinking from one bottle nipple or eating from a spoon in a certain way), you may have a hard time changing the way she does this. This is a very common characteristic of children with poor muscle tone. Once they find a motor plan (ie, sequence of movements) that works for them, they resist trying a different way, even if it is a more effective way. The information in this book will assist you in systematically helping your child with Down syndrome make these changes. Adjusting to change and practicing activities in a variety of ways (systematically, not haphazardly) can help your baby's brain work in a more flexible manner. This is an important life skill for everyone to learn.

One in 800 children is born with Down syndrome,[518] according to the U.S. Centers for Disease Control and Intervention. As with babies born prematurely, I find that we have far greater success in the treatment of children with Down syndrome if we:

- Start treatment as soon as possible (ie, at birth)
- Provide appropriate stimulation during critical learning periods

This book will help you. Through the use of the techniques outlined here, you will see that your baby with Down syndrome is really not very different from other babies when treatment begins at birth and when you capitalize on natural, critical learning periods.

I have always enjoyed working with babies with Down syndrome, because they are usually happy babies and just plain fun. I am not quite sure what my world would be like without them.

Woodbine House Publishers *(www.woodbinehouse.com)* specializes in books for parents of children with Down syndrome. In addition to Patricia Winder's book on gross motor skills (mentioned previously), I also suggest:

- *Babies with Down Syndrome: A New Parent's Guide,* edited by Karen Stray-Gundersen[519]

- *Medical & Surgical Care for Children with Down Syndrome: A Guide for Parents,* edited by D.C. Van Dyke, MD; Philip Mattheis, MD; Susan Schoon Eberly, MA; and Janet Williams, RN, PhD[520]

- *Early Communication Skills for Children with Down Syndrome: A Guide for Parents and Professionals* (2nd edition), by Dr Libby Kumin[521] (Note: I had the pleasure of working and teaching with Dr Kumin at Loyola College in Maryland for a number of years)

Blueberry Shoes Productions, LLC *(www.blueberryshoes.com),* has several DVDs available for parents. I have also had the pleasure of working with Will Schermerhorn, who wrote, edited, and produced these films:

- *Down Syndrome: The First 18 Months,* by Will Schermerhorn[522]

- *Discovery: Pathways to Better Speech for Children with Down Syndrome,* by Will Schermerhorn[523]

- *What Did You Say? A Guide to Speech Intelligibility in People with Down Syndrome,* by Dr Libby Kumin and Will Schermerhorn[524] (published by Woodbine House, Inc)

- *Kids with Down Syndrome: Staying Healthy and Making Friends,* by Will Schermerhorn[525]

TalkTools carries a DVD called *Developing Oral-Motor and Feeding Skills in the Down Syndrome Population.* This DVD was assembled by Lori Overland, whose work was discussed in chapter 6.

Children with Autism

Autism, by definition, includes a spectrum of disorders (found in the *Diagnostic and Statistical Manual of Mental Disorders,* published by the American Psychiatric Association). One type is called *pervasive developmental disorder (nonspecified).* Individuals with this disorder have many developmental difficulties, including feeding and communication problems. There is another form of autism called *childhood disintegrative disorder.* These children develop well until 18 to 24 months of age, when suddenly they lose many of their previously acquired skills, particularly the ability to communicate. Asperger syndrome is yet another form of autism spectrum disorder. Individuals with this disorder are usually very intelligent but have a difficult time with social interaction, emotional control, and some everyday activities you and I take for granted.

According to Scully, some characteristics of children with autism include brain growth abnormality, communication impairments, social impairments, self-stimulation behaviors, self-injurious behaviors, play deficits, behavioral problems, and sensory differences.[526] Nash reports that people with autism can have sensory disturbances, food allergies, gastrointestinal problems, depression, obsessive compulsiveness, seizure disorders, attention deficit disorder, and extreme anxiety.[527]

Here is a list of the physical differences or problems I consistently observe in children with autism:

- Muscle tone (often poor or on the low side of normal)
- Strength (often mild to moderate weakness, poorly graded)
- Stability and mobility (often out of sync, poorly graded)
- Movement (often out of sync, poorly graded, significant motor planning problems)
- Sensory systems (out of sync, poorly graded)

The areas listed here are supposed to work together, so a child can effectively move different parts of the body, including the mouth. Children with autism seem to have difficulties in all the areas listed.

Poor muscle tone or tone on the low side of normal means the child may not have enough stiffness in muscles to hold or move the bones effectively in relation to gravity.[528] Children with autism often have mild to moderate muscle weakness and difficulty using the right amount of strength (ie, graded strength) for activities. With regard to stability and mobility, they have difficulty holding one body part still enough (eg, the jaw) so that another can move (eg, the tongue).

The complex process called *motor planning* is a particular challenge for children with autism. This is where the brain tells the muscles the sequence and rhythm of movements, how far to move, and in what direction to move. Motor planning is needed for every intentional movement in the body.

The many different sensory systems (particularly the ones sensing touch and movement) need to be in good working order for the processes of feeding and speech to occur. Children with autism have difficulty coordinating information from the many sensory systems. The book entitled, *The Out-of-Sync Child: Recognizing and Coping with Sensory Integration Dysfunction,* by Carol Stock Kranowitz, is a book for parents that discusses sensory processing difficulties in children.

I have been around and worked with many individuals with autism throughout my life and career. It began when I was a child. I did not know that my sister was on the autism spectrum. My sister would probably be identified as having pervasive developmental disorder (nonspecified) if she were alive today. My sister lived in an institution, or a group home, most of her life.

When I worked for the Maryland School for the Blind in the 1980s and 1990s, I worked with many individuals who would now be identified as having autism. Most of these children had been born prematurely and had many complications. When I was a clinical supervisor at Loyola College in Maryland in the 1990s, we saw the population of children with autism grow at an extremely rapid pace. Most of the children I have treated in private practice since 2001 have had some form of autism.

Currently, the number of children with autism has soared to one in 150 children in the United States.[529] These children are different from the group of children I treated at the Maryland School for the Blind many years ago. As a group, they are not born prematurely and do not have a lot of medical complications at birth. They have problems with feeding and communication development, which often go undiagnosed until the child is beyond the critical learning periods for these processes. Because of this problem, I have provided a checklist of potential autism characteristics seen in infants.

ACTIVITY 10.2: CHARACTERISTICS OF INFANTS WITH AUTISM[530-531]

You can use this checklist to see if your baby has any of these characteristics. With the rising numbers of children being diagnosed with autism, it is important that all children be screened for autism from birth. Pediatricians and other professionals are developing processes for this type of screening. If your child is having difficulty in any area of development, please work with your child's pediatrician. If your child's pediatrician cannot help you, it may be wise to contact the local early intervention team.

Date	Age	Characteristics
	Birth to 3 months and beyond	Very passive, requires little attention[532]
	Birth to 3 months and beyond	Extremely irritable, hard to feed, has irregular sleep patterns, resists cuddling[533]
	3–6 Months	Has little to no response to name, your smile, speech sounds, or social play

Date	Age	Characteristics
	3–6 Months	Problems with eye contact may be seen
	3–6 Months	May seem hearing impaired at times
	9–12 Months	Exhibits excessive mouthing (not discriminative mouthing)
	9–12 Months	Child exhibits delayed response when hearing her own name; may respond if prompted or cued
	9–12 Months	No babbling, pointing, or meaningful gestures are heard or seen by 12 months
	9–12 Months	Demonstrates aversion to social touch
	1–2 Years	Demonstrates limited or no eye contact or smiling
	1–2 Years	Demonstrates poor or no imitation
	1–2 Years	No words are heard by 16 months
	1–2 Years	Demonstrates loss of speech, language, babbling, or social skills
	1–2 Years	May have an unusual-sounding voice or make unusual sounds
	1–2 Years	No two-word combinations are heard by age 2[534]
	1–2 Years	Demonstrates limited toy interactions (may get overly attached to an object or line up toys excessively)

Individuals with autism have difficulty modulating sensory information. As infants, they may be extremely passive babies who require little attention, or they may be very irritable and difficult to feed, demonstrating irregular sleep patterns and a resistance to cuddling.[535] Between 3 and 6 months of age, babies with autism often show little to no response to their name, your smile, speech sounds, or social play. A parent may notice problems with eye contact at this time. The child may also seem hearing impaired at times (ie, inconsistently responding to sound).

Note: All children need to have hearing screenings from birth. You can find the hearing screening guidelines of the American Academy of Pediatrics (The National Center of Medical Home Initiatives for Children with Special Needs) at *www.aap.org*.[536]

Between 9 and 12 months, parents often see a delayed response from the child when calling her name. However, a parent may be able to prompt or cue the child to respond to her name by using a visual and/or touch cue. Communication skills such as babbling, pointing, and gesturing (meaningfully) are often noticeably absent by 12 months. The child may have social touch aversions (ie, doesn't like to be touched by others) and demonstrate excessive mouthing. This excessive mouthing is qualitatively different from the important discriminative mouthing that typically begins around 5 to 6 months of age. It is obsessive and not particularly discriminative. See chapter 4 for information about appropriate discriminative mouthing, which is very important for your child's mouth development.

Between 1 and 2 years of age, the child's limited eye contact is usually apparent. Eye contact is fleeting at best. Children with autism often do not smile in response to others' smiles. Imitation of body movements, use of everyday objects (eg, a comb or spoon), and appropriate actions with toys are frequently limited or virtually nonexistent. In fact, toy interaction is usually very limited. The child may become overly attached to one particular object (not necessarily a toy) and throw a tantrum if it is taken away. She may excessively place toys or objects into rows or lines.

A child with autism usually demonstrates little to no word imitation between 1 and 2 years of age. By 16 months, the child often says no words. However, some children with autism take a slightly different path and lose speech, language, babbling, and social skills they previously had. This is frequently seen between 18 months and 2 years of age and is called *childhood disintegrative disorder*. Children with autism often produce unusual vocal sounds. They seem to have difficulty modulating and coordinating their breathing with their voices. Two-word combinations are usually not heard in 2-year-olds with autism.

Any baby who is at risk for autism needs good assessment, follow-up, and intervention. Intervention usually involves intense work with an early intervention team (ie, 20 to 25 hours per week).[537–538]

Autism can co-occur with other disorders (eg, Down syndrome, cerebral palsy, and hearing loss). A thorough medical assessment will help identify any other conditions.

It is also crucial for you to have your child's hearing screened on a regular basis. A hearing loss can mimic other disorders, such as autism. It will compound your child's problems if she does have autism. As mentioned previously, you can find the hearing screening guidelines of the American Academy of Pediatrics (The National Center of Medical Home Initiatives for Children with Special Needs) at *www.aap.org*.[539]

If you are the parent of a young baby who is at risk for autism, you will need to do some special activities with your baby at home, in your natural environment, under the guidance of therapists and other specialists. These therapists and specialists are your team. See chapter 9 for information on the early intervention team. Since it is normal to interact with a baby many hours each day, you will already have the intensity level of 20 to 25 hours per week in place.

However, a baby who is at risk for autism often does not provide the interactive feedback that other children provide. This can be very difficult for parents. Your therapists and other specialists will help you learn your child's unique ways of interacting and how to encourage more typical interactions.

Here are some ideas to encourage more typical interactions in children who are at risk for autism:

1. A child who is at risk for autism may not like to be held, so you can do activities while she is on her belly on the floor, sitting in a chair, or sitting on the floor. Belly time (when awake) is extremely important for all young children, particularly those with any problems with muscle tone. As mentioned previously, I have consistently observed that children with autism appear to have muscle tone that is on the low side of normal.

2. When interacting with your baby or toddler, use activities that promote alertness and calmness. Too many activities that excite your child may cause her to become out of control and overexcited. Mix exciting activities with calming ones. You can change your child's environment to help calm her. A change in lighting, music, or the amount of stimulation in the room can often do the trick.

3. When working with a sensitive child (ie, any child with sensory processing difficulties), make small changes in your routine over time, and prepare your child by talking about and showing her changes ahead of time. Children with sensory processing concerns often have difficulty with changes but

can make changes with time, consistency, and patience. Your daily routines should be predictable, yet somewhat flexible. You can use pictures to prepare your child for new ideas or changes, to give activity choices, and to show what will happen next. The Mayer Johnson Boardmaker software is often used for this purpose *(www.mayer-johnson.com)*.

4. Give your baby appropriate choices whenever possible. This is good advice for all parents. For example, show your baby two choices (eg, a soft cookie and an open cup containing breast milk around 6 months of age). Give her the one she reaches toward or looks at. This gives her the chance to communicate. It also makes her a partner in feeding or any other process. You can use picture or sign language communication for choice making, as well. We will discuss this after Kathie Harrington's list in just a moment.

5. As your child grows older and becomes more interested in the television, you can record things you want your child to do on your camcorder and show it to him on TV. I had one child who needed but resisted the oral massage discussed in chapter 5. After we videotaped his brother participating in oral massage and allowed him to watch the video a few times, he was ready to begin oral massage. Children with autism often need to see processes before they are ready to do them, since they are often visual learners. (See Kathie Harrington's list of success tips for children with autism.)

Note: Use the television sparingly. Some children are calmed when they look at the TV (some even space out), while others become overstimulated. If your child becomes overexcited or spaces out with any activity, you want to do that activity for only a short period of time. Babies and toddlers should not watch TV for long periods of time. The American Academy of Pediatrics, or AAP, recommends no TV viewing for children under age 2 and no more than 2 hours per day for children over the age of 2.[540] See the AAP Web site for updates and more information *(www.aap.org)*.

Kathie Harrington (a speech-language pathologist and mom of a child with autism) provides some excellent advice for working with children with autism. Kathie's "Ten Laws of Success for Children with Autism" are quoted here (I think they represent good advice for parents of children in general.)[541–542]

- Autism is a *reason,* never an excuse
- *Success* builds success
- Nobody ever rose to a low *expectation*
- *Fear* is not an option
- Small *steps* grow into giant leaps
- *Interaction* across and within environments is essential

- *Visual learners* need to see
- Blended *therapies* mix well
- *Laughter* is not a detriment to learning
- The top line is *independence*[543–544]

If your baby or toddler is at risk for autism spectrum disorder, consider the use of picture communication and/or sign language. This is consistent with Kathie Harrington's recommendation that visual learners need to see. Some parents are concerned that the use of pictures or signs will limit the child's motivation to speak. However, research says the opposite. See the section "What to Do If Your Child Is Not on Track with Speech and Communication" in chapter 7 for more information.

Here are some suggestions to promote communication with your baby by using pictures and/or signs:

1. Around 6 months of age, begin to introduce pictures and/or signs to go along with activities (eg, beginning the Picture Exchange Communication System, or PECS, and/or the K & K Sign and Say Verbal Language Kit, by Tamara Kasper and Nancy Kaufman). Community hospitals offer sign-language courses for parents and babies. Many Web sites are also available on this topic.

2. Introduce pictures and/or signs to your baby gradually (ie, not too many at one time).

3. Work toward joint attention (ie, where you and your baby look at pictures and objects together).

4. Make activities fun for you and your baby (eg, nonchalantly looking at and labeling pictures or signing). Don't stress yourself or your baby. Children with special needs are particularly sensitive to stress, and you don't need any extra stress as a parent.

5. After you have introduced pictures or signs a few times, you may see your baby look toward the concept you are mentioning.

6. Working with pictures is a nice early literacy activity for any child. Babies with Down syndrome also tend to be very visual learners and have fun with this type of activity. I often introduce the first set of pictures from the Kaufman Speech Praxis Treatment Kit: Basic Level around 6 months of age to my little clients who are at risk for speech problems.

If you have a child with autism, there are also many treatment options offered in the home and/or in a school or clinic setting. Some are listed here:

- Dr Greenspan's Floor time
- Dr Gutstein's Relationship Development Intervention, or RDI

- The Son-Rise Program (Autism Treatment Center of America)
- Dr Robin Allen's Behavioral Services and Products
- Dr Lovaas's Applied Behavioral Analysis, or ABA
- Treatment and Education for Autistic and Other Communicatively Handicapped Children, or TEACCH

Children with Cerebral Palsy

According to the U.S. Center for Disease Control and Prevention, 10,000 babies are born in the United States each year with cerebral palsy.[545] When I worked for the Maryland School for the Blind, I treated many children with cerebral palsy. Some children have a mild form of this disorder and are not easily diagnosed.

Cerebral palsy is believed to be caused by a brain injury before or during birth. It results in orthopedic, movement, and postural disorders that often lead to feeding and communication problems. Treatment usually involves physical, occupational, and speech-language therapy, as well as other therapies.

Parents of children with cerebral palsy will benefit from the information provided in this book because the book educates parents about critical learning periods for feeding and communication development. Therapists working with the family can help parents adjust activities as needed and develop reasonable goals based on these critical learning periods.

It is easiest to begin treatment at birth or as soon as the disorder is recognized for the best possible outcome. Without proactive intervention (eg, working with critical learning periods for skill development), children with cerebral palsy may not develop adequate feeding and communication skills. The earlier the intervention, the easier it is to make changes and sustain skills.

Children with cerebral palsy need treatment. Neurodevelopmental and sensory processing treatments are often treatments of choice. See *www.ndta.org* for information on neurodevelopmental treatment and *www.thesensoryworld.com* for information on sensory processing.

Physical therapist Lois Bly has written a number of books based on neurodevelopmental principles that illustrate the facilitation of more typical movement patterns in babies. These books were primarily written for physical therapists. However, the illustrations, explanations, and ideas help others understand the recommendations made by physical therapists. Another current resource for parents and professionals is *The Child with Traumatic Brain Injury or Cerebral Palsy: A Context-Sensitive Family-based Approach to Development,* by Lucia Willadino Braga and Alyosio Campos da Paz, Jr.

Children with Hearing Loss

According to the American Academy of Pediatrics (The National Center of Medical Home Initiatives for Children with Special Needs), 33 infants are born daily with some amount of hearing loss, making this the most common congenital disorder in the United States.[546] I have worked with many children who had some degree of hearing loss. These include children with fluctuating hearing loss (eg, middle-ear problems) and children with permanent hearing loss.

The parents of these children can greatly benefit from the information provided about critical learning periods for feeding and communication development in this book. Since many children with hearing impairment do not have concurrent developmental or motor disorders, the developmental information presented in chapters 1 through 6 may be easily applied. The information in chapters 7 through 9 will be useful for communication development, mouth development, and working with the necessary professionals. This is very important information for parents of children with hearing impairment, since these children often have significant communication difficulties.

Have your child's hearing screened according to the guidelines of the American Academy of Pediatrics *(www.aap.org).*[547] If your child has any amount of hearing loss, it is crucial for you and your child to work with a pediatric audiologist (see chapter 9). Many children with other developmental problems also have hearing loss (eg, children with Down syndrome and children with cleft palates). We have already talked about children with Down syndrome. Now let's talk about children with other types of developmental delays.

Children with Other Developmental Delay

In addition to working with children with Down syndrome, autism, cerebral palsy, hearing loss, and complications from premature birth, I have treated children with many other disorders. The parents of these children can benefit from this book because they need good developmental information. Much of the information in the book was derived from my therapeutic experience with the processes of feeding and communication when working with children who had special needs.

The following chart outlines many disorders, their characteristics, professionals who work with these disorders, and what to do. The chart can help you problem solve with other team members regarding appropriate assessment and treatment strategies for your child. You will also notice that many of the disorders have cleft lip and/or palate as a characteristic. If your child has any form of a cleft, please see the comments below this chart. The disorders are listed in alphabetical order.[548]

ACTIVITY 10.3: DISORDERS IN CHILDREN WITH OTHER DEVELOPMENTAL DELAY

Problem	Face and Mouth Characteristics	Person(s) to See	What to Do
Apert Syndrome	Cranial sutures grow together early; midface not well developed; cleft palate; hyponasality; mouth breathing; tongue forward in the mouth; eating, drinking, and speech problems	Pediatrician; pediatric ear, nose, and throat specialist; audiologist; pediatric craniofacial specialist; pediatric dentist; cleft palate team; speech-language pathologist; occupational therapist; others as appropriate	Evaluate for surgical repair of structures; treatment to develop most typical patterns possible
Cornelia de Lange Syndrome	Small, oddly shaped nose; thin, turned down top lip; cleft palate; poorly developed lower jaw; eating, drinking, and speech problems	Pediatrician; pediatric ear, nose, and throat specialist; audiologist; pediatric craniofacial specialist; pediatric dentist; cleft palate team; speech-language pathologist; occupational therapist; others as appropriate	Evaluate for surgical repair of structures; treatment to develop most typical patterns possible
Ectrodactyly-Ectodermal Dysplasia-Clefting Syndrome	Cleft lip and palate; problems with soft-palate function; dental problems; poorly developed top jaw; eating, drinking, and speech problems	Pediatrician; pediatric ear, nose, and throat specialist; audiologist; pediatric craniofacial specialist; pediatric dentist; cleft palate team; speech-language pathologist; occupational therapist; others as appropriate	Evaluate for surgical repair of structures; treatment to develop most typical patterns possible

Fetal Alcohol Syndrome	Short, turned up nose; poorly developed top and/or bottom jaw; poor muscle tone; problems with motor coordination; high number of individuals with cleft palate; eating, drinking, and speech problems	Pediatrician; pediatric ear, nose, and throat specialist; audiologist; pediatric craniofacial specialist; pediatric dentist; cleft palate team; speech-language pathologist; occupational therapist; others as appropriate	Evaluate for surgical repair of structures if needed; treatment to develop most typical patterns possible
Fragile X Syndrome	Large forehead; long, narrow lower jaw; eating, drinking, speech, and other motor development problems	Pediatrician; pediatric dentist; pediatric ear, nose, and throat specialist; audiologist; speech-language pathologist; occupational therapist; others as appropriate	Evaluation and treatment to develop most typical patterns possible
Goldenhar Syndrome	Poorly developed face and/or head; facial features different from one side of the face to the other; poorly developed lower jaw; weakness or paralysis of facial muscles; cleft palate; weakness or paralysis of soft palate; eating, drinking, speech, and resonance problems	Pediatrician; pediatric ear, nose, and throat specialist; audiologist; pediatric craniofacial specialist; pediatric dentist; cleft palate team; speech-language pathologist; occupational therapist; others as appropriate	Evaluate for surgical repair of structures; treatment to develop most typical patterns possible

ACTIVITY 10.3: (cont.)

Problem	Face and Mouth Characteristics	Person(s) to See	What to Do
Moebius Syndrome	Paralysis on both sides of the face; problems with tongue movement in all directions; eating, drinking, and speech problems; high number of individuals with cleft palate and poorly developed lower jaw	Pediatrician; pediatric ear, nose, and throat specialist; audiologist; pediatric craniofacial specialist; pediatric dentist; cleft palate team; speech-language pathologist; occupational therapist; others as appropriate	Evaluate for surgical repair of structures if needed; treatment to develop most typical patterns possible
Noonan Syndrome	Wide-set eyes; tongue and mouth differences; small, turned-up nose; wide mouth; lips look like "cupid's bow;"[549] narrow top and bottom jaw with high, arched palate; problems with occlusion and/or bite; other dental problems; eating, drinking, and speech problems	Pediatrician; pediatric dentist; pediatric ear, nose, and throat specialist; audiologist; speech-language pathologist; occupational therapist; others as appropriate	Evaluation and treatment to develop most typical patterns possible
Oro-Facial-Digital Syndromes	Cleft lip or cleft lip and palate; restricted lips (frenulums); missing center top or bottom teeth; poorly developed lower jaw; tongue differences; eating, drinking, and speech problems	Pediatrician; pediatric ear, nose, and throat specialist; audiologist; pediatric craniofacial specialist; pediatric dentist; cleft palate team; speech-language pathologist; occupational therapist; others as appropriate	Evaluate for surgical repair of structures; treatment to develop most typical patterns possible

Syndrome	Characteristics	Specialists	Treatment
Oto-Palatal-Digital Syndrome	Small jaw; upper airway blockage; cleft palate; teeth missing; eating, drinking, and speech problems	Pediatrician; pediatric ear, nose, and throat specialist; audiologist; pediatric craniofacial specialist; pediatric dentist; cleft palate team; speech-language pathologist; occupational therapist; others as appropriate	Evaluate for surgical repair of structures; treatment to develop most typical patterns possible
Pierre-Robin Sequence	Poorly developed lower jaw; tongue placed in the bottom of the mouth; cleft palate; soft palate in half, eating, drinking, speech, and resonance problems	Pediatrician; pediatric ear, nose, and throat specialist; audiologist; pediatric craniofacial specialist; pediatric dentist; cleft palate team; speech-language pathologist; occupational therapist; others as appropriate	Evaluate for surgical repair of structures; treatment to develop most typical patterns possible
Prader-Willi Syndrome	Poor muscle tone; eating, drinking, and speech problems	Pediatrician; pediatric dentist; pediatric ear, nose, and throat specialist; audiologist; speech-language pathologist; occupational therapist; others as appropriate	Evaluation and treatment to develop most typical patterns possible
Stickler Syndrome	Poorly developed midface and jaw; submucosal or complete cleft palate; eating, drinking, speech, and resonance problems	Pediatrician; pediatric ear, nose, and throat specialist; audiologist; pediatric craniofacial specialist; pediatric dentist; cleft palate team; speech-language pathologist; occupational therapist; others as appropriate	Evaluate for surgical repair of structures; treatment to develop most typical patterns possible

ACTIVITY 10.3: (cont.)

Problem	Face and Mouth Characteristics	Person(s) to See	What to Do
Treacher Collins Syndrome	Poorly developed top and/or bottom jaw; submucosal or complete cleft palate; short or unmoving soft palate; problems with occlusion and/or bite; poorly developed teeth; nose shaped like a beak; eating, drinking, and speech problems	Pediatrician; pediatric ear, nose, and throat specialist; audiologist; pediatric craniofacial specialist; pediatric dentist; cleft palate team; speech-language pathologist; occupational therapist; others as appropriate	Evaluate for surgical repair of structures; treatment to develop most typical patterns possible
Turner Syndrome	Narrow top jaw and palate; small lower jaw; eating, drinking, and speech problems	Pediatrician; pediatric dentist; pediatric ear, nose, and throat specialist; audiologist; speech-language pathologist; occupational therapist; others as appropriate	Evaluation and treatment to develop most typical patterns possible
Van der Woude Syndrome	Mounds or pits on bottom lip; cleft lip or palate; top lip shaped like "cupid's bow,"[550] problems with soft-palate function; eating, drinking, speech, and resonance problems	Pediatrician; pediatric ear, nose, and throat specialist; audiologist; pediatric craniofacial specialist; pediatric dentist; cleft palate team; speech-language pathologist; occupational therapist; others as appropriate	Evaluate for surgical repair of structures; treatment to develop most typical patterns possible

My Child with Particular Special Needs

Velocardiofacial Syndrome	Poor muscle tone; long face; prominent nasal bridge; long, tubular nose; narrow palpebral fissures; small mouth; turned-down top lip; cleft lip and/or palate; soft palate in half; eating, drinking, speech (dysarthria and dyspraxia), and resonance problems[551]	Pediatrician; pediatric ear, nose, and throat specialist; audiologist; pediatric craniofacial specialist; pediatric dentist; cleft palate team; speech-language pathologist; occupational therapist; others as appropriate	Evaluate for surgical repair of structures; treatment to develop most typical patterns possible
Waardenburg Syndrome	Cleft lip and/or palate; lower jaw protruded forward; eating, drinking, and speech problems	Pediatrician; pediatric ear, nose, and throat specialist; audiologist; pediatric craniofacial specialist; pediatric dentist; cleft palate team; speech-language pathologist; occupational therapist; others as appropriate	Evaluate for surgical repair of structures; treatment to develop most typical patterns possible
Williams Syndrome	Short palpebral fissures; depressed nasal bridge; small, upturned nose; long philtrum; prominent lips; open-mouth posture; small, missing, or poorly aligned teeth;[552] eating, drinking, and speech problems	Pediatrician; pediatric dentist; pediatric ear, nose, and throat specialist; audiologist; speech-language pathologist; occupational therapist; others as appropriate	Evaluation and treatment to develop most typical patterns possible

A Few Comments Regarding Treatment of Children with Cleft Lip and Palate

With regard to the clefting that is a characteristic of many of these disorders, significant care must be taken when working with children who have repaired cleft lips or cleft palates. While these children can benefit from oral massage and other appropriately selected and applied facilitation techniques, great care must be taken to work with the cleft palate team on when to apply these techniques. The surgeon must give the therapist permission (ie, a written order) to use massage and other forms of hands-on manipulation techniques with children who have undergone surgical repairs. Once the surgeon gives this permission, properly applied massage and hands-on facilitation can help reduce scar tissue, as well as increase sensation and movement.

Also, I believe that activities causing changes in intraoral pressure (ie, the pressure within the mouth) must be applied carefully with children who have had repaired hard palates. This would include any blowing activities and drinking from a straw. While some of these activities could be beneficial if done properly, significant changes in intraoral pressure may cause a new hole to form in a repaired hard palate. This is called a *fistula*. All activities that change intraoral pressure need to be applied carefully or not applied if the therapist is unsure of the work. A physician's order must also be given for this work.

While this book mentions the special care needed when feeding or treating a child with a cleft lip and/or palate, there are entire books and other resources dedicated to this topic. If your child has a cleft lip and/or palate, ask your cleft palate team for information on the best resources for you and your child. See Appendices A and B for the resources mentioned in this book.

Appendix A: Resources for Parents and Care Providers

Here are many of the resources mentioned within the book and a few others.

Articles, Books, Materials, and DVDs

Agin MC, Geng LF, Micholl MJ. *The Late Talker: What to Do If Your Child Isn't Talking Yet.* New York, NY: St. Martin's Press; 2003. This book (written by a developmental pediatrician, parent, and professional writer) helps parents navigate the large amount of (often conflicting) information surrounding the topic of "late-talking children," so parents and children can get the help they need.

American Academy of Pediatrics. Changing concepts of sudden infant death syndrome: implications for infant sleeping environment and sleep position. *Pediatrics.* 2000;105:650–656. Sudden infant death syndrome, or SIDS, report and guidelines.

Apel K, Masterson JJ. *Beyond Baby Talk: From Sounds to Sentences—A Parent's Complete Guide to Language Development.* Rockville, MD: American Speech-Language Hearing Association; 2001. This book is a parent-friendly book that covers speech and language development from infancy to preschool.

Banker B. *Silly Songs for Phonology and Sound Awareness.* Eau Claire, WI: Thinking Publications; 1998. These songs are slowed down, contain words that young children use, and can be matched with a "bottom-up" approach to speech treatment.

Batmanghelidj F. *Your Body's Many Cries for Water.* Vienna, VA: Global Health Solutions; 1997. This book presents research on the relationship between dehydration and illness.

Braga LW, da Paz AC Jr. *The Child with Traumatic Brain Injury or Cerebral Palsy: A Context-sensitive Family-based Approach to Development.* New York, NY: Taylor & Francis; 2006. This book provides step-by-step instructions for important everyday activities based on five important principles that are easy for teams and families to apply.

Brideson L. *As a Parent What Can I Do to Improve My Child's Feeding and Speaking?* [DVD]. Tucson, AZ: TalkTools; 2008. This 3-hour DVD teaches home use of feeding and oral-motor therapy techniques.

Cave S. *What Your Doctor May Not Tell You about Children's Vaccinations.* New York, NY: Grand Central Publishing; 2001. This book is a popular resource on vaccines written for parents.

Dougherty DP. *Teach Me How to Say It Right: Helping Your Child with Articulation Problems.* Oakland, CA: New Harbinger Publications Inc; 2005. This book provides parents of children (newborn to age 8) with information on speech development and disorders.

Dyer L. *Look Who's Talking! How to Enhance Your Child's Language Development from Birth.* Minnetonka, MN: Meadowbrook Press; 2004. This book provides parents with ideas to encourage good speech and language development from birth.

Eisenberg A, Murkoff HE, Hathaway SE. *What to Expect the First Year.* New York, NY: Workman Publishing; 1989. This book has specific child development information for parents.

Eisenberg A, Murkoff HE, Hathaway SE. *What to Expect: The Toddler Years.* New York, NY: Workman Publishing; 1994. This book has specific child development information for parents.

Ernsperger L, Stegen-Hanson T. *Just Take a Bite: Easy, Effective Answers to Food Aversions and Eating Challenges.* Arlington, TX: Future Horizons Inc; 2004. This resource helps parents look at the many aspects of picky eating.

Franz K. *Baby-Led Breastfeeding . . . The Mother-Baby Dance [DVD].* Los Angeles, CA: Geddes Productions; 2007. This DVD helps mothers learn to breast-feed naturally.

Greenspan SI, Weider S. *The Child with Special Needs: Encouraging Intellectual and Emotional Growth.* Reading, MA: Perseus Books; 1998. This book helps parents and therapists look at each child with special needs as unique and then create a systematic approach to helping the child reach developmental milestones.

Harrington, K. *For Parents and Professionals: Autism.* East Moline, IL: LinguiSystems Inc; 1998. This book was written by a speech-language pathologist who is a parent of a child with autism. She specializes in the treatment of individuals with autism.

Heitler S. *David Decides about Thumbsucking: A Story for Children; A Guide for Parents.* Denver, CO: Reading Matters; 1996. This book contains a story for older children who still suck their thumbs, as well as information on thumb-sucking for parents.

Huggins K. *The Nursing Mother's Companion.* 4th ed. Boston, MA: The Harvard Common Press; 1999. This is a thorough and easy-to-read resource on breast-feeding. It also has a section on nursing babies born prematurely.

Huggins K, Ziedrich L. *The Nursing Mother's Guide to Weaning.* Boston, MA: The Harvard Common Press; 1994. This resource provides nursing moms with ideas for weaning at different ages.

Jelm JM. *A Parent Guide to Verbal Dyspraxia.* DeKalb, IL: Janelle Publications Inc; 2000. This book provides parents with information on childhood apraxia of speech (a speech motor planning disorder) and includes a visual cueing system that can be used to promote improved speech.

Karp H. *The Happiest Baby on the Block.* New York, NY: Bantam Dell; 2003. This book is a resource on calming babies during the first 3 months of life.

Kaufman NR. *Kaufman Speech Praxis Treatment Kit for Children: Basic Level.* Gaylord, MI: Northern Speech Services; 1997. This kit contains child-friendly pictures of words children can often begin to say if used according to the curriculum.

Klaus MH, Klaus PH. *Your Amazing Newborn.* Boston, MA: Merloyd Lawrence; 1998. This book is beautifully photographed and contains detailed information for parents about the newborn.

Kranowitz CS. *The Out-of-Sync Child: Recognizing and Coping with Sensory Integration Dysfunction.* New York, NY: A Perigee Book; 1998. This is a parent-friendly book on sensory processing problems in children.

Kumin L. *Early Communication Skills for Children with Down Syndrome: A Guide for Parents and Professionals.* 2nd ed. Bethesda, MD: Woodbine House Inc; 2003. This book looks at speech and language development in children with Down syndrome from birth through the three-word stage.

Kumin L, Schermerhorn W. *What Did You Say? A Guide to Speech Intelligibility in People with Down Syndrome [DVD].* Bethesda, MD: Woodbine House Inc; 2006. This DVD takes viewers step-by-step through factors that affect speech clarity in youngsters and adults with Down syndrome.

Linden DW, Paroli ET, Doron MW. *Preemies: The Essential Guide for Parents of Premature Babies.* New York, NY: Pocket Books; 2000. This book has information on breast-feeding a preemie, as well as bottle-feeding tips.

Madden SL. *The Preemie Parents' Companion: The Essential Guide to Caring for Your Premature Baby in the Hospital, at Home, and through the First Years.* Boston, MA: The Harvard Common Press; 2000. This book contains sections on feeding.

Marshalla P. *Becoming Verbal with Childhood Apraxia: New Insights on Piaget for Today's Therapy.* Mill Creek, WA: Marshalla Speech & Language; 2007. This book helps therapists and parents learn to assist children with becoming more vocal, verbal, communicative, imitative, and interactive.

Marshalla P. *Breastfeeding Blues: Advice from a Dairy Queen.* Mill Creek, WA: Marshalla Speech & Language; 2006. This is a funny book to lighten a mom's day about the "hidden experiences" of breast-feeding.

Marshalla P. *How to STOP Drooling.* Mill Creek, WA: Marshalla Speech & Language; 2006. This is a practical, easy-to-follow parents' guide on how to stop drooling.

Marshalla P. *How to STOP Thumbsucking and Other Oral Habits.* Mill Creek, WA: Marshalla Speech & Language; 2004. This is a practical, easy-to-follow parents' guide on how to stop thumb-sucking and other detrimental oral habits.

Martin KL. *Does My Child Have a Speech Problem?* Chicago, IL: Chicago Review Press Inc; 1997. This book answers parents' top 50 questions regarding speech and language development.

McClure VS. *Infant Massage: A Handbook for Loving Parents.* Rev ed. New York, NY: Bantam Books; 1989. This book provides parents with step-by-step instruction on full-body infant massage.

Meek MM. *Motokinesthetic Approach [DVD].* Albuquerque, NM: Clinician's View; 1994. These DVDs teach parents and professionals to use hands-on facilitation techniques to promote speech movements. Visit *www.cliniciansview .com* for more information.

Mohrbacher N, Kendall-Tackett K. *Breastfeeding Made Simple: Seven Natural Laws for Nursing Mothers.* Oakland, CA: New Harbinger Publications, Inc; 2005. This book has research-based information on breast-feeding.

Montagu A. *Touching: The Human Significance of the Skin.* 3rd ed. New York, NY: Harper & Row; 1986. This book is for anyone interested in the significance of human touch and interaction. It also has a chapter on the importance of breast-feeding.

Morris SE, Klein MD. *Pre-Feeding Skills: A Comprehensive Resource for Mealtime Development.* San Antonio, TX: Therapy Skill Builders; 2000. This book is a complete resource on feeding development and treatment. It is for parents, therapists, and others who work with children that have significant feeding problems.

Nathanson LW. *The Portable Pediatrician: A Practicing Pediatrician's Guide to Your Child's Growth, Development, Health and Behavior, from Birth to Age Five.* New York, NY: HarperCollins; 2002. This book was written by a pediatrician and is a well-organized reference for parents.

Northrup C. *Mother-Daughter Wisdom: Creating a Legacy of Physical and Emotional Health.* New York, NY: Bantam Dell; 2005. This book is focused on mothers, and daughters and contains a significant amount of child-development information.

Overland L. *Oral-Motor and Feeding Skills in the Down Syndrome Population [DVD].* Tucson, AZ: TalkTools; 1999. This is a 6-hour DVD seminar.

Page DC. *Your Jaws–Your Life.* Baltimore, MD: SmilePage Publishing; 2003. This book was written by a dentist. It discusses the relationship between the condition of the mouth (specifically the jaw) and health in a lively and entertaining yet factual manner.

Pepper J, Weitzman E. *It Takes Two to Talk: A Practical Guide for Parents of Children with Language Delays.* 3rd ed. Toronto, ON, Canada; Hanen Centre; 2004. This book teaches parents to follow their child's lead and communicate naturally.

Rapp D. *Is This Your Child? Discovering and Treating Unrecognized Allergies in Children and Adults.* New York, NY: William Morrow & Co Inc; 1991. This book is a thorough resource on allergies and sensitivities in children.

Rivard JM, Rivard J. *Noisy Stories: Language Activities for Children of All Communicative Abilities.* Solana Beach, CA: Mayer-Johnson Inc; 2000. These stories have a lot of simple speech repetition in them to help children practice speech.

Rosenfeld-Johnson S. *Drooling Remediation Program for Children and Adults.* Tucson, AZ: TalkTools; 2008. This is an oral-motor approach to drooling, for both parents and therapists.

Rothenbury A. *Breastfeeding Is Not a Spectator Sport: Strategies for the Domestic Coaching Team.* Available at: www.breastfeedinghelpdesk.com. This book explains "how to fix" the three most common breast-feeding problems mothers face in the first weeks after giving birth.

Samuels M, Samuels N. *The Well Baby Book: A Comprehensive Manual of Baby Care, from Conception to Age Four.* New York, NY: Summit Books; 1991. While this book was written a while ago, it is still a resource for parents with unique information.

Satter E. *Child of Mine: Feeding with Love and Good Sense.* Boulder, CO: Bull Publishing Co; 2000. This is a resource on nutrition, with "good-sense" feeding tips for children from birth to 5 years of age.

Satter E. *How to Get Your Kid to Eat . . . But Not Too Much.* Palo Alto, CA: Bull Publishing Co; 1987. This is a resource on nutrition, with "good-sense" feeding tips for children of all ages.

Schermerhorn W. *Kids with Down Syndrome: Staying Healthy and Making Friends [DVD].* Vienna, VA: Blueberry Shoes Productions LLC; 2008. This DVD is an up-to-date and comprehensive guide to the social and health issues of children with Down syndrome. It includes a chapter on fostering friendships and encouraging conversation.

Schermerhorn W. *Discovery: Pathways to Better Speech for Children with Down Syndrome [DVD].* Vienna, VA: Blueberry Shoes Productions LLC; 2005. This DVD outlines the latest thinking on developing and improving talking skills in children with Down syndrome.

Schermerhorn W. *Down Syndrome: The First 18 Months [DVD].* Vienna, VA: Blueberry Shoes Productions LLC; 2003. This DVD presents an overview of what to expect and what to do for babies and children with Down syndrome from birth to 18 months of age. It has chapters on topics related to speech development.

Sears RW. *The Vaccine Book: Making the Right Decision for Your Child.* New York, NY: Little, Brown and Co; 2007. This book helps parents sort through often-conflicting information and make informed decisions when vaccinating their children.

Stray-Gundersen K, ed. *Babies with Down Syndrome: A New Parents' Guide.* Bethesda, MD: Woodbine House Inc; 1995. This book is a resource for parents of babies with Down syndrome.

Tenpenny SJ. *Vaccines: The Risks, the Benefits, the Choices, a Resource Guide for Parents.* USA: Insight Publishing; 2006. This book is a well-researched resource on vaccines.

Van Dyke DC, Mattheis P, Everly SS, Williams J, eds. *Medical & Surgical Care for Children with Down Syndrome: A Guide for Parents.* Bethesda, MD: Woodbine House Inc; 1995. This book is thorough and understandable.

Virginia Smiles Inc. *A Beautiful Child: Welcoming a Baby with Cleft Lip and Palate [video].* Vienna, VA: Blueberry Shoes Productions LLC; 2002. This film can be seen on the Virginia Smiles Web site at *www.virginia-smiles.org*.

West D, Marasco L. *The Breastfeeding Mother's Guide to Making More Milk.* Columbus, OH: McGraw Hill; 2009. This book focuses on a common problem for breast-feeding mothers (ie, milk supply).

Winders PC. *Gross Motor Skills in Children with Down Syndrome: A Guide for Parents and Professionals.* Bethesda, MD: Woodbine House Inc; 1997. This book is an essential guide to good gross motor development in children with Down syndrome.

Web Sites

Ages and Stages, LLC:
www.agesandstages.net (Diane Bahr's workshops)

American Academy of Pediatrics:
www.aap.org (breast-feeding, hearing screening, SIDS, etc)

American Dental Association:
www.ada.org

American Massage Therapy Association:
www.amtamassage.org

American Occupational Therapy Association:
www.aota.org

American Physical Therapy Association:
www.apta.org

American Speech-Language-Hearing Association:
www.asha.org

ARK Therapeutic Services:
www.arktherapeuticservices.com (feeding and mouth development products)

Autism Coalition:
www.autismcoalition.org

Autism Research Centre:
www.autismresearchcentre.com (Cambridge University, Simon Baron-Cohen)

Autism Society of America:
www.autism-society.org

Autism Speaks:
www.autismspeaks.org

Autism Treatment Center of America:
www.autismtreatmentcenter.org

Beckman and Associates:
www.beckmanoralmotor.com (Beckman Facilitation Techniques)

Behavioral Services and Products, Inc:
www.robinallen.com (Dr Robin Allen, focus on autism)

Breast Feeding Help Desk:
www.breastfeedinghelpdesk.com

Breastfeeding Techniques That Work:
www.geddesproduction.com

Blueberry Shoes Productions, LLC:
www.blueberryshoes.com (DVDs on Down syndrome)

Brian Palmer, dentist:
www.brianpalmerdds.com (breast-feeding, tongue tie information)

Cherab Foundation:
www.cherab.org (Childhood apraxia/dyspraxia of speech)

Childhood Apraxia of Speech Association:
www.apraxia-kids.org

Cleft Palate Foundation:
www.cleftline.org

CleftPals:
www.cleftpals.org.au (in Australia)

Clinician's View:
www.clinicians-view.com (DVDs on motokinesthetic cueing and feeding)

Cure Autism Now:
www.cureautismnow.org

Evidence-based Treatment Alternatives:
www.teachtown.com (per Good Speech, Inc)

First Signs:
www.firstsigns.org (sign language for babies)

"First Stories" Project
www.whatsthestorybaby.com (infant communication)

Floortime Foundation:
www.floortime.org (autism)

Future Horizons, Inc:
www.fhautism.com (information on autism)

Good Speech, Inc:
www.kathiesgoodspeech.com (Kathy Harrington's Web site, autism)

The Hanen Centre:
www.hanen.org (child-led communication)

The Happiest Baby on the Block:
www.thehappiestbaby.org (calming)

International Association of Infant Massage Instructors:
www.iaim.ws

International Association of Orofacial Myology:
www.iaom.com (see "Parent's Page")

International Lactation Consultant Association:
www.ilca.org

The Kaufman Children's Center for Speech, Language, Sensory-Motor, and Social Connections, Inc:
www.kidspeech.com (Nancy Kaufman's work)

Marshalla Speech and Language:
www.pammarshalla.com

Mayer-Johnson:
www.mayer-johnson.com (Boardmaker)

Mealtime Notions, LLC:
www.mealtimenotions.com (information on feeding, Marsha Dunn Klein)

Mothering Magazine:
www.mothering.com (breast-feeding)

Myofascial Release:
www.myofascialrelease.com (John Barnes, PT)

National Alliance for Autism Research:
www.naar.org

National Autism Center:
www.nationalautismcenter.org

National Down Syndrome Congress:
www.ndsccenter.org

National Down Syndrome Society:
www.ndss.org

Neuro-Developmental Treatment Association:
www.ndta.org

New Visions:
www.new-vis.com (information on music and feeding, Suzanne Evans Morris)

One Step Ahead:
www.onestepahead.com

Oral Motor Information:
www.oral-motor.com (Diane Bahr's Web site); *www.oralmotorinstitute.org* (Oral Motor Institute Study Group)

Playful Puppets, Inc:
www.playfulpuppets.com (feeding puppets)

PROMPT Institute, Inc:
www.promptinstitute.com (hands-on speech)

Relationship Development Intervention:
www.rdiconnect.com (autism)

Sears Family of Medical Professionals:
www.askdrsears.com (allergies, vaccines, etc)

Smiles:
www.cleft.org (cleft palate)

Speech Bin, Inc:
www.speechbin.com (feeding and mouth development products)

Speech Pathology Associates:
www.chewytubes.com (Chewy Tubes)

STOKKE:
www.stokke.com (STOKKE Tripp Trapp chair)

TalkTools:
www.talktools.net (feeding and mouth development products and workshops)

Therapro:
www.theraproducts.com (feeding and mouth development products)

Tips from Moms:
www.cafemom.com (per Good Speech, Inc)

The Upledger Institute:
www.upledger.com (craniosacral treatment)

U.S. Centers for Disease Control and Prevention on Autism:
www.ckc.gov/ncbddd/autism/actearly

U.S. National Institutes of Health Autism Research Network:
www.autismresearchnetwork.org

U.S. National Institute of Mental Health:
www.nimh.nih.gov/publicat/autism.cfm (autism)

Virginia Smiles, Inc:
www.virginia-smiles.org (cleft palate)

The Weaning Room:
www.theweaningroom.com (Gill Rapley's "baby-led" feeding)

Woodbine House Publishers:
www.woodbinehouse.com (information for parents of children with special needs)

World Health Organization:
www.who.int

Your Jaws—Your Life:
www.SmilePage.com (David C. Page and functional jaw orthopedics)

COMPANIES THAT CARRY PRODUCTS FOR CHILDREN THAT CANNOT BE FOUND IN MOST STORES

Feeding products, Chewy Tubes, ARK's Grabbers, and other safe chewing toys (eg, Debra Beckman's Tri-Chews)

COMPANY	PHONE NUMBER	WEB SITE
ARK Therapeutic Services, Inc	(803) 438-9779	www.arktherapeutic.com
New Visions	(800) 606-7112	www.new-vis.com
The Speech Bin	(800) 850-8602	www.speechbin.com
SuperDuper Publications	(800) 277-8737	www.superduperinc.com
TalkTools	(888) 529-2879	www.talktools.net
Therapro	(800) 257-5376	www.theraproducts.com

Appendix B:
Additional Resources for Professionals

Resources used by both parents and professionals are listed in Appendix A. Some additional professional resources are listed here. A more thorough listing of professional references can be found in *Oral Motor Assessment and Treatment: Ages and Stages,* by Diane Chapman Bahr.

Arvedson JC, Brodsky L. *Pediatric Swallowing and Feeding: Assessment and Management.* San Diego, CA: Singular Publishing Group; 1993. This book discusses medical and therapeutic management of children with feeding and swallowing disorders and includes nutrition, drooling, and craniofacial concerns.

Bahr DC. *Oral Motor Assessment and Treatment: Ages and Stages.* Boston, MA: Allyn & Bacon; 2001. This book is a complete resource on oral motor assessment and treatment for therapists and other professionals. It covers essential anatomy and physiology, development, and the many aspects of oral motor assessment and treatment by age group (ie, feeding, motor speech, orofacial myofunctional treatment, oral massage and facilitation, oral activities and exercises).

Ball MJ, Gibbon FE. *Vowel Disorders.* Boston, MA: Butterworth-Heinemann; 2002. This book contains very specific information and research on vowel disorders in children.

Barnes SM. *Taming the Tongue Thrust [DVD].* Arcadia, CA: Suzanne M. Barnes; 1994. This program is on DVD for clients to use for home practice when working with a speech-language pathologist trained in orofacial myology.

Bly L. *Baby Treatment: Based on NDT Principles.* San Antonio, TX: Therapy Skill Builders; 1999. This book helps therapists and others learn to facilitate more typical movement patterns in babies via photographs and clearly written descriptions.

Bly L. *Motor Skills Acquisition in the First Year: An Illustrated Guide to Normal Development.* San Antonio, TX: Therapy Skill Builders; 1994. This is a must-have book for therapists and others learning about normal movement development.

Boshart CA. *Oral-Facial Flip Book and Reference Guide.* Temecula, CA: Speech Dynamics; 1999. This book contains pictures of facial measurements and descriptions found in chapter 8.

Boshart CA. *Oral-Motor Seminar: "Hard Tissue Analysis" Supplement [video].* Temecula, CA: Speech Dynamics; 1995. This video teaches the measurements discussed in the section of this book titled, "What Your Child's

Face and Mouth Should Look Like" in chapter 8. Char Boshart and Patricia Balthazor have also written an orofacial myofunctional therapy program entitled *Swalloworks*.

Caruso AJ, Strand EA. *Clinical Management of Motor Speech Disorders in Children.* New York, NY: Thieme; 1999. This is a comprehensive, research-based resource on assessment and treatment of motor speech problems in children. You will find the work of Dr Raymond D. Kent in this book.

Fernando C. *Tongue Tie–From Confusion to Clarity: A Guide to the Diagnosis and Treatment of Ankyloglossia.* Australia: Tandem Publications; 1998. This is a book on tongue-tie, with photographs, assessment information, and research to assist with clinical decision-making.

Field T. *Touch Therapy.* New York, NY: Churchill Livingstone; 2000. This book is for anyone interested in research related to human touch, interaction, and health in a variety of populations (including babies).

Genna CW. *Supporting Sucking Skills in Breastfeeding Infants.* Sudbury, MA: Jones & Bartlett Publishers; 2008. This is a resource for healthcare professionals working with mothers and infants on breast-feeding. The information can be used with mothers of full-term healthy infants and infants with special needs.

Golding-Kushner KJ. *Therapy Techniques for Cleft Palate Speech & Related Disorders.* San Diego, CA: Singular; 2001. This book discusses treatment of speech disorders in children with cleft palates, from preschool to adolescence.

Hall KD. *Pediatric Dysphagia Resource Guide.* San Diego, CA: Singular; 2001. This book has information on pediatric feeding and swallowing and includes information on working in neonatal and pediatric intensive-care-unit environments.

Hanson ML, Mason RM. *Orofacial Myology: International Perspectives.* Springfield, IL: Charles C. Thomas; 2003. This book on orofacial myology was written by Hanson, an orofacial myologist and speech-language pathologist, and Mason, an orthodontist and speech-language pathologist.

Hayden DA, Square PA. *Verbal Motor Production Assessment for Children.* San Antonio, TX: Psychological Corporation; 1999. This tool assesses muscle tone, respiration, phonation, reflexes, muscle function (jaw, lips, and tongue), and motor planning. It was developed for children aged 3 to 12 years and has speech and nonspeech normative information.

Hill RR. Apraxia Kit. Tucson, AZ: TalkTools; 2005. This kit contains three sets of tools (Bilabial Shapes, Tactile Tubes, and Speech Blocks) to cue clients who cannot attain appropriate articulator placement with traditional therapeutic methods. A DVD entitled *A Muscle-based Approach to Apraxia of Speech in Children* is also available.

Jelm JM. *Oral-Motor/Feeding Rating Scale.* Tucson, AZ: Therapy Skill Builders; 1990. This assessment tool looks at jaw, lip, and tongue function during feeding, from 1 year of age to adulthood.

Jelm JM. *Verbal Dyspraxia Profile.* DeKalb, IL: Janelle Publications; 2001. This test assesses automatic versus imitative oral movements by comparing feeding with nonfeeding movement patterns. Materials include an overview of oral motor development, tables comparing movement patterns used in feeding versus those used in speech, a diagnostic checklist, and sample treatment goals.

Kamhi AG, Pollock KE (eds). *Phonological Disorders in Children: Clinical Decision Making in Assessment and Intervention.* Baltimore, MD: Paul H. Brooks Publishing Co; 2005. This is an updated resource for speech-language pathologists on the assessment and treatment of phonological disorders in children.

Kaufman NR. *Kaufman Speech Praxis Test for Children.* Detroit, MI: Wayne State University Press; 1995. This tool assesses simple to complex motor speech tasks (ie, pure vowels to polysyllabic sound combinations) by using imitation. It has normative information for ages 2 years to 5 years 11 months.

Lynch JI, Brookshire BL, Fox DR. *A Curriculum for Infants and Toddlers with Cleft Palate.* Chapel Hill, NC: Cleft Palate Foundation; 1993. This is a speech and language curriculum for birth to age 3.

Marshalla P. *Apraxia Uncovered: The Seven Stages of Phoneme Development.* Mill Creek, WA: Marshalla Speech & Language; 2005. This is a book and audio seminar on speech sound development and treatment of speech intelligibility problems.

Marshalla P. *Oral Motor Techniques in Articulation and Phonological Therapy.* Mill Creek, WA: Marshalla Speech & Language; 2000. This book teaches therapists and others how to facilitate jaw, lip, and tongue movements for speech production and how to work with oral sensation.

Marshalla P. *Vowel Tracks: For Improving Intelligibility.* Mill Creek, WA: Marshalla Speech & Language; 2007. This is a recorded lecture and notes on improving vowel production and, consequently, speech intelligibility.

Merenstein GB, Gardner SL (eds). *Handbook of Neonatal Intensive Care.* 5th ed. St Louis, MO: Mosby; 2002. This book has a chapter on breast-feeding neonates with special needs.

Merkel R. *SMILE (SysteMatic Intervention for Lingual Elevation).* Tucson, AZ: TalkTools; 2002. This is a tongue-thrust remediation program, designed for children aged 7 to 12 years.

Oetter P, Richter EW, Frick SM. *M.O.R.E.: Integrating the Mouth with Sensory and Postural Functions.* 2nd ed. Hugo, MN: PDP Press Inc; 1995. This book helps with understanding the importance of suck-swallow-breathe synchrony and many sensory aspects of mouth development.

Peterson-Falzone SJ, Hardin-Jones MA, Karnell MP. *Cleft Palate Speech.* 3rd ed. Philadelphia, PA: Mosby; 2001. This book focuses on the evaluation and treatment of speech disorders in individuals with cleft palates.

Peterson-Falzone SJ, Hardin-Jones MA, Karnell MP, Trost-Cardamone J. *The Clinician's Guide to Treating Cleft Palate Speech.* Philadelphia, PA: Mosby; 2006. This is a pocket guide that provides quick and easy references for treating individuals with cleft palate speech.

Pierce, RB. *Swallow Right: An Exercise Program to Correct Swallowing Patterns.* Tucson, AZ: Communication Skill Builders; 1993. This is an affordable and easy-to-use program to correct tongue-thrust swallow, low tongue-resting posture, and detrimental oral habits.

Riordan J, Auerbach KG. *Breastfeeding and Human Lactation.* 2nd ed. Sudbury, MA: Jones & Bartlett Publishers; 1998. This book has a chapter on breast-feeding the preterm infant.

Rosenfeld-Johnson S. *Assessment and Treatment of the Jaw: Putting It All Together: Sensory, Feeding, and Speech.* Tucson, AZ: TalkTools; 2007. This book and DVD contain a systematic approach to jaw work using a variety of tools (eg, Chewy Tubes and bite blocks). It also has a section on tooth-grinding and other detrimental oral habits.

Rosenfeld-Johnson S. *Oral Placement Therapy for Speech Clarity and Feeding.* 4th rev ed. Tucson, AZ: Innovative Therapists International; 2009. This book contains a variety of systematic oral activities using tools such as horns, straws, bubbles, and others to obtain grading, dissociation, and direction of movement in the mouth. This work is used with people who cannot attain appropriate movements during traditional feeding and speech treatment.

Rossetti LM. *Communication Intervention: Birth to Three.* 2nd ed. United States: Singular/Thomson Learning; 2001. This book provides professionals with information on communication intervention with children from birth to 3 years by the author of *The Rossetti Infant-Toddler Language Scale.*

Russell J, Albery L. *Practical Intervention for Cleft Palate Speech.* Great Britain: Speechmark Publishing Ltd; 1999. This book contains information on prespeech and early speech development, as well as speech remediation.

Schiavoni ME. *Jaw Rehabilitation Program.* South Portland, ME: Speech Pathology Associates LLC; 2000. This program systematically facilitates appropriate grading, dissociation, and direction of movement in the jaw. The jaw elevator and depressor muscles are used in eating, drinking, and speaking.

Tuchman DN, Walter RS (eds). *Disorders of Feeding and Swallowing in Infants and Children: Pathophysiology, Diagnosis, and Treatment.* San Diego, CA: Singular Publishing Group; 1994. This book provides clinicians with medically based pediatric feeding and swallowing information. I have had the great pleasure of working with both Dr David Tuchman and Dr Maureen Lefton-Greif, who wrote chapters in this book.

Vulpe SG. *Vulpe Assessment Battery: Developmental Assessment, Performance Analysis, Individualized Programming.* Toronto, ON, Canada: National Institute on Mental Retardation; 1977. This tool contains detailed information on speech and communication development.

Wetherby AM, Prizant BM (eds). *Autism Spectrum Disorders: A Transactional Developmental Perspective.* Baltimore, MD: Brookes Publishing; 2000. This research-based text on autism spectrum disorders focuses on understanding and addressing social and communication challenges, enhancing assessment and treatment, and supporting families in facilitating their child's development.

Williams L, McCauley R, MacLeod S (eds). *Treatment of Speech Sound Disorders in Children.* Baltimore, MD: Brookes Publishing. In press. This book promises to be the most up-to-date, evidence-based resource on the treatment of speech disorders in children. It has a chapter by Dr Megan Hodge from the University of Alberta, Canada.

Notes

1. Karp H. *The Happiest Baby on the Block.* New York, NY: Bantam Dell; 2002:4.

2. Morris SE, Klein MD. *Pre-Feeding Skills: A Comprehensive Resource for Mealtime Development.* 2nd ed. San Antonio, TX: Therapy Skill Builders; 2000:51–52.

3. Oetter P, Richter EW, Frick SM. *M.O.R.E.: Integrating the Mouth with Sensory and Postural Functions.* 2nd ed. Hugo, MN: PDP Press Inc; 1995:8, 18, 20, 27.

4. Page DC. "Real" early orthodontic treatment: from birth to age 8. *Funct Orthod: J Funct Jaw Orthop.* 2003;20(1–2):48–58.

5. Upledger JE, Vredevoogd JD. *Craniosacral Therapy.* Seattle, WA: East-land Press; 1983:185–199, 256–258.

6. Upledger JE. *A Brain Is Born: Exploring the Birth and Development of the Central Nervous System.* Berkeley, CA: North Atlantic Book; and Palm Beach Gardens, FL: The Upledger Institute Inc; 1996:216–217.

7. Geddes DT, Kent JC, Mitoulas LR, Hartmann PE. Tongue movement and intra-oral vacuum in breastfeeding infants. *J Early Hum Dev.* 2008;10:1016.

8. Coryllos E, Genna CW, Salloum AC. Congenital tongue-tie and its impact on breastfeeding. American Academy of Pediatrics: Section on Breastfeeding. http://www.aap.org. Accessed August 24, 2009.

9. Page DC. *Your Jaws—Your Life.* Baltimore, MD: SmilePage Publishing; 2003:28–29.

10. Montagu A. *Touching: The Human Significance of the Skin.* 3rd ed. New York, NY: Harper & Row Publishers; 1986:84.

11. Oetter P, Richter EW, Frick SM. *M.O.R.E.: Integrating the Mouth with Sensory and Postural Functions.* 2nd ed. Hugo, MN: PDP Press Inc; 1995:18.

12. Metson RB. *The Harvard Medical School Guide to Healing Your Sinuses.* New York, NY: McGraw-Hill; 2005:161–162.

13. Northrup C. *Mother-Daughter Wisdom: Creating a Legacy of Physical and Emotional Health.* New York, NY: Bantam Dell; 2005:242.

14. Stein R. As babies are born earlier, they risk problems later. *Washington Post.* May 20, 2006:A1.

15. Bahr DC. *Oral Motor Assessment and Treatment: Ages and Stages.* Boston, MA: Allyn & Bacon; 2001:4–7.

16. Love RJ, Webb WG. *Neurology for the Speech-Language Pathologist.* 3rd ed. Boston, MA: Butterworth-Heinemann; 1996:287–293.

17. Morris SE, Klein MD. *Pre-Feeding Skills: A Comprehensive Resource for Feeding Development.* Tucson, AZ: Therapy Skill Builders; 1987:26–27.

18. Morris SE, Klein MD. *Pre-Feeding Skills: A Comprehensive Resource for Mealtime Development.* 2nd ed. San Antonio, TX: Therapy Skill Builders; 2000:71, 697–711.

19. Samuels M, Samuels N. *The Well Baby Book: A Comprehensive Manual of Baby Care, from Conception to Age Four.* New York, NY: Summit Books; 1991:142.

20. Tuchman DN, Walter RS. *Disorders of Feeding and Swallowing in Infants and Children: Pathophysiology, Diagnosis, and Treatment.* San Diego, CA: Singular Publishing Group; 1994:29–31.

21. Montagu A. *Touching: The Human Significance of the Skin.* 3rd ed. New York, NY: Harper & Row Publishers; 1986:69–95.

22. Stevenson RD, Allaire JH. The development of normal feeding and swallowing. *Pediatr Clin North Am.* 1991;38(6):1439–1453.

23. Montagu A. *Touching: The Human Significance of the Skin*. 3rd ed. New York, NY: Harper & Row Publishers; 1986:82.

24. Oetter P, Richter EW, Frick SM. *M.O.R.E.: Integrating the Mouth with Sensory and Postural Functions*. 2nd ed. Hugo, MN: PDP Press Inc; 1995:21.

25. Karp H. *The Happiest Baby on the Block*. New York, NY: Bantam Dell; 2002:4.

26. Geddes DT, Kent JC, Mitoulas LR, Hartmann PE. Tongue movement and intra-oral vacuum in breastfeeding infants. *J Early Hum Dev*. 2008;10:1016.

27. Coryllos E, Genna CW, Salloum AC. Congenital tongue-tie and its impact on breastfeeding. American Academy of Pediatrics: Section on Breastfeeding. http://www.aap.org. Accessed August 24, 2009.

28. Coryllos E, Genna CW, Salloum AC. Congenital tongue-tie and its impact on breastfeeding. American Academy of Pediatrics: Section on Breastfeeding. http://www.aap.org. Accessed August 24, 2009.

29. Written communication with P. Merrill, Greater Baltimore Medical Center, Baltimore, MD; March 2008.

30. West D, Marasco L. *The Breastfeeding Mother's Guide to Making More Milk*. Columbus, OH: McGraw Hill; 2009.

31. Written communication with P. Merrill, Greater Baltimore Medical Center, Baltimore, MD; March 2008.

32. Cummings NP, Neifert MR, Pabst MJ, Johnston RB. Oxidative metabolic response and microbicidal activity of human milk macrophages: effect of lipopolysaccharide and muramyl dipeptide. *Infect Immun*. 1985;49(2):435–439.

33. Colson SD, Meek JH, Hawdon JM. Optimal positions for the release of primitive neonatal reflexes stimulating breastfeeding. *Early Hum Dev*. 2008;84:441–449.

34. Colson S. Maternal breastfeeding positions: have we got it right? (1). *Pract Midwife.* 2005;8(10):24, 26–27.

35. Colson S. Maternal breastfeeding positions: have we got it right? (2). *Pract Midwife.* 2005;8(11):29–32.

36. Zemlin WR. *Speech and Hearing Science: Anatomy and Physiology.* 4th ed. Boston, MA: Allyn & Bacon; 1998:547.

37. Ginsberg IA, White TP. Otological considerations in audiology. In: Katz J, ed. *Handbook of Clinical Audiology.* 2nd ed. Baltimore, MD: Williams &Wilkins; 1978:13.

38. Goetzinger CP. Word discrimination testing. In Katz J, ed. *Handbook of Clinical Audiology.* 2nd ed. Baltimore, MD: Williams & Wilkins; 1978:151.

39. Sachs J. The emergence of intentional communication. In: Gleason JB, ed. *The Development of Language.* 3rd ed. New York, NY: Macmillan Publishing Co; 1993:40.

40. Montagu A. *Touching: The Human Significance of the Skin.* 3rd ed. New York, NY: Harper & Row Publishers; 1986:69–95.

41. Page DC. *Your Jaws–Your Life.* Baltimore, MD: SmilePage Publishing; 2003:46–47.

42. Page DC. "Real" early orthodontic treatment: from birth to age 8. *Funct Orthod: J Funct Jaw Orthop.* 2003;20(1–2):48–58.

43. Huggins K. *The Nursing Mother's Companion.* 4th ed. Boston, MA: The Harvard Common Press; 1999.

44. Montagu A. *Touching: The Human Significance of the Skin.* 3rd ed. New York, NY: Harper & Row Publishers; 1986:83.

45. Pottenger FM, Krohn B. Influence of breast feeding on facial development. *Arch Pediatr.* 1950;67:454–461.

46. Robinson S, Naylor SR. The effects of late weaning on the deciduous teeth. *Br Dent J.* 1963;115:250.

47. Nizel A. Nursing-bottle syndrome: rampant dental caries in young children. *Nutr News.* 1975;38:1.

48. Broad FE. The effects of infant feeding on speech quality. *N Z Med J.* 1972;76:28–31.

49. Broad FE. Further studies on the effects of infant feeding on speech quality. *N Z Med J.* 1975;82:373–376.

50. Bertrand FM. The relationship of prolonged breastfeeding to facial features. *Cent Afr J Med.* 1968;14:226–227.

51. Montagu A. *Touching: The Human Significance of the Skin.* 3rd ed. New York, NY: Harper & Row Publishers; 1986:85.

52. Page DC. "Real" early orthodontic treatment: from birth to age 8. *Funct Orthod: J Funct Jaw Orthop.* 2003;20(1–2):48–58.

53. Page DC. "Real" early orthodontic treatment: from birth to age 8. *Funct Orthod: J Funct Jaw Orthop.* 2003;20(1–2):54.

54. Paunio P, Rautava P, Sillanpaa M. Sucking habits in 3 year old children and the association between these habits and dental occlusion. *Acta Odont Scand.* 1993;51(1):23–29.

55. Davis DW, Bell PA. Infant feeding practices and occlusal outcomes: a longitudinal study. *J Can Dent Assoc.* 1991;57(7):593–594.

56. Paunio P, Rautava P, Sillanpaa M. The Finnish family competence study: the effects of living conditions on sucking habits in 3-year-old Finnish children and the association between these habits and dental occlusion. *Acta Odont Scand.* 1993:51(1):23–29.

57. Ogarrd B, Larsson E, Lindsten R. The effect of sucking habits, cohort, sex, inter-canine arch widths, and breast or bottle feeding on posterior crossbite in Norwegian and Swedish 3-year-old children. *Am J Orthod Dentofacial Orthop.* 1994;106(2):161–166.

58. Page DC. "Real" early orthodontic treatment: from birth to age 8. *Funct Orthod: J Funct Jaw Orthop.* 2003;20(1–2):56.

59. Aniansson G, Alm B, Andersson B, et al. A prospective cohort study on breast-feeding and otitis media in Swedish infants. *Pediatr Infect Dis J.* 1994;13:183–188.

60. Watkins CJ, Leeder SR, Corkhill RT. The relationship between breast and bottle-feeding and respiratory illness in the first year of life. *J Epidemiol Community Health.* 1979;33:180–182.

61. Gerstein HC. Cow's milk exposure and type 1 diabetes mellitus. *Diabetes Care.* 1994;17:13–19.

62. Barlow B, Santulli TV, Heird WC, et al. An experimental study of acute neonatal entercolotis: the importance of breastmilk. *J Pediatr Surg.* 1974;9:587–595.

63. Saarinen UM, Kajossari M. Breast-feeding as prophylaxis against atopic disease: prospective follow-up study until 17 years old. *Lancet.* 1995;346:1065–1069.

64. Cullinan TR, Saunder DI. Prediction of infant hospital admission risk. *Arch Dis Child.* 1983;68:423–427.

65. Mitchell EA, Scragg R, Stewart AW, et al. Results from the first year of the New Zealand cot-death study. *N Z Med J.* 1991;104:71–75.

66. Palmer B. The influence of breastfeeding on the development of the oral cavity: a commentary. *J Hum Lactation.* 1998;14(2):93–98.

67. Montagu A. *Touching: The Human Significance of the Skin.* 3rd ed. New York, NY: Harper & Row Publishers; 1986:69–95.

68. Kimball ER. How I get mothers to breastfeed. *Physician's Manage.* June 1968 (OB/GYN's suppl).

69. Hoefer C, Hardy MC. Later development of breast fed and artificially fed infants. *JAMA.* 1929;96:615–619.

70. Horwood LJ, Ferguson DM. Breastfeeding and later cognitive and academic outcomes. *Pediatrics.* Jan 1998;101(1):E8.

71. Hoefer C, Hardy MC. Later development of breast fed and artificially fed infants. *JAMA.* 1929;96:615–619.

72. Enlow DH, Hans MG. *Essentials of Facial Growth.* Philadelphia, PA: W. B. Saunders; 1996.

73. Yamada T, Tanne K, Miyamoto K, Yamauchi K. Influences of nasal respiratory obstruction on craniofacial growth in young Macaca fuscata monkeys. *Am J Orthod Dentofacial Orthop.* 1997;111(1):38–43.

74. Wright JL. Diseases of the small airways. *Lung.* 2001;179(6):375–396.

75. Page DC. *Your Jaws—Your Life.* Baltimore, MD: SmilePage Publishing; 2003:33.

76. Written communication with P. Merrill, Greater Baltimore Medical Center, Baltimore, MD; March 2008.

77. Satter E. *Child of Mine: Feeding with Love and Good Sense.* Boulder, CO: Bull Publishing Co; 2000.

78. Satter E. *How to Get Your Kid to Eat…But Not Too Much.* Palo Alto, CA: Bull Publishing Co; 1987.

79. Written communication with P. Merrill, Greater Baltimore Medical Center, Baltimore, MD; March 2008.

80. Satter E. *Child of Mine: Feeding with Love and Good Sense.* Boulder, CO: Bull Publishing Co; 2000:162.

81. Written communication with P. Merrill, Greater Baltimore Medical Center, Baltimore, MD; March 2008.

82. Satter E. *Child of Mine: Feeding with Love and Good Sense.* Boulder, CO: Bull Publishing Co; 2000:165–166, 206–207.

83. Satter E. *Child of Mine: Feeding with Love and Good Sense.* Boulder, CO: Bull Publishing Co; 2000:218.

84. Satter E. *Child of Mine: Feeding with Love and Good Sense.* Boulder, CO: Bull Publishing Co; 2000:219.

85. Satter E. *Child of Mine: Feeding with Love and Good Sense.* Boulder, CO: Bull Publishing Co; 2000:231.

86. Written communication with P. Merrill, Greater Baltimore Medical Center, Baltimore, MD; March 2008.

87. Northrup C. *Mother-Daughter Wisdom: Creating a Legacy of Physical and Emotional Health.* New York, NY: Bantam Dell; 2005:212–214.

88. Batmanghelidj F. *Your Body's Many Cries for Water.* Vienna, VA: Global Health Solutions; 1997:8.

89. Morris SE, Klein MD. *Pre-Feeding Skills: A Comprehensive Resource for Mealtime Development.* 2nd ed. San Antonio, TX: Therapy Skill Builders; 2000:327.

90. Batmanghelidj F. *Your Body's Many Cries for Water.* Vienna, VA: Global Health Solutions; 1997:13.

91. Northrup C. *Mother-Daughter Wisdom: Creating a Legacy of Physical and Emotional Health.* New York, NY: Bantam Dell; 2005:212–214.

92. Morris SE, Klein MD. *Pre-Feeding Skills: A Comprehensive Resource for Mealtime Development.* 2nd ed. San Antonio, TX: Therapy Skill Builders; 2000:327.

93. Batmanghelidj F. *Your Body's Many Cries for Water.* Vienna, VA: Global Health Solutions; 1997.

94. Satter E. *Child of Mine: Feeding with Love and Good Sense.* Boulder, CO: Bull Publishing Co; 2000:176–177.

95. Satter E. *Child of Mine: Feeding with Love and Good Sense.* Boulder, CO: Bull Publishing Co; 2000:509.

96. Bahr DC. *Oral Motor Assessment and Treatment: Ages and Stages.* Boston, MA: Allyn & Bacon; 2001:5, 17–20, 44–45, 121–133, 147.

97. Morris SE, Klein MD. *Pre-Feeding Skills: A Comprehensive Resource for Feeding Development.* Tucson, AZ: Therapy Skill Builders; 1987:306.

98. Morris SE, Klein MD. *Pre-Feeding Skills: A Comprehensive Resource for Mealtime Development.* 2nd ed. San Antonio, TX: Therapy Skill Builders; 2000:51–53, 71, 697–711.

99. Morris SE. Developmental implications for the management of feeding problems in neurologically impaired infants. *Semin Speech Lang.* 1985;6(4):293–315.

100. Oetter P, Richter EW, Frick SM. *M.O.R.E.: Integrating the Mouth with Sensory and Postural Functions.* 2nd ed. Hugo, MN: PDP Press Inc; 1995:8, 20, 27.

101. Winstock A. *Eating & Drinking Difficulties in Children: A Guide for Practitioners.* Oxon, UK: Speechmark Publishing Ltd; 2005.

102. Bly L. *Motor Skills Acquisition Checklist.* San Antonio, TX: Therapy Skill Builders; 2000:20–21.

103. Montagu A. *Touching: The Human Significance of the Skin.* 3rd ed. New York, NY: Harper & Row Publishers; 1986:84.

104. Eisenberg A, Murkoff HE, Hathaway SE. *What to Expect the First Year.* New York, NY: Workman Publishing; 1989.

105. Written communication with P. Merrill, Greater Baltimore Medical Center, Baltimore, MD; March 2008.

106. Northrup C. *Mother-Daughter Wisdom: Creating a Legacy of Physical and Emotional Health.* New York, NY: Bantam Dell; 2005:242.

107. Page DC. "Real" early orthodontic treatment: from birth to age 8. *Funct Orthod: J Funct Jaw Orthop.* 2003;20(1–2):56.

108. Gray LP. Relationship of septal deformity to snuffly noses, poor feeding, sticky eyes and blocked nasolacrimal ducts. *Int J Pediatr Otorhinolaryngol.* 1980;2(3):201–215.

109. Page DC. *Your Jaws—Your Life.* Baltimore, MD: SmilePage Publishing; 2003:33.

110. Page DC. *Your Jaws—Your Life.* Baltimore, MD: SmilePage Publishing; 2003:33.

111. Page DC. *Your Jaws—Your Life.* Baltimore, MD: SmilePage Publishing; 2003:34–37.

112. Lundberg JO, Farkas-Szallasi T, Weitzberg E, et al. High nitric oxide production in human paranasal sinuses. *Nat Med.* 1995;April 1(4): 370–373.

113. Schedin U, Norman M, Gustafsson LE, Herin P, Frostell C. Endogenous nitric oxide in the upper airways of healthy newborn infants. *Pediatr Res.* 1996;40(1):148–151.

114. McCann SM, Licinio J, Wong ML, Yu WH, Karanth S, Rettorri V. The nitric oxide hypothesis of aging. *Exp Gerontol.* 1998;33(7–8):813–826.

115. Northrup C. *The Wisdom of Menopause: Creating Physical and Emotional Health and Healing During the Change.* New York, NY: Bantam Books; 2001:162.

116. McCann SM, Licinio J, Wong ML, Yu WH, Karanth S, Rettorri V. The nitric oxide hypothesis of aging. *Exp Gerontol.* 1998;33(7–8):813–826.

117. Lundberg JO, Settergren G, Gelinder S, Lundberg JM, Alving K, Weitzberg E. Inhalation of nasally derived nitric oxide modulates pulmonary function in humans. *Acta Physiol Scand.* 1996;158(4):343–347.

118. Northrup C. *Mother-Daughter Wisdom: Creating a Legacy of Physical and Emotional Health.* New York, NY: Bantam Dell; 2005:548.

119. Northrup C. *Mother-Daughter Wisdom: Creating a Legacy of Physical and Emotional Health.* New York, NY: Bantam Dell; 2005:539.

120. Alexander R. Oral-motor treatment for infants and young children with cerebral palsy. *Semin Speech Lang.* 1987;8(1):87–100.

121. Written communication with P. Merrill, Greater Baltimore Medical Center, Baltimore, MD; March 2008.

122. Rapp D. *Is This Your Child? Discovering and Treating Unrecognized Allergies in Children and Adults.* New York, NY: William Morrow & Co Inc; 1991:99–131.

123. Rapp D. *Is This Your Child? Discovering and Treating Unrecognized Allergies in Children and Adults.* New York, NY: William Morrow & Co Inc; 1991:99–131.

124. Rapp D. *Is This Your Child? Discovering and Treating Unrecognized Allergies in Children and Adults.* New York, NY: William Morrow & Co Inc; 1991:102.

125. Crook WG. *Detecting Your Hidden Allergies.* Jackson, TN: Professional Books Inc; 1988.

126. Rapp D. *Is This Your Child? Discovering and Treating Unrecognized Allergies in Children and Adults.* New York, NY: William Morrow & Co Inc; 1991.

127. Rapp D. *Is This Your Child? Discovering and Treating Unrecognized Allergies in Children and Adults.* New York, NY: William Morrow & Co Inc; 1991:103–111.

128. Karp H. *The Happiest Baby on the Block.* New York, NY: Bantam Dell; 2002:26–27.

129. Rapp D. *Is This Your Child? Discovering and Treating Unrecognized Allergies in Children and Adults.* New York, NY: William Morrow & Co Inc; 1991:103–111.

130. Rapp D. *Is This Your Child? Discovering and Treating Unrecognized Allergies in Children and Adults.* New York, NY: William Morrow & Co Inc; 1991:125–128.

131. Rapp D. *Is This Your Child? Discovering and Treating Unrecognized Allergies in Children and Adults.* New York, NY: William Morrow & Co Inc; 1991:125–128.

132. Sears W, Sears M, Sears J, Sears R. Tracking Down Food Allergies. http://www.askdrsears.com. Accessed August 26, 2009.

133. Karp H. *The Happiest Baby on the Block.* New York, NY: Bantam Dell; 2002.

134. Orenstein SR, Whitington PF. Positioning for prevention of gastroesophageal reflux. *J Pediatr.* 1983;103:534–537.

135. Meyers WF, Herbst JJ. Effectiveness of positioning therapy for gastroesophageal reflux. *Pediatrics.* 1982;69:768–772.

136. Vandenplas Y, Sacre-Smits L. Seventeen-hour continuous esophageal pH monitoring in the newborn: evaluation of the influence of position in asymptomatic and symptomatic babies. *J Pediatr Gastroenterol Nutr.* 1985;4:356–361.

137. American Academy of Pediatrics. Changing concepts of sudden infant death syndrome: implications for infant sleeping environment and sleep position. *Pediatrics.* 2000;105(3):650–656.

138. American Academy of Pediatrics. Changing concepts of sudden infant death syndrome: implications for infant sleeping environment and sleep position. *Pediatrics.* 2000;105(3):650–656.

139. Fleming PJ, Blair PS, Bacon C. Environment of infants during sleep and risk of the sudden infant death syndrome: results of 1993–5 case-control study for confidential inquiry into still births and deaths in infancy. *BMJ.* 1996;313:191–195.

140. L'Hoir MP, Engleberts AC, Van Well GTJ, et al. Risk and preventive factors for cot death in the Netherlands, a low incidence country. *Eur J Pediatr.* 1998;157:681–688.

141. Arnestad M, Andersen M, Rognum TO. Is the use of a dummy or carry-cot of importance for sudden infant death? *Eur J Pediatr.* 1997;156:968–970.

142. Mitchell EA, Taylor BJ, Ford RPK. Dummies and sudden infant death syndrome. *Arch Dis Child.* 1993;68:501–504.

143. American Academy of Pediatrics. Changing concepts of sudden infant death syndrome: implications for infant sleeping environment and sleep position. *Pediatrics.* 2000;105(3):650–656.

144. American Academy of Pediatrics. Changing concepts of sudden infant death syndrome: implications for infant sleeping environment and sleep position. *Pediatrics.* 2000;105(3):650–656.

145. Tenpenny SJ. *Vaccines: The Risks, the Benefits, the Choices, a Resource Guide for Parents.* USA: Insight Publishing; 2006.

146. Cave S. *What Your Doctor May Not Tell You about Children's Vaccinations.* New York, NY: Grand Central Publishing; 2001.

147. Sears RW. *The Vaccine Book: Making the Right Decision for Your Child.* New York, NY: Little, Brown and Co; 2007.

148. Rapp D. *Is This Your Child? Discovering and Treating Unrecognized Allergies in Children and Adults.* New York, NY: William Morrow & Co Inc; 1991:115.

149. Morris SE, Klein MD. *Pre-Feeding Skills: A Comprehensive Resource for ealtime Development.* 2nd ed. San Antonio, TX: Therapy Skill Builders; 2000:69.

150. Bahr DC. *Oral Motor Assessment and Treatment: Ages and Stages.* Boston, MA: Allyn & Bacon; 2001:4–7.

151. Morris SE, Klein MD. *Pre-Feeding Skills: A Comprehensive Resource for Feeding Development.* Tucson, AZ: Therapy Skill Builders; 1987:26–27.

152. Tuchman DN, Walter RS. *Disorders of Feeding and Swallowing in Infants and Children: Pathophysiology, Diagnosis, and Treatment.* San Diego, CA: Singular Publishing Group; 1994:29–31.

153. Morris SE, Klein MD. *Pre-Feeding Skills: A Comprehensive Resource for Feeding Development.* Tucson, AZ: Therapy Skill Builders; 1987:306.

154. Eisenberg A, Murkoff HE, Hathaway SE. *What to Expect the First Year.* New York, NY: Workman Publishing; 1989.

155. Montagu A. *Touching: The Human Significance of the Skin.* 3rd ed. New York, NY: Harper & Row Publishers; 1986:84.

156. Bahr DC. *Oral Motor Assessment and Treatment: Ages and Stages.* Boston, MA: Allyn & Bacon; 2001:5, 17–20, 44–45, 121–133, 147.

157. Morris SE, Klein MD. *Pre-Feeding Skills: A Comprehensive Resource for Feeding Development.* Tucson, AZ: Therapy Skill Builders; 1987:306.

158. Morris SE, Klein MD. *Pre-Feeding Skills: A Comprehensive Resource for Mealtime Development.* 2nd ed. San Antonio, TX: Therapy Skill Builders; 2000:51–53, 71, 697–711.

159. Morris SE. Developmental implications for the management of feeding problems in neurologically impaired infants. *Semin Speech Lang.* 1985;6(4):293–315.

160. Oetter P, Richter EW, Frick SM. *M.O.R.E.: Integrating the Mouth with Sensory and Postural Functions.* 2nd ed. Hugo, MN: PDP Press Inc; 1995:8, 20, 27.

161. Winstock A. *Eating & Drinking Difficulties in Children: A Guide for Practitioners.* Oxon, UK: Speechmark Publishing Ltd; 2005.

162. Perkins WH, Kent RD. *Functional Anatomy of Speech, Language, and Hearing: A Primer.* Boston, MA: Allyn & Bacon; 1986:131.

163. Pierce RB. *Tongue Thrust: A Look at Oral Myofunctional Disorders.* Lincoln, NE: Cliffs Notes Inc; 1978:31.

164. Bly L. *Motor Skills Acquisition Checklist.* San Antonio, TX: Therapy Skill Builders; 2000:20–21.

165. Boshart CA. Essential oral-motor techniques: a one-day seminar [workshop]. Temecula, CA: Speech Dynamics Inc; 1998.

166. Kent RD. Motor control: neurophysiology and functional development. In: Caruso AJ, Strand EA, eds. *Clinical Management of Motor Speech Disorders in Children.* New York, NY: Thieme Medical Publishers; 1999:29–71.

167. Montagu A. *Touching: The Human Significance of the Skin.* 3rd ed. New York, NY: Harper & Row Publishers; 1986:84.

168. Eisenberg A, Murkoff HE, Hathaway SE. *What to Expect the First Year.* New York, NY: Workman Publishing; 1989.

169. Eisenberg A, Murkoff HE, Hathaway SE. *What to Expect: The Toddler Years.* New York, NY: Workman Publishing; 1994.

170. Morris SE, Klein MD. *Pre-Feeding Skills: A Comprehensive Resource for Mealtime Development.* 2nd ed. San Antonio, TX: Therapy Skill Builders; 2000:70.

171. Stevenson RD, Allaire JH. The development of normal feeding and swallowing. *Pediatr Clin N Am.* 1991;38(6):1439–1453.

172. Moore CA, Smith A, Ringel RL. Task-specific organization of activity in human jaw muscles. *J Speech Hear Res.* 1988;31:670–680.

173. Karp H. *The Happiest Baby on the Block.* New York, NY: Bantam Dell; 2002:176.

174. American Academy of Pediatrics. Changing concepts of sudden infant death syndrome: implications for infant sleeping environment and sleep position. *Pediatrics.* 2000;105(3):650–656.

175. Li D, Willinger M, Petitti DB, Odouli R, Hoffman HJ. Use of dummy (pacifier) during sleep and risk of sudden infant death syndrome (SIDS): population based case-control study. *BMJ.* 2006;332(7532):18–22.

176. Karp H. *The Happiest Baby on the Block.* New York, NY: Bantam Dell; 2002:177.

177. Duncan B, Ey J, Holberg CJ, Wright AL, Martinez FD, Taussig LM. Exclusive breast-feeding for at least 4 months protects against otitis media. *Pediatrics*. 1993;91:867–872.

178. Niemela M, Pihakari O, Pokka T, Uhari M, Uhari M. Pacifier as a risk factor for acute otitis media: a randomized, controlled trial of parental counseling. *Pediatrics*. 2000;106(3):483–488.

179. Niemela M, Pihakari O, Pokka T, Uhari M, Uhari M. Pacifier as a risk factor for acute otitis media: a randomized, controlled trial of parental counseling. *Pediatrics*. 2000;106(3):483–488.

180. Niemela M, Pihakari O, Pokka T, Uhari M, Uhari M. Pacifier as a risk factor for acute otitis media: a randomized, controlled trial of parental counseling. *Pediatrics*. 2000;106(3):483–488.

181. Karp H. *The Happiest Baby on the Block*. New York, NY: Bantam Dell; 2002:177.

182. Montagu A. *Touching: The Human Significance of the Skin*. 3rd ed. New York, NY: Harper & Row Publishers; 1986:69–95.

183. Page DC. *Your Jaws—Your Life*. Baltimore, MD: SmilePage Publishing; 2003:46–47.

184. Page DC. "Real" early orthodontic treatment: from birth to age 8. *Funct Orthod: J Funct Jaw Orthop*. 2003;20(1–2):48–58.

185. Kramer MS, Barr RG, Dagenais S, et al. Pacifier use, early weaning, and cry/fuss behavior. *JAMA*. 2001;286:322–326.

186. O'Neill P. Acute otitis media. *BMJ*. 1999;319(7213):833–835.

187. Niemela M, Pihakari O, Pokka T, Uhari M, Uhari M. Pacifier as a risk factor for acute otitis media: a randomized, controlled trial of parental counseling. *Pediatrics*. 2000;106(3):483–488.

188. American Academy of Pediatrics. Changing concepts of sudden infant death syndrome: implications for infant sleeping environment and sleep position. *Pediatrics*. 2000;105(3):650–656.

189. Li D, Willinger M, Petitti DB, Odouli R, Hoffman HJ. Use of dummy (pacifier) during sleep and risk of sudden infant death syndrome (SIDS): population based case-control study. *BMJ*. 2006;332(7532):18–22.

190. Niemela M, Pihakari O, Pokka T, Uhari M, Uhari M. Pacifier as a risk factor for acute otitis media: a randomized, controlled trial of parental counseling. *Pediatrics*. 2000;106(3):483–488.

191. Karp H. *The Happiest Baby on the Block*. New York, NY: Bantam Dell; 2002:178.

192. Rosenfeld-Johnson S. A three-part treatment plan for oral-motor therapy [workshop]. Baltimore, MD: Innovative Therapists International; 1999.

193. Rosenfeld-Johnson S. A three-part treatment plan for oral-motor therapy [workshop]. Baltimore, MD: Innovative Therapists International; 1999.

194. Marshalla P. *How to STOP Thumbsucking and Other Oral Habits*. Mill Creek, WA: Marshalla Speech & Language; 2004.

195. Heitler S. *David Decides about Thumbsucking: A Story for Children; a Guide for Parents*. Denver, CO: Reading Matters; 1996.

196. Bahr DC. *Oral Motor Assessment and Treatment: Ages and Stages*. Boston, MA: Allyn & Bacon; 2001:147.

197. Morris SE, Klein MD. *Pre-Feeding Skills: A Comprehensive Resource for Mealtime Development*. 2nd ed. San Antonio, TX: Therapy Skill Builders; 2000:697–711.

198. Oetter P, Richter EW, Frick SM. *M.O.R.E.: Integrating the Mouth with Sensory and Postural Functions*. 2nd ed. Hugo, MN: PDP Press Inc; 1995:8, 20, 27.

199. Perkins WH, Kent RD. *Functional Anatomy of Speech, Language, and Hearing: A Primer*. Boston, MA: Allyn & Bacon; 1986:131.

200. Pierce RB. *Tongue Thrust: A Look at Oral Myofunctional Disorders*. Lincoln, NE: Cliffs Notes Inc; 1978:31.

201. Nathanson LW. *The Portable Pediatrician for Parents: A Month-by-Month Guide to Your Child's Physical and Behavioral Development from Birth to Age Five.* New York, NY: Harper Perennial; 1994:59–60.

202. Morris SE, Klein MD. *Pre-Feeding Skills: A Comprehensive Resource for Mealtime Development.* 2nd ed. San Antonio, TX: Therapy Skill Builders; 2000:697.

203. Marshalla P. *How to STOP Drooling.* Mill Creek, WA: Marshalla Speech & Language; 2006.

204. Field T. *Touch Therapy.* New York, NY: Churchill Livingstone; 2000.

205. Montagu A. *Touching: The Human Significance of the Skin.* 3rd ed. New York, NY: Harper & Row Publishers; 1986.

206. Gunzenhauser N. *Advances in Touch: New Implications in Human Development.* USA: Johnson & Johnson Consumer Products Inc; 1990.

207. McClure VS. *Infant Massage: A Handbook for Loving Parents.* Rev ed. New York, NY: Bantam Books; 1989.

208. Bahr DC. *Oral Motor Assessment and Treatment: Ages and Stages.* Boston, MA: Allyn & Bacon; 2001:102–142.

209. Bahr DC. *Oral Motor Assessment and Treatment: Ages and Stages.* Boston, MA: Allyn & Bacon; 2001:250–251.

210. Wayson S. Oral normalization protocol. Workshop and handout presented at: Maryland School for the Blind; 1983.

211. Bahr DC. *Oral Motor Assessment and Treatment: Ages and Stages.* Boston, MA: Allyn & Bacon; 2001:115–121.

212. Morris SE, Klein MD. *Pre-Feeding Skills: A Comprehensive Resource for Feeding Development.* 2nd ed. San Antonio, TX: Therapy Skill Builders; 2000.

213. Bahr DC. *Oral Motor Assessment and Treatment: Ages and Stages.* Boston, MA: Allyn & Bacon; 2001:45.

214. Boehme R. Integration of neuro-developmental treatment and myofascial release in adult orthopedics. In: Barnes JF, ed. *Myofascial Release: The Search for Excellence: A Comprehensive Evaluatory and Treatment Approach.* Paoli, PA: Rehabilitation Services, Inc; 1990:209–217.

215. Rosenfeld-Johnson S. A three-part treatment plan for oral-motor therapy [workshop]. Baltimore, MD: Innovative Therapists International; 1999.

216. Upledger JE. *Craniosacral Therapy II: Beyond the Dura.* Seattle, WA: Eastland Press; 1987:197–207.

217. Rosenfeld-Johnson S. *Oral-Motor Exercises for Speech Clarity.* Tucson, AZ: Innovative Therapists International; 1999.

218. Rosenfeld-Johnson S. *Oral-Motor Exercises for Speech Clarity.* Tucson, AZ: Innovative Therapists International; 1999.

219. Rosenfeld-Johnson S. *Oral-Motor Exercises for Speech Clarity.* Tucson, AZ: Innovative Therapists International; 1999.

220. Karp H. *The Happiest Baby on the Block.* New York, NY: Bantam Dell; 2002:4.

221. Rosenfeld-Johnson S. A three-part treatment plan for oral-motor therapy [workshop]. Baltimore, MD: Innovative Therapists International; 1999.

222. Satter E. *Child of Mine: Feeding with Love and Good Sense.* Boulder, CO: Bull Publishing Co; 2000:250–251.

223. Stoppard M. *First Foods.* New York, NY: DK Publishing Inc; 1998:14–15.

224. Morris SE, Klein MD. *Pre-Feeding Skills: A Comprehensive Resource for Feeding Development.* 2nd ed. San Antonio, TX: Therapy Skill Builders; 2000:697–711.

225. Samuels M, Samuels N. *The Well Baby Book: A Comprehensive Manual of Baby Care, from Conception to Age Four.* New York, NY: Summit Books; 1991:162.

226. Huggins K. *The Nursing Mother's Companion.* 4th ed. Boston, MA: The Harvard Common Press; 1999:31.

227. Satter E. *Child of Mine: Feeding with Love and Good Sense.* Boulder, CO: Bull Publishing Co; 2000:293–294, 338–339.

228. Morris SE, Klein MD. *Pre-Feeding Skills: A Comprehensive Resource for Feeding Development.* 2nd ed. San Antonio, TX: Therapy Skill Builders; 2000:323–325.

229. Morris SE, Klein MD. *Pre-Feeding Skills: A Comprehensive Resource for Feeding Development.* 2nd ed. San Antonio, TX: Therapy Skill Builders; 2000:323–325.

230. Satter E. *Child of Mine: Feeding with Love and Good Sense.* Boulder, CO: Bull Publishing Co; 2000:293–294, 338–339.

231. Morris SE, Klein MD. *Pre-Feeding Skills: A Comprehensive Resource for Feeding Development.* 2nd ed. San Antonio, TX: Therapy Skill Builders; 2000:323–325.

232. Satter E. *Child of Mine: Feeding with Love and Good Sense.* Boulder, CO: Bull Publishing Co; 2000:293–294, 338–339.

233. Morris SE, Klein MD. *Pre-Feeding Skills: A Comprehensive Resource for Mealtime Development.* 2nd ed. San Antonio, TX: Therapy Skill Builders; 2000:323–325.

234. Batmanghelidj F. *Your Body's Many Cries for Water.* Vienna, VA: Global Health Solutions; 1997:13.

235. Northrup C. *Mother-Daughter Wisdom: Creating a Legacy of Physical and Emotional Health.* New York, NY: Bantam Dell; 2005:212–214.

236. Morris SE, Klein MD. *Pre-Feeding Skills: A Comprehensive Resource for Feeding Development.* 2nd ed. San Antonio, TX: Therapy Skill Builders; 2000:327.

237. Rosenfeld-Johnson S. A three-part treatment plan for oral-motor therapy [workshop]. Baltimore, MD: Innovative Therapists International; 1999.

238. Field T. *Touch Therapy.* New York, NY: Churchill Livingstone; 2000.

239. Satter E. *Child of Mine: Feeding with Love and Good Sense.* Boulder, CO: Bull Publishing Co; 2000.

240. Satter E. *How to Get Your Kid to Eat...But Not Too Much.* Palo Alto, CA: Bull Publishing Co; 1987.

241. Ernsperger L, Stegen-Hanson T. *Just Take a Bite: Easy, Effective Answers to Food Aversions and Eating Challenges.* Arlington, TX: Future Horizons Inc; 2004.

242. Morris SE, Klein MD. *Pre-Feeding Skills: A Comprehensive Resource for Feeding Development.* Tucson, AZ: Therapy Skill Builders; 1987:305.

243. Morris SE, Klein MD. *Pre-Feeding Skills: A Comprehensive Resource for Feeding Development.* 2nd ed. San Antonio, TX: Therapy Skill Builders; 2000:51–53, 71, 697–711.

244. Morris SE. Developmental implications for the management of feeding problems in neurologically impaired infants. *Semin Speech Lang.* 2004;6(4):293–315.

245. Oetter P, Richter EW, Frick SM. *M.O.R.E.: Integrating the Mouth with Sensory and Postural Functions.* 2nd ed. Hugo, MN: PDP Press Inc; 1995:8, 20, 27.

246. Winstock A. *Eating & Drinking Difficulties in Children: A Guide for Practitioners* Oxon, UK: Speechmark Publishing Ltd; 2005.

247. Perkins WH, Kent RD. *Functional Anatomy of Speech, Language, and Hearing: A Primer.* Boston, MA: Allyn & Bacon; 1986:131.

248. Pierce RB. *Tongue Thrust: A Look at Oral Myofunctional Disorders.* Lincoln, NE: Cliffs Notes Inc; 1978:31.

249. Boshart CA. Essential oral-motor techniques: a one-day seminar [workshop]. Temecula, CA: Speech Dynamics Inc; 1998.

250. Kent RD. Motor control: neurophysiology and functional development. In: Caruso AJ, Strand EA, eds. *Clinical Management of Motor Speech Disorders in Children.* New York, NY: Thieme Medical Publishers; 1999:29–71.

251. Eisenberg A, Murkoff HE, Hathaway SE. *What to Expect the First Year.* New York, NY: Workman Publishing; 1989.

252. Eisenberg A, Murkoff HE, Hathaway SE. *What to Expect: The Toddler Years.* New York, NY: Workman Publishing; 1994.

253. Stevenson RD, Allaire JH. The development of normal feeding and swallowing. *Pediatr Clin N Am.* 1991;38(6):1439–1453.

254. Boynton S. *Moo, Baa, La La La!* New York, NY: Little Simon; 1995.

255. Kent RD. Motor control: neurophysiology and functional development. In: Caruso AJ, Strand EA, eds. *Clinical Management of Motor Speech Disorders in Children.* New York, NY: Thieme Medical Publishers; 1999:29–71.

256. Rossetti L. *The Rossetti Infant-Toddler Language Scale.* East Moline, IL: LinguiSystems Inc; 1990:2–9.

257. Vulpe SG. *Vulpe Assessment Battery: Developmental Assessment, Performance Analysis, Individualized Programming.* Toronto, ON: National Institute on Mental Retardation; 1977:151–165.

258. Hedrick DL, Prather EM, Tobin AR. *The Sequenced Inventory of Communication Development.* Seattle, WA: University of Washington Press; 1984.

259. Reidlich CE, Herzfeld ME. *0 to 3 Years: An Early Language Curriculum.* Moline, IL: LinguiSystems Inc; 1983.

260. Dyer L. *Look Who's Talking: How to Enhance Your Child's Language Development Starting at Birth.* Minnetonka: MN: Meadowbrook Press; 2004.

261. Retherford KS. *Normal Development: A Database of Communication and Related Behaviors, Birth to 12+ Years.* Eau Claire, WI: Thinking Publications; 2003.

262. Kent R. Articulatory and acoustic perspectives on speech development. In: Reilly AP, ed. *The Communication Game: Perspectives on*

the Development of Speech, Language, and Nonverbal Communication Skills. Skillman, NJ: Johnson & Johnson Baby Products Co; 1980:38–43.

263. Oller DK. The emergence of speech sounds in infancy. In: Yeni-Komshian G, Kavanagh JA, Ferguson CA, eds. *Child Phonology: Volume 1. Production.* New York, NY: Academic Press; 1980:93–112.

264. Locke J. *Phonological Acquisition and Change.* New York, NY: Academic Press; 1983:10.

265. Grunwell P. *Clinical Phonology.* 2nd ed. Rockville, MD: Aspen Publishers; 1987:231.

266. Stoel-Gammon C, Cooper J. Patterns of early lexical and phonological development. *J Child Lang.* 1984;11:247–271.

267. Owens RE. *Language Development: An Introduction.* 4th ed. Needham Heights, MA: Allyn & Bacon; 1996:95–105, 162–195.

268. Chen H, Irwin O. Infant speech vowel and consonant types. *J Speech Disord.* 1946;11(1):27–29.

269. Irwin O. Infant speech: development of vowel sounds. *J Speech Hear Disord.* 1948;13:31–34.

270. Vulpe SG. *Vulpe Assessment Battery: Developmental Assessment, Performance Analysis, Individualized Programming.* Toronto, ON: National Institute on Mental Retardation; 1977:152.

271. Vulpe SG. *Vulpe Assessment Battery: Developmental Assessment, Performance Analysis, Individualized Programming.* Toronto, ON: National Institute on Mental Retardation; 1977:153.

272. Irwin O. Infant speech: development of vowel sounds. *J Speech Hear Disord.* 1948;13:31–34.

273. Vulpe SG. *Vulpe Assessment Battery: Developmental Assessment, Performance Analysis, Individualized Programming.* Toronto, ON: National Institute on Mental Retardation; 1977:154.

274. Miller JF, Rosin P, Netsell R. *Differentiating Productive Language Deficits and Speech Motor Control Problems in Children.* Paper presented at: Annual convention of the Wisconsin Speech and Hearing Association; April 1979; Madison, WI.

275. Oller DK. Infant vocalization and the development of speech. *Allied Health Behav Sci.* 1978;1:523–549.

276. Miller JF, Rosin P, Netsell R. *Differentiating Productive Language Deficits and Speech Motor Control Problems in Children.* Paper presented at: Annual convention of the Wisconsin Speech and Hearing Association; April 1979; Madison, WI.

277. Ingram D. *Procedures for the Phonological Analysis of Children's Language.* Baltimore, MD: University Park Press; 1981.

278. Ingram D. *Phonological Disability in Children.* 2nd ed. New York, NY: American Elsevier; 1989.

279. Donegan P. Normal vowel development. In: Ball MJ, Gibbon FE, eds. *Vowel disorders.* Boston, MA: Butterworth-Heinemann; 2002.

280. Wachs T. Utilization of a Piagetian approach to the investigation of early experience effects: a research strategy and some illustrative data. *Merrill-Palmer Q;* 1976;22(1):11–30.

281. Coplan J. *Early Language Milestone Scale.* Tulsa, OK: Modern Education Corporation; 1987.

282. Miller JF, Rosin P, Netsell R. *Differentiating Productive Language Deficits and Speech Motor Control Problems in Children.* Paper presented at: Annual convention of the Wisconsin Speech and Hearing Association; April 1979; Madison, WI.

283. Stoel-Gammon C. Phonetic inventories, 15–24 months: a longitudinal study. *J Speech Hear Res.* 1985;28:505–512.

284. Dyson A. Phonetic inventories of 2- and 3-year old children. *J Speech Hear Disord.* 1988;53:89–93.

285. Robb M, Bleile K. Consonant inventories of young children from 8 to 25 months. *J Clin Linguistics Phonetics;* 1994;8:295–320.

286. Stoel-Gammon C. Phonetic inventories, 15–24 months: a longitudinal study. *J Speech Hear Res.* 1985;28:505–512.

287. Dyson A. Phonetic inventories of 2- and 3-year old children. *J Speech Hear Disord.* 1988;53:89–93.

288. Robb M, Bleile K. Consonant inventories of young children from 8 to 25 months. *J Clin Linguistics Phonetics.* 1994;8:295–320.

289. Retherford KS. *Normal Development: A Database of Communication and Related Behaviors, Birth to 12+ Years.* Eau Claire, WI: Thinking Publications; 2003.

290. Grunwell P. *Clinical Phonology.* 2nd ed. Rockville, MD: Aspen Publishers; 1987:231.

291. Lipsitt L. Learning processes of human newborns. *Merrill-Palmer Q.* 1966;12:45–71.

292. Mehrabian A. Measures of vocabulary and grammatical skills for children up to age six. *Dev Psychol.* 1970;2:439–446.

293. Donegan P. Normal vowel development. In: Ball MJ, Gibbon FE, eds. *Vowel disorders.* Boston, MA: Butterworth-Heinemann; 2002:2.

294. Owens RE. *Language Development: An Introduction.* 4th ed. Boston, MA: Allyn & Bacon; 1996:99.

295. Grunwell P. *Clinical Phonology.* 2nd ed. Rockville, MD: Aspen Publishers; 1987:231.

296. Sander E. When are speech sounds learned? *J Speech Hear Disord.* 1972;37:55–63.

297. Grunwell P. *Clinical Phonology.* 2nd ed. Rockville, MD: Aspen Publishers; 1987:231.

298. Lipsitt L. Learning processes of human newborns. *Merrill-Palmer Q.* 1966;12,:45–71.

299. Mehrabian A. Measures of vocabulary and grammatical skills for children up to age six. *Dev Psychol.* 1970;2:439–446.

300. Sander E. When are speech sounds learned? *J Speech Hear Disord.* 1972;37:55–63.

301. Sander E. When are speech sounds learned? *J Speech Hear Disord.* 1972;37:55–63.

302. Sander E. When are speech sounds learned? *J Speech Hear Disord.* 1972;37:55–63.

303. Van Riper C. *Speech Correction: Principles and Methods.* 6th ed. Englewood Cliffs, NJ: Prentice-Hall Inc; 1978:107.

304. Sander E. When are speech sounds learned? *J Speech Hear Disord.* 1972;37:55–63.

305. Boshart CA. Essential oral-motor techniques: a one-day seminar [workshop]. Temecula, CA: Speech Dynamics Inc; 1998.

306. Kent RD. Motor control: neurophysiology and functional development. In: Caruso AJ, Strand EA, eds. *Clinical Management of Motor Speech Disorders in Children.* New York, NY: Thieme Medical Publishers; 1999:34.

307. Kent RD. Motor control: neurophysiology and functional development. In: Caruso AJ, Strand EA, eds. *Clinical Management of Motor Speech Disorders in Children.* New York, NY: Thieme Medical Publishers; 1999:31.

308. Kent RD. Motor control: neurophysiology and functional development. In: Caruso AJ, Strand EA, eds. *Clinical Management of Motor Speech Disorders in Children.* New York, NY: Thieme Medical Publishers; 1999:32.

309. Oetter P, Richter EW, Frick SM. *M.O.R.E.: Integrating the Mouth with Sensory and Postural Functions.* 2nd ed. Hugo, MN: PDP Press Inc; 1995:27.

310. Oetter P, Richter EW, Frick SM. *M.O.R.E.: Integrating the Mouth with Sensory and Postural Functions.* 2nd ed. Hugo, MN: PDP Press Inc; 1995:47.

311. Oetter P, Richter EW, Frick SM. *M.O.R.E.: Integrating the Mouth with Sensory and Postural Functions.* 2nd ed. Hugo, MN: PDP Press Inc; 1995:48.

312. Oetter P, Richter EW, Frick SM. *M.O.R.E.: Integrating the Mouth with Sensory and Postural Functions.* 2nd ed. Hugo, MN: PDP Press Inc; 1995:27.

313. Kent RD. Motor control: neurophysiology and functional development. In: Caruso AJ, Strand EA, eds. *Clinical Management of Motor Speech Disorders in Children.* New York, NY: Thieme Medical Publishers; 1999:33.

314. Oetter P, Richter EW, Frick SM. *M.O.R.E.: Integrating the Mouth with Sensory and Postural Functions.* 2nd ed. Hugo, MN: PDP Press Inc; 1995:27.

315. Oetter P, Richter EW, Frick SM. *M.O.R.E.: Integrating the Mouth with Sensory and Postural Functions.* 2nd ed. Hugo, MN: PDP Press Inc; 1995:26.

316. Nicolosi L, Harryman E, Kresheck J. *Terminology of Communication Disorders: Speech-Language-Hearing.* 3rd ed. Baltimore, MD: Williams & Wilkins; 1989:227.

317. Rosenfeld-Johnson S. *Oral-Motor Exercises for Speech Clarity.* Tucson, AZ: Innovative Therapists International; 1999.

318. Oetter P, Richter EW, Frick SM. *M.O.R.E.: Integrating the Mouth with Sensory and Postural Functions.* 2nd ed. Hugo, MN: PDP Press Inc; 1995:47.

319. Bahr DC. *Oral Motor Assessment and Treatment: Ages and Stages.* Boston, MA: Allyn & Bacon; 2001:5, 17–20, 44–45, 121–133, 147.

320. Morris SE, Klein MD. *Pre-Feeding Skills: A Comprehensive Resource for Mealtime Development.* 2nd ed. San Antonio, TX: Therapy Skill Builders; 2000:51–53, 71, 697–711.

321. Oetter P, Richter EW, Frick SM. *M.O.R.E.: Integrating the Mouth with Sensory and Postural Functions.* 2nd ed. Hugo, MN: PDP Press Inc; 1995:8, 20, 27.

322. Perkins WH, Kent RD. *Functional Anatomy of Speech, Language, and Hearing: A Primer.* Boston, MA: Allyn & Bacon; 1986:131.

323. Pierce RB. *Tongue Thrust: A Look at Oral Myofunctional Disorders.* Lincoln, NE: Cliffs Notes Inc; 1978:31.

324. Boshart CA. Essential oral-motor techniques: a one-day seminar [workshop]. Temecula, CA: Speech Dynamics Inc; 1998.

325. Kent RD. Motor control: neurophysiology and functional development. In: Caruso AJ, Strand EA, eds. *Clinical Management of Motor Speech Disorders in Children.* New York, NY: Thieme Medical Publishers; 1999:29–71.

326. Rossetti L. *The Rossetti Infant-Toddler Language Scale.* East Moline, IL: LinguiSystems Inc; 1990:2–13.

327. Vulpe SG. *Vulpe Assessment Battery: Developmental Assessment, Performance Analysis, Individualized Programming.* Toronto, ON: National Institute on Mental Retardation; 1977:151–177.

328. Hedrick DL, Prather EM, Tobin AR. *The Sequenced Inventory of Communication Development.* Seattle, WA: University of Washington Press; 1984.

329. Reidlich CE, Herzfeld ME. *0 to 3 Years: An Early Language Curriculum.* Moline, IL: LinguiSystems Inc; 1983:63–122.

330. Dyer L. *Look Who's Talking: How to Enhance Your Child's Language Development Starting at Birth.* Minnetonka: MN: Meadowbrook Press; 2004.

331. Retherford KS. *Normal Development: A Database of Communication and Related Behaviors, Birth to 12+ Years.* Eau Claire, WI: Thinking Publications; 2003.

332. Kent R. Articulatory and acoustic perspectives on speech development. In: Reilly AP, ed. *The Communication Game: Perspectives on the Development of Speech, Language, and Nonverbal Communication Skill.* Skillman, NJ: Johnson & Johnson Baby Products Co; 1980:38–43.

333. Oller DK. The emergence of speech sounds in infancy. In: Yeni-Komshian G, Kavanagh JA, Ferguson CA, eds. *Child Phonology: Volume 1. Production.* New York, NY: Academic Press; 1980:93–112.

334. Locke J. *Phonological Acquisition and Change.* New York, NY: Academic Press; 1983:10.

335. Grunwell P. *Clinical Phonology.* 2nd ed. Rockville, MD: Aspen Publishers; 1987:231.

336. Stoel-Gammon C, Cooper J. Patterns of early lexical and phonological development. *J Child Lang.* 1984;11:247–271.

337. Owens RE. *Language Development: An Introduction.* 4th ed. Needham Heights, MA: Allyn & Bacon; 1996:162–195.

338. Miller JF, Chapman R. The relation between age and mean length of utterance in morphemes. *J Speech Hear Res.* 1981;24:151–161.

339. Page DC. "Real" early orthodontic treatment: from birth to age 8. *Funct Orthod: J Funct Jaw Orthop.* 2003;20(1–2):54.

340. Van der Liden F. *Facial Growth and Facial Orthopedics.* Hanover Park, IL: Quintessence Publishing Co Inc; 1986.

341. Enlow D. *Handbook of Facial Growth.* New York, NY: W. B. Saunders Book Publishers; 1982.

342. Widmer RP. The normal development of teeth. *Aust Fam Physician.* 1992;21:1251–1261.

343. Smith A, Weber CM, Newton J, Denny M. Developmental and age-related changes in reflexes of the human jaw-closing system. *Electroencephalogr Clin Neurophysiol.* 1991;81:118–128.

344. Langlois A, Baken R. Development of respiratory time factors in infant cry. *Dev Med Child Neurol.* 1976;18:732–737.

345. Wasz-Hockert O, Lind J, Vuorenkoski V, Partanen T, Valanne E. *The Infant Cry.* London, England: Spastics International Medical Publications; 1968.

346. Wolff P. The natural history of crying and other vocalization in early infancy. In: Foss B, ed. *Determinants of Infant Behavior IV.* London, England: Methuen; 1969:81–109.

347. Trevarthen C. Communication and cooperation in early infancy: a description of primary intersubjectivity. In: Bullowa M, ed. *Before Speech.* New York, NY: Cambridge University Press; 1979:321–347.

348. Chen H, Irwin O. Infant speech vowel and consonant types. *J Speech Disord.* 1946;11(1):27–29.

349. Irwin O. Infant speech: development of vowel sounds. *J Speech Hear Disord.* 1948;13:31–34.

350. Vulpe SG. *Vulpe Assessment Battery: Developmental Assessment, Performance Analysis, Individualized Programming.* Toronto, ON: National Institute on Mental Retardation; 1977:152.

351. Vulpe SG. *Vulpe Assessment Battery: Developmental Assessment, Performance Analysis, Individualized Programming.* Toronto, ON: National Institute on Mental Retardation; 1977:153.

352. Irwin O. Infant speech: Development of vowel sounds. *J Speech Hear Disord.* 1948;13:31–34.

353. Vulpe SG. *Vulpe Assessment Battery: Developmental Assessment, Performance Analysis, Individualized Programming.* Toronto, ON: National Institute on Mental Retardation; 1977:154.

354. Vulpe SG. *Vulpe Assessment Battery: Developmental Assessment, Performance Analysis, Individualized Programming.* Toronto, ON: National Institute on Mental Retardation; 1977:154.

355. Stevenson RD, Allaire JH. The development of normal feeding and swallowing. *Pediatr Clin N Am.* 1991;38(6):1439–1453.

356. Miller JF, Rosin P, Netsell R. *Differentiating Productive Language Deficits and Speech Motor Control Problems in Children.* Paper presented at: Annual convention of the Wisconsin Speech and Hearing Association; April 1979; Madison, WI.

357. Oller DK. Infant vocalization and the development of speech. *Allied Health Behav Sci.* 1978;1:523–549.

358. Miller JF, Rosin P, Netsell R. *Differentiating Productive Language Deficits and Speech Motor Control Problems in Children.* Paper presented at: Annual convention of the Wisconsin Speech and Hearing Association; April 1979; Madison, WI.

359. White B. *The First Three Years of Life.* Englewood Cliffs, NJ: Prentice-Hall; 1975.

360. Kaye K. Thickening thin data: the maternal role in developing communication and language. In: Bullowa M, ed. *Before Speech.* New York, NY: Cambridge University Press; 1979:191–206.

361. Wetherby A, Prizant B. *Communication and Symbolic Behavior Scales-Normed Edition.* Baltimore, MD: Brookes Publishing; 1993.

362. Retherford KS. *Normal Development: A Database of Communication and Related Behaviors, Birth to 12+ Years.* Eau Claire, WI: Thinking Publications; 2003:7.

363. Bruner JS. From communication to language: a psychological perspective. *Cognition.* 1974/1975;3(3):255–287.

364. Marcos H. Communicative functions of pitch range and pitch direction in infants. *J Child Lang.* 1987;14:255–268.

365. White B. *The First Three Years of Life.* Englewood Cliffs, NJ: Prentice-Hall; 1975.

366. White B. *The First Three Years of Life.* Englewood Cliffs, NJ: Prentice-Hall; 1975.

367. Fletcher S. Palatometry principles and practice. Session presented at the annual meeting of the American Speech-Language-Hearing Association; November 2008; Chicago, IL.

368. Dorais A. Palatometry: an approach for treating articulation problems. *Word of Mouth.* 2009;20(5):1–4.

369. Kent RD. Motor control: neurophysiology and functional development. In: Caruso AJ, Strand EA, eds. *Clinical Management of Motor Speech Disorders in Children.* New York, NY: Thieme Medical Publishers; 1999:38.

370. Coggins T, Carpenter R. The communicative intention inventory. *J Appl Psycholinguist.* 1981;2:235–251.

371. Dore J. A pragmatic description of early language development. *J Psycholinguist Res.* 1974;3(4):343–350.

372. Marcos H. Communicative functions of pitch range and pitch direction in infants. *J Child Lang.* 1987;14:255–268.

373. Ingram D. *Procedures for the Phonological Analysis of Children's Language.* Baltimore, MD: University Park Press; 1981.

374. Ingram D. *Phonological Disability in Children.* 2nd ed. New York, NY: American Elsevier; 1989.

375. Marcos H. Communicative functions of pitch range and pitch direction in infants. *J Child Lang.* 1987;14:255–268.

376. Retherford KS. *Normal Development: A Database of Communication and Related Behaviors, Birth to 12+ Years.* Eau Claire, WI: Thinking Publications; 2003:2–3.

377. Donegan P. Normal vowel development. In: Ball MJ, Gibbon FE, eds. *Vowel disorders.* Boston, MA: Butterworth-Heinemann; 2002.

378. Snow C, Ninio A. The contract of literacy: what children learn from learning to read books. In: Teale W, Sulzby E, eds. *Emergent Literacy: Writing and Reading.* Norwood, NJ: Ablex; 1986:116–138.

379. Retherford KS. *Normal Development: A Database of Communication and Related Behaviors, Birth to 12+ Years.* Eau Claire, WI: Thinking Publications; 2003:2–3.

380. Wachs T. Utilization of a Piagetian approach to the investigation of early experience effects: a research strategy and some illustrative data. *Merrill-Palmer Q.* 1976;22(1):11–30.

381. Coplan J. *Early Language Milestone Scale.* Tulsa, OK: Modern Education Corporation; 1987.

382. Miller JF, Rosin P, Netsell R. *Differentiating Productive Language Deficits and Speech Motor Control Problems in Children.* Paper presented at: Annual convention of the Wisconsin Speech and Hearing Association; April 1979; Madison, WI.

383. Stoel-Gammon C. Phonetic inventories, 15–24 months: a longitudinal study. *J Speech Hear Res.* 1985;28:505–512.

384. Dyson A. Phonetic inventories of 2- and 3-year old children. *J Speech Hear Disord.* 1988;53:89–93.

385. Robb M, Bleile K. Consonant inventories of young children from 8 to 25 months. *J Clin Linguistics Phonetics.* 1994;8:295–320.

386. Stoel-Gammon C. Phonetic inventories, 15–24 months: a longitudinal study. *J Speech Hear Res.* 1985;28:505–512.

387. Dyson A. Phonetic inventories of 2- and 3-year old children. *J Speech Hear Disord.* 1988;53:89–93.

388. Robb M, Bleile K. Consonant inventories of young children from 8 to 25 months. *J Clin Linguistics Phonetics.* 1994;8:295–320.

389. Bloom L, Rocissano L, Hood L. Adult-child discourse: Developmental interaction between information processing and linguistic interaction. *Cogn Psychol.* 1976;8(4):521–552.

390. Bloom L, Rocissano L, Hood L. Adult-child discourse: developmental interaction between information processing and linguistic interaction. *Cogn Psychol.* 1976;8(4):521–552.

391. White B. *The First Three Years of Life.* Englewood Cliffs, NJ: Prentice-Hall; 1975.

392. Rossetti L. *The Rossetti Infant-Toddler Language Scale.* East Moline, IL: LinguiSystems Inc; 1990:10.

393. White B. *The First Three Years of Life.* Englewood Cliffs, NJ: Prentice-Hall; 1975.

394. Rossetti L. *The Rossetti Infant-Toddler Language Scale.* East Moline, IL: LinguiSystems Inc; 1990:11.

395. White B. *The First Three Years of Life.* Englewood Cliffs, NJ: Prentice-Hall; 1975.

396. Vulpe SG. *Vulpe Assessment Battery: Developmental Assessment, Performance Analysis, Individualized Programming.* Toronto, ON: National Institute on Mental Retardation; 1977:168.

397. Rossetti L. *The Rossetti Infant-Toddler Language Scale.* East Moline, IL: LinguiSystems Inc; 1990:12.

398. White B. *The First Three Years of Life.* Englewood Cliffs, NJ: Prentice-Hall; 1975.

399. Kamhi AG. Summary, reflections, and future directions. In: Kamhi AG, Pollock KE, eds. *Phonological Disorders in Children: Clinical Decision Making in Assessment and Intervention.* Baltimore, MD: Paul H. Brooks Publishing Co; 2005:215.

400. Dougherty DP. *Teach Me How to Say It Right: Helping Your Child with Articulation Problems.* Oakland, CA: New Harbinger Publications Inc; 2005.

401. Marshalla P. *Becoming Verbal with Childhood Apraxia: New Insights on Piaget for Today's Therapy.* Mill Creek, WA: Marshalla Speech & Language; 2007.

402. Martin KL. *Does My Child Have a Speech Problem?* Chicago, IL: Chicago Review Press Inc; 1997.

403. Kaufman NR. Kaufman Speech Praxis Treatment Kit for Children. Gaylord, MI: Northern Speech Services; 1997.

404. Hayden DA. The PROMPT model: use and application for children with mixed phonological-motor impairment. *Adv Speech-Lang Pathol.* 2006;8(3):265–281.

405. Hayden DA. PROMPT: A tactually grounded treatment approach to speech production disorders. In: Stockman I, ed. *Movement and Action in Learning and Development: Clinical Implications for Pervasive Developmental Disorders.* San Diego, CA: Elsevier-Academic Press; 2004:255–297.

406. Meek MM. *Motokinesthetic Approach* [videotape]. Albuquerque, NM: Clinician's View; 1994.

407. Jelm JM. *A Parent Guide to Verbal Dyspraxia.* DeKalb, IL: Janelle Publications Inc; 2000.

408. Banker B. *Silly Songs for Phonology and Sound Awareness.* Eau Claire, WI: Thinking Publications; 1998.

409. Rivard JM, Rivard J. *Noisy Stories: Language Activities for Children of All Communicative Abilities.* Solana Beach, CA: Mayer-Johnson Inc; 2000.

410. Rosenbeck J, Lemme M, Ahern M, Harris E, Wertz T. A treatment for apraxia of speech in adults. *J Speech Hear Disord.* 1973;38:462–472.

411. Strand E, Stoeckel R, Baas B. Treatment of severe childhood apraxia of speech: a treatment efficacy study. *J Med Speech Pathol.* 2006;14: 297–307.

412. Bahr D, Rosenfeld-Johnson S. Treatment of children with speech oral placement disorders (OPDS): a paradigm emerges. *Commun Disord Q.* In press.

413. DeThorne LS, Johnson CJ, Walder L, Mahurin-Smith J. When "Simon Says" doesn't work: alternatives to imitation for facilitating early speech development. *Am J Speech Lang Pathol.* 2009;18(2):133–145.

414. Kent RD. Motor control: neurophysiology and functional development. In: Caruso AJ, Strand EA, eds. *Clinical Management of Motor Speech Disorders in Children.* New York, NY: Thieme Medical Publishers; 1999:42.

415. Evans CA. Postnatal facial growth, birth through adolescence. In: Avery JK, ed. *Oral Dev Histol.* 2nd ed. New York, NY: Thieme Medical Publishers; 1994:58–67.

416. Solberg WK, Woo MW, Houston JB. Prevalence of mandibular dysfunction in young adults. *J Am Dent Assoc.* 1979;98:25–34.

417. Boshart CA. *Oral-Motor Seminar: "Hard Tissue Analysis" Supplement* [videotape]. Temecula, CA: Speech Dynamics; 1995.

418. Boshart CA. *Oral-Motor Seminar: "Hard Tissue Analysis" Supplement* [videotape]. Temecula, CA: Speech Dynamics; 1995.

419. Bahr DC. *Oral Motor Assessment and Treatment: Ages and Stages.* Boston, MA: Allyn & Bacon; 2001:146–147.

420. Page DC. *Your Jaws—Your Life.* Baltimore, MD: SmilePage Publishing; 2003.

421. Mason RM. A retrospective and prospective view of orofacial myology. *Int J Orofacial Myology.* 2005;31:1, 5–14.

422. Morris SE, Klein MD. *Pre-Feeding Skills: A Comprehensive Resource for Mealtime Development.* 2nd ed. San Antonio, TX: Therapy Skill Builders; 2000:123.

423. Mason RM. A retrospective and prospective view of orofacial myology. *Int J Orofacial Myology.* 2005;31:1, 5–14.

424. Written communication with P. Taylor, Bloomsburg, PA; May 2008.

425. Kent RD. Motor control: neurophysiology and functional development. In: Caruso AJ, Strand EA, eds. *Clinical Management of Motor Speech Disorders in Children*. New York, NY: Thieme Medical Publishers; 1999:29–30.

426. Kent RD. Motor control: neurophysiology and functional development. In: Caruso AJ, Strand EA, eds. *Clinical Management of Motor Speech Disorders in Children*. New York, NY: Thieme Medical Publishers; 1999:29.

427. Bahr DC. *Oral Motor Assessment and Treatment: Ages and Stages*. Boston, MA: Allyn & Bacon; 2001:5, 17–20, 44–45, 121–133, 147.

428. Morris SE, Klein MD. *Pre-Feeding Skills: A Comprehensive Resource for Mealtime Development*. 2nd ed. San Antonio, TX: Therapy Skill Builders; 2000:51–53, 71, 697–711.

429. Morris SE. Developmental implications for the management of feeding problems in neurologically impaired infants. *Semin Speech Lang*. 1985;6(4):293–315.

430. Oetter P, Richter EW, Frick SM. *M.O.R.E.: Integrating the Mouth with Sensory and Postural Functions*. 2nd ed. Hugo, MN: PDP Press Inc; 1995:8, 18, 20, 27.

431. Winstock A. *Eating & Drinking Difficulties in Children: A Guide for Practitioners* Oxon, UK: Speechmark Publishing Ltd; 2005.

432. Perkins WH, Kent RD. *Functional Anatomy of Speech, Language, and Hearing: A Primer*. Boston, MA: Allyn & Bacon; 1986:131.

433. Pierce RB. *Tongue Thrust: A Look at Oral Myofunctional Disorders*. Lincoln, NE: Cliffs Notes Inc; 1978:31.

434. Boshart CA. Essential oral-motor techniques: a one-day seminar [workshop]. Temecula, CA: Speech Dynamics Inc; 1998.

435. Kent RD. Motor control: neurophysiology and functional development. In: Caruso AJ, Strand EA, eds. *Clinical Management of Motor Speech*

Disorders in Children. New York, NY: Thieme Medical Publishers; 1999:29–71.

436. Dyer L. *Look Who's Talking: How to Enhance Your Child's Language Development Starting at Birth.* Minnetonka: MN: Meadowbrook Press; 2004.

437. Montagu A. *Touching: The Human Significance of the Skin.* 3rd ed. New York, NY: Harper & Row Publishers; 1986:84.

438. Page DC. "Real" early orthodontic treatment: from birth to age 8. *Funct Orthod: J Funct Jaw Orthop.* 2003;20(1–2):48–58.

439. Page DC. *Your Jaws—Your Life.* Baltimore, MD: SmilePage Publishing; 2003.

440. Rossetti L. *The Rossetti Infant-Toddler Language Scale* [test form]. East Moline, IL: LinguiSystems Inc; 1990:2–9.

441. Vulpe SG. *Vulpe Assessment Battery: Developmental Assessment, Performance Analysis, Individualized Programming.* Toronto, ON: National Institute on Mental Retardation; 1977:151–165.

442. Hedrick DL, Prather EM, Tobin AR. *The Sequenced Inventory of Communication Development.* Seattle, WA: University of Washington Press; 1984.

443. Reidlich CE, Herzfeld ME. *0 to 3 Years: An Early Language Curriculum.* Moline, IL: LinguiSystems Inc; 1983.

444. Retherford KS. *Normal Development: A Database of Communication and Related Behaviors, Birth to 12+ Years.* Eau Claire, WI: Thinking Publications; 2003.

445. Kent R. Articulatory and acoustic perspectives on speech development. In: Reilly AP, ed. *The Communication Game: Perspectives on the Development of Speech, Language, and Nonverbal Communication Skills.* Skillman, NJ: Johnson & Johnson Baby Products Co; 1980:38–43.

446. Bahr DC. *Oral Motor Assessment and Treatment: Ages and Stages.* Boston, MA: Allyn & Bacon; 2001:5, 17–20.

447. Morris SE, Klein MD. *Pre-Feeding Skills: A Comprehensive Resource for Feeding Development.* Tucson, AZ: Therapy Skill Builders; 1987:8–10.

448. Morris SE, Klein MD. *Pre-Feeding Skills: A Comprehensive Resource for Mealtime Development.* 2nd ed. San Antonio, TX: Therapy Skill Builders; 2000:51–53.

449. Page DC. *Your Jaws—Your Life.* Baltimore, MD: SmilePage Publishing; 2003:28–29.

450. Page DC. "Real" early orthodontic treatment: from birth to age 8. *Funct Orthod: J Funct Jaw Orthop.* 2003;20(1–2):54.

451. Van der Liden F. *Facial Growth and Facial Orthopedics.* Hanover Park, IL: Quintessence Publishing Co Inc; 1986.

452. Enlow D. *Handbook of Facial Growth.* New York, NY: W. B. Saunders Book Publishers; 1982.

453. Widmer RP. The normal development of teeth. *Aust Family Physician.* 1992;21:1251–1261.

454. Smith A, Weber CM, Newton J, Denny M. Developmental and age-related changes in reflexes of the human jaw-closing system. *Electroencephalogr Clin Neurophysiol.* 1991;81:118–128.

455. Trevarthen C. Communication and cooperation in early infancy: a description of primary intersubjectivity. In: Bullowa M, ed. *Before Speech.* New York, NY: Cambridge University Press; 1979:321–347.

456. Page DC. "Real" early orthodontic treatment: from birth to age 8. *Funct Orthod: J Funct Jaw Orthop.* 2003;20(1–2):54.

457. Van der Liden F. *Facial Growth and Facial Orthopedics.* Hanover Park, IL: Quintessence Publishing Co Inc; 1986.

458. Enlow D. *Handbook of Facial Growth.* New York, NY: W. B. Saunders Book Publishers; 1982.

459. Widmer RP. The normal development of teeth. *Aust Family Physician.* 1992;21:1251–1261.

460. Smith A, Weber CM, Newton J, Denny M. Developmental and age-related changes in reflexes of the human jaw-closing system. *Electroencephalogr Clin Neurophysiol.* 1991;81:118–128.

461. Widmer RP. The normal development of teeth. *Aust Family Physician.* 1992;21:1251–1261.

462. Smith A, Weber CM, Newton J, Denny M. Developmental and age-related changes in reflexes of the human jaw-closing system. *Electroencephalogr Clin Neurophysiol.* 1991;81:118–128.

463. Page DC. "Real" early orthodontic treatment: from birth to age 8. *Funct Orthod: J Funct Jaw Orthop.* 2003;20(1–2):54.

464. Van der Liden F. *Facial Growth and Facial Orthopedics.* Hanover Park, IL: Quintessence Publishing Co Inc; 1986.

465. Enlow D. *Handbook of Facial Growth.* New York, NY: W. B. Saunders Book Publishers; 1982.

466. Widmer RP. The normal development of teeth. *Aust Family Physician.* 1992;21:1251–1261.

467. Smith A, Weber CM, Newton J, Denny M. Developmental and age-related changes in reflexes of the human jaw-closing system. *Electroencephalogr Clin Neurophysiol.* 1991;81:118–128.

468. Widmer RP. The normal development of teeth. *Aust Family Physician.* 1992;21:1251–1261.

469. Smith A, Weber CM, Newton J, Denny M. Developmental and age-related changes in reflexes of the human jaw-closing system. *Electroencephalogr Clin Neurophysiol.* 1991;81:118–128.

470. Stevenson RD, Allaire JH. The development of normal feeding and swallowing. *Pediatr Clin N Am.* 1991;38(6):1439–1453.

471. Page DC. "Real" early orthodontic treatment: from birth to age 8. *Funct Orthod: J Funct Jaw Orthop.* 2003;20(1–2):54.

472. Van der Liden F. *Facial Growth and Facial Orthopedics.* Hanover Park, IL: Quintessence Publishing Co Inc; 1986.

473. Enlow D. *Handbook of Facial Growth.* New York, NY: W. B. Saunders Book Publishers; 1982.

474. Widmer RP. The normal development of teeth. *Aust Family Physician.* 1992;21:1251–1261.

475. Smith A, Weber CM, Newton J, Denny M. Developmental and age-related changes in reflexes of the human jaw-closing system. *Electroencephalogr Clin Neurophysiol.* 1991;81:118–128.

476. Kent RD. Motor control: neurophysiology and functional development. In: Caruso AJ, Strand EA, eds. *Clinical Management of Motor Speech Disorders in Children.* New York, NY: Thieme Medical Publishers; 1999: 38.

477. Marcos H. Communicative functions of pitch range and pitch direction in infants. *J Child Lang.* 1987;14:255–268.

478. Marcos H. Communicative functions of pitch range and pitch direction in infants. *J Child Lang.* 1987;14:255–268.

479. Kent RD. Motor control: neurophysiology and functional development. In: Caruso AJ, Strand EA, eds. *Clinical Management of Motor Speech Disorders in Children.* New York, NY: Thieme Medical Publishers; 1999:38.

480. Marcos H. Communicative functions of pitch range and pitch direction in infants. *J Child Lang.* 1987;14:255–268.

481. Kent RD. Motor control: neurophysiology and functional development. In: Caruso AJ, Strand EA, eds. *Clinical Management of Motor Speech*

Disorders in Children. New York, NY: Thieme Medical Publishers; 1999:29–71.

482. Page DC. "Real" early orthodontic treatment: from birth to age 8. *Funct Orthod: J Funct Jaw Orthop.* 2003;20(1–2):48–58.

483. Bahr DC. *Oral Motor Assessment and Treatment: Ages and Stages.* Boston, MA: Allyn & Bacon; 2001:147.

484. Page DC. How to promote & provide functional jaw orthopedics. *Funct Orthod: J Funct Jaw Orthop.* 2001;18(1):27.

485. Van der Linden F. *Facial Growth and Facial Orthopedics.* Hanover Park, IL: Quintessence Publishing Co; 1986.

486. Kent RD. Motor control: neurophysiology and functional development. In: Caruso AJ, Strand EA, eds. *Clinical Management of Motor Speech Disorders in Children.* New York, NY: Thieme Medical Publishers; 1999:29–71.

487. Bahr DC. *Oral Motor Assessment and Treatment: Ages and Stages.* Boston, MA: Allyn & Bacon; 2001:147.

488. Kent RD. Motor control: neurophysiology and functional development. In: Caruso AJ, Strand EA, eds. *Clinical Management of Motor Speech Disorders in Children.* New York, NY: Thieme Medical Publishers; 1999:38.

489. Page DC. "Real" early orthodontic treatment: from birth to age 8. *Funct Orthod: J Funct Jaw Orthop.* 2003;20(1–2):48–58, 50.

490. Subtelny JD. *Early Orthodontic Treatment.* Hanover Park, IL: Quintessence Publishing Co; 2000:271.

491. Bahr DC. *Oral Motor Assessment and Treatment: Ages and Stages.* Boston, MA: Allyn & Bacon; 2001:20.

492. Bahr DC. *Oral Motor Assessment and Treatment: Ages and Stages.* Boston, MA: Allyn & Bacon; 2001:20.

493. Kent RD. Motor control: neurophysiology and functional development. In: Caruso AJ, Strand EA, eds. *Clinical Management of Motor Speech*

Disorders in Children. New York, NY: Thieme Medical Publishers; 1999:29–71.

494. Bahr DC. *Oral Motor Assessment and Treatment: Ages and Stages*. Boston, MA: Allyn & Bacon; 2001:147.

495. Kent RD. Motor control: neurophysiology and functional development. In: Caruso AJ, Strand EA, eds. *Clinical Management of Motor Speech Disorders in Children*. New York, NY: Thieme Medical Publishers; 1999:29–71.

496. Kent RD. Motor control: neurophysiology and functional development. In: Caruso AJ, Strand EA, eds. *Clinical Management of Motor Speech Disorders in Children*. New York, NY: Thieme Medical Publishers; 1999:29–71.

497. Bahr DC. *Oral Motor Assessment and Treatment: Ages and Stages*. Boston, MA: Allyn & Bacon; 2001:147.

498. Bias CL, Chick S, Morgan B. Oral motor skills and breastfeeding: finding the help you need. MOBI Motherhood International Web site. http://www.mobimotherhood.org. Accessed August 26, 2009.

499. Prematurity: a national health crisis. March of Dimes Web site. http://www.marchofdimes.com. Accessed August 26, 2009.

500. Stein R. As babies are born earlier, they risk problems later. *Washington Post*. May 20, 2006:A1.

501. Madden SL. *The Preemie Parents' Companion: The Essential Guide to Caring for Your Premature Baby in the Hospital, at Home, and Through the First Years*. Boston, MA: The Harvard Common Press; 2000:5.

502. Morris SE, Klein MD. *Pre-Feeding Skills: A Comprehensive Resource for Mealtime Development*. 2nd ed. San Antonio, TX: Therapy Skill Builders; 2000:554.

503. Morris SE, Klein MD. *Pre-Feeding Skills: A Comprehensive Resource for Mealtime Development*. 2nd ed. San Antonio, TX: Therapy Skill Builders; 2000:554.

504. Merenstein GB, Gardner SL, eds. *Handbook of Neonatal Intensive Care.* 5th ed. St Louis, MO: Mosby Inc; 2002:394–395.

505. Field T. *Touch Therapy.* New York, NY: Churchill Livingstone; 2000.

506. Morris SE, Klein MD. *Pre-Feeding Skills: A Comprehensive Resource for Mealtime Development.* 2nd ed. San Antonio, TX: Therapy Skill Builders; 2000:537–554.

507. Huggins K. *The Nursing Mother's Companion.* 4th ed. Boston, MA: Harvard Common Press; 1999:97–104.

508. Madden SL. *The Preemie Parents' Companion: The Essential Guide to Caring for Your Premature Baby in the Hospital, at Home, and through the First Years.* Boston, MA: The Harvard Common Press; 2000.

509. Linden DW, Paroli ET, Doron MW. *Preemies: The Essential Guide for Parents of Premature Babies.* New York, NY: Pocket Books; 2000.

510. Merenstein GB, Gardner SL, eds. *Handbook of Neonatal Intensive Care.* 5th ed. St Louis, MO: Mosby Inc; 2002.

511. Riordan J, Auerbach KG. *Breastfeeding and Human Lactation.* 2nd ed. Sudbury, MA: Jones & Bartlett Publishers; 1998.

512. Bahr DC. *Oral Motor Assessment and Treatment: Ages and Stages.* Boston, MA: Allyn & Bacon; 2001:36.

513. Winders PC. *Gross Motor Skills in Children with Down Syndrome: A Guide for Parents and Professionals.* Bethesda, MD: Woodbine House Inc; 1997.

514. Bahr DC. *Oral Motor Assessment and Treatment: Ages and Stages.* Boston, MA: Allyn & Bacon; 2001:36.

515. Bahr DC. *Oral Motor Assessment and Treatment: Ages and Stages.* Boston, MA: Allyn & Bacon; 2001:36.

516. Boshart CA. Essential oral-motor techniques: a one-day seminar [workshop]. Temecula, CA: Speech Dynamics Inc; 1998.

517. Newborn and infant hearing screening activities .The National Center of Medical Home Initiatives for Children with Special Needs 2008. American Academy of Pediatrics Web site. http://www.aap.org. Accessed August 26, 2009.

518. Risk factors for Down syndrome. U.S. Centers for Disease Control and Prevention Web site. http://www.cdc.gov/ncbddd/bd/ds.htm. Accessed October 5, 2005.

519. Stray-Gundersen K, ed. *Babies with Down Syndrome: A New Parents' Guide.* Bethesda, MD: Woodbine House Inc; 1995.

520. Van Dyke DC, Mattheis P, Everly SS, Williams J, eds. *Medical & Surgical Care for Children with Down Syndrome: A Guide for Parents.* Bethesda, MD: Woodbine House Inc; 1995.

521. Kumin L. *Early Communication Skills for Children with Down Syndrome: A Guide for Parents and Professionals.* 2nd ed. Bethesda, MD: Woodbine House Inc; 2003.

522. Schermerhorn W. *Down Syndrome: The First 18 Months* [DVD]. Vienna, VA: Blueberry Shoes Productions LLC; 2003.

523. Schermerhorn W. *Discovery: Pathways to Better Speech for Children with Down Syndrome* [DVD]. Vienna, VA: Blueberry Shoes Productions LLC; 2005.

524. Kumin L, Schermerhorn W. *What Did You Say? A Guide to Speech Intelligibility in People with Down Syndrome* [DVD]. Bethesda, MD: Woodbine House Inc; 2006.

525. Schermerhorn W. *Kids with Down Syndrome: Staying Healthy and Making Friends* [DVD]. Vienna, VA: Blueberry Shoes Productions LLC; 2008.

526. Scully J. Autism: tools for recognizing, differentiating, and intervening [workshop]. Las Vegas, NV: Medical Educational Services Inc; 2005.

527. Nash JM. The secrets of autism: the number of children diagnosed with autism and Asperger's is exploding. Why? *Time.* http://www.time.com/time/covers/1101020506/scautism.html. Accessed August 26, 2009.

528. Boehme R. Integration of neuro-developmental treatment and myofascial release in adult orthopedics. In: Barnes JF, ed. *Myofascial Release: The Search for Excellence: A Comprehensive Evaluatory and Treatment Approach.* Paoli, PA: Rehabilitation Services, Inc; 1990:209–217.

529. Morbidity and mortality weekly report. U.S. Centers for Disease Control and Prevention Web site. http://cdc.gov/. Accessed February 8, 2007.

530. Bauman ML. Autism: clinical features and neurobiological observations. In: The Interdisciplinary Council on Developmental and Learning Disorders (ICDL) Clinical Practice Guidelines. Bethesda, MD: ICDL Press; 2000:689–703.

531. Scully J. Autism: tools for recognizing, differentiating, and intervening [workshop]. Las Vegas, NV: Medical Educational Services Inc; 2005.

532. Bauman ML. Autism: clinical features and neurobiological observations. In: The Interdisciplinary Council on Developmental and Learning Disorders (ICDL) Clinical Practice Guidelines. Bethesda, MD: ICDL Press; 2000:689–703.

533. Bauman ML. Autism: clinical features and neurobiological observations. In: The Interdisciplinary Council on Developmental and Learning Disorders (ICDL) Clinical Practice Guidelines. Bethesda, MD: ICDL Press; 2000:689–703.

534. Newschaffer CJ. Autism among us: rising concerns and the public health response [video]. Johns Hopkins Bloomberg School of Public Health. Public Health Training Network Web site. http://www.publichealthgrandrounds.unc.edu/autism/webcast.htm. Accessed August 26, 2009.

535. Bauman ML. Autism: clinical features and neurobiological observations. In: The Interdisciplinary Council on Developmental and Learning Disorders (ICDL) Clinical Practice Guidelines. Bethesda, MD: ICDL Press; 2000:689–703.

536. Newborn and infant hearing screening activities .The National Center of Medical Home Initiatives for Children with Special Needs 2008.

American Academy of Pediatrics Web site. http://www.aap.org. Accessed August 26, 2009.

537. Lord C, McGee JP. *Educating Children with Autism.* Washington, DC: National Academics Press; 2001:219.

538. Prelock P. Understanding autism spectrum disorders: the role of speech-language pathologists and audiologists in service delivery. *ASHA Leader.* 2001;617:5–7.

539. Newborn and infant hearing screening activities .The National Center of Medical Home Initiatives for Children with Special Needs 2008. American Academy of Pediatrics Web site. http://www.aap.org. Accessed August 26, 2009.

540. Pulling the plug on TV violence. American Academy of Pediatrics Web site. http://www.aap.org. Accessed August 26, 2009.

541. Harrington K. *For Parents and Professionals: Autism.* East Moline, IL: LinguiSystems Inc; 1998.

542. Harrington K. *For Parents and Professionals: Autism in Adolescents and Adults.* East Moline, IL: LinguiSystems Inc; 2000.

543. Harrington K. *For Parents and Professionals: Autism.* East Moline, IL: LinguiSystems Inc; 1998.

544. Harrington K. *For Parents and Professionals: Autism in Adolescents and Adults.* East Moline, IL: LinguiSystems Inc; 2000.

545. U.S. Centers for Disease Control and Prevention National Center on Birth Defects and Developmental Disabilities Web site. http://cdc.gov/ncbddd. Accessed October 29, 2004.

546. Newborn and infant hearing screening activities. The National Center of Medical Home Initiatives for Children with Special Needs 2008. American Academy of Pediatrics Web site. http://www.aap.org. Accessed August 26, 2009.

547. Newborn and infant hearing screening activities. The National Center of Medical Home Initiatives for Children with Special Needs 2008. American Academy of Pediatrics Web site. http://www.aap.org. Accessed August 26, 2009.

548. Bahr DC. *Oral Motor Assessment and Treatment: Ages and Stages.* Boston, MA: Allyn & Bacon; 2001:36–37.

549. Bahr DC. *Oral Motor Assessment and Treatment: Ages and Stages.* Boston, MA: Allyn & Bacon; 2001:36.

550. Bahr DC. *Oral Motor Assessment and Treatment: Ages and Stages.* Boston, MA: Allyn & Bacon; 2001:37.

551. Bahr DC. *Oral Motor Assessment and Treatment: Ages and Stages.* Boston, MA: Allyn & Bacon; 2001:37.

552. Bahr DC. *Oral Motor Assessment and Treatment: Ages and Stages.* Boston, MA: Allyn & Bacon; 2001:37.

Index

Note: Page numbers followed by *f, t,* or *i* refer to figures, tables, or illustrations, respectively.

Movement, 105–107. *See also* Tongue
  movement
  belly time and, 56
  dissociation of, 48, 50
  grading of, 145–146, 329, 333
  independent, 97
Mucus, 27, 28
Muscles, 57, 87–88, 131–132, 135, 287
Muscle tone, low, 121, 129
  autism and, 333, 337
  Down syndrome and, 326, 327, 331
Mutism, 272
Mylohyoid muscles, 132, 287
Myofascial release, 285, 327

N

Narrow palate, 8
Nasal and sinus areas, 4*f*
Nasal obstruction, 8, 54
Nasopharynx, 4*f*, 26, 109
National Board for Certification in Occupational
  Therapy, 317
National Certification Board for Therapeutic
  Massage and Body Work, 318
Natural language, 274
Near-term babies, 10, 21, 40, 322
Neck hyperextension, 22, 25
Neck reflexes. *See* Asymmetric tonic neck reflex
Newborns, 3*i*, 6–7, 10
Nipples, bottle. *See* Bottle nipples
Nitric oxide, 54–55
Noisy Stories kit, 273
Nonverbal communication, 200, 233, 234*i*
Noonan syndrome, 344*t*
Nose. *See* Nasal and sinus areas
Nose breathing, 8, 30, 54–56, 55*i*
  feeding and, 10, 25
  problems with, 67
Nurse practitioners, 67
Nurses, and breast-feeding, 312
Nursing. *See* Breast-feeding
Nursing Mother's Companion, The, 29, 325
Nutrition, 41–44, 81
  mother's, 72
Nutritionists, 313. *See also* Dietitians, pediatric

O

Obstetricians, 72
Occlusal contact, 300
Occlusion, 22, 280

Occupational therapists, 62, 196, 315, 317–318
Open bite, 287, 328
Open cup, 45, 168*i*
Ophthalmologists, pediatric, 318
Oral awareness, 125, 130, 135, 145, 196*i*, 285
Oral habits, detrimental, 288
Oral hygiene, 135–136. *See also* Tooth brushing
  swallowing and, 176, 287
Oral massage, 125–126, 129–136, 131*i*, 132*i*,
  134–136*i*, 196*i*
*Oral Motor Assessment and Treatment: Ages and
  Stages,* 272
Oral motor treatment, 284–285
Orbicularis oris muscle, 131
Organizations
  American Academy of Pediatrics, 23, 30, 44,
    331, 338
  American Massage Therapy Association, 318
  American Occupational Therapy Association,
    34, 317
  American Physical Therapy Association, 318
  American Speech-Language-Hearing
    Association, 34, 313
  International Association of Infant Massage,
    124, 125, 129, 324
  International Association of Orofacial
    Myology, 287, 289
  International Board Certified Lactation
    Consultants, 31–32, 312–313
  International Lactation Consultant
    Association, 34
  National Board for Certification in
    Occupational Therapy, 317
  National Certification Board for Therapeutic
    Massage and Body Work, 318
Oro-facial-digital syndromes, 344*t*
Orofacial myofunctional disorder, 287
Orofacial myofunctional therapy, 67, 284, 285
Orofacial myologists, 277, 285
Orthodontic nipples, 33
Orthodontic pacifiers, 110
Orthodontic problems, 30, 276
Orthodontic treatment, xv, 281
Orthopedic disorders, 318
Orthopedics, functional jaw, 67
Otitis media, 30, 109. *See also* Ear infections
Otolaryngologists, 313. *See also* Ear, nose, and
  throat specialists
Oto-palatal-digital syndrome, 345*t*
*Out-of-Sync Child, The: Recognizing and
  Coping with Sensory Integration
  Dysfunction,* 333

Overbite, 280, 281, 328
Overfeeding, 42–43, 79
Overjet, 280, 281
Overweight, 30, 42

P

Paced bottle-feeding, 25–26
Pacifiers, 82, 108–110
    fit of. See Activity 2.3
    modifying, 113
    vocalizing and, 217
    weaning from, 98, 100–101, 111t, 112–115
Pacing (cueing), 272
Palate, 4f. See also Hard palate; High, narrow
    palate
Palatometry, 252
Palmomental reflex, 87, 88
Parent Guide to Verbal Dyspraxia, A, 272
Parroting, 249, 261
Partnership with professionals, 311, 320
Pediatricians. See also Specialists
    allergies and, 74, 76
    coughing and, 80
    cup drinking and, 45
    diet and, 64, 74, 81
    ear infection and, 68
    foods, pureed/solid and, 50, 316
    growth and, 42, 316
    iron and, 43, 50
    latch and, 34
    massage and, 125, 130
    mucus suctioning and, 67
    nasal obstruction and, 54, 67
    preemies and, 325
    rashes and, 62
    referrals and, 310, 319
    reflexes and, 11, 46
    reflux and, 61, 79, 81
    side effects and, 288
    sleeping position and, 80
    speech and, 218, 268, 315
    toddlers and, 76
    voice box and, 70
Perspiration, 74
Pervasive developmental disorder, 332
Pet dander, 62, 74
Philtrum, 281
Phonological disorder, 269
Physical therapists, 318, 340
Physicians. See Dentists, pediatric; Pediatricians;
    Specialists

Picky eating, 194–197, 195t
Picture books, 218
Picture Exchange Communication System, 339
Pictures and early literacy, 249i, 271, 339
Pierre-Robin sequence, 345t
Pitch, 230, 292
Pneumonia, 69, 70
Portion sizes, 44, 186, 187–188t
Positioning, 316i
    after breast/bottle-feeding, 68, 81
    during breast/bottle-feeding, 25–26, 27i,
        28–29t, 35
    liquid flowing too fast, 37–38
    for oral massage, 126, 127i, 196i
Posture/postural control, 50, 230
Prader-Willi syndrome, 345t
Praise, 114, 201
Preemie Parents' Companion: The Essential
    Guide to Caring for Your Premature Baby
    in the Hospital, at Home, and Through the
    First Years, 325
Preemies, 270, 315, 322–326. See also Preterm
    babies
Preemies: The Essential Guide for Parents of
    Premature Babies, 325
Pre-feeding skills, 45
Pre-Feeding Skills: A Comprehensive Resource
    for Mealtime Development, 45, 126, 323,
    325
Preservatives, 178
Preterm babies, 9, 82, 124
Products not found in stores, 92t, 139–140t, 163t
Professionals, other, 318–320. See also Lactation
    consultants; Nurse practitioners; Therapists
PROMPT (Prompts for Restructuring Oral
    Muscular Phonetic Targets), 271
Prone position, 81
Proprioceptive system, 227
Prosodic features, 230, 242
Psychologists, pediatric, 319
Pulse, fast, 74
Punishment, 114
Pureed foods, 50

R

Rashes, 62, 125, 130. See also Eczema
Rate of speech/feeding. See Feeding: rate of;
    Speech: rate of
Reading, 218, 273
Recessed-lid cups, 170i
Referrals to professionals, 310–311

Sensory Focus

UNDERSTANDING THE ISSUES BEHIND THE BEHAVIOR

Get Four Seasons of the Best Special Needs Information Available!

Receive the latest information on sensory and behavior issues delivered to your mailbox or inbox every three months. To subscribe today, or for sample articles, visit **www.sensoryfocusmagazine.com** or call us at **888•507•2193**.

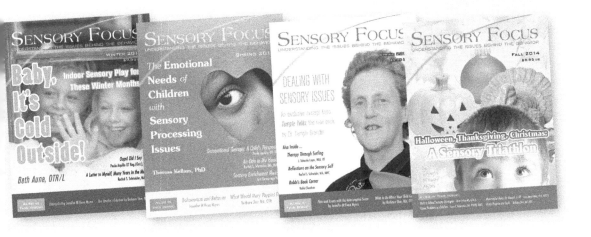

Lightning Source UK Ltd.
Milton Keynes UK
UKHW031021131120
373260UK00004BA/258